# BESTMEDICINE

# Hypertension
## Angiotensin receptor blockers

Dr George Kassianos
Professor Bryan Williams
Dr Mark Davis

*Foreword by Claire Rayner*
*President of the Patients Association*

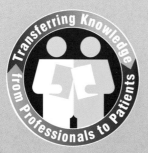

Managing Editor: Dr Scott Chambers
Medical Writers: Dr Eleanor Bull, Dr Richard Clark
Editorial Controller: Emma Catherall
Operations Manager: Julia Potterton
Designer: Chris Matthews
Typesetter: Julie Smith
Indexer: Laurence Errington
Director – Online Business: Peter Llewellyn
Publishing Director: Julian Grover
Publisher: Stephen I'Anson

1 Bankside
Lodge Road
Long Hanborough
Oxfordshire
OX29 8LJ, UK
Tel: +44 (0)1993 885370
Fax: +44 (0)1993 881868
Email: *enquiries@bestmedicine.com*

*www.bestmedicine.com*
*www.csfmedical.com*

The content of *BESTMEDICINE* is the work of a number of authors and has been produced in line with our standard editorial procedures, including the peer review of the disease overview and the drug reviews, and the passing of the final manuscript for publication by the Managing Editor and the Editor-in-Chief or the Medical Editor. Whilst every effort has been made to ensure the accuracy of the information at the date of approval for publication, the Authors, the Publisher, the Editors and the Editorial Board accept no responsibility whatsoever for any errors or omissions or for any consequences arising from anything included in or excluded from *BESTMEDICINE*.

All reasonable effort is made to avoid infringement of copyright law, including the redrawing of figures adapted from other sources. Where copyright permission has been deemed necessary, attempts are made to gain appropriate permission from the copyright holder. However, the Authors, the Publisher, the Editors and the Editorial Board accept no personal responsibility for any infringement of copyright law howsoever made. Any queries regarding copyright approvals or permissions should be addressed to the Managing Editor.

**You are strongly urged to consult your doctor before taking, stopping or changing any of the products reviewed or referred to in *BESTMEDICINE* or any other medication that has been prescribed or recommended by your doctor.**

A catalogue record for this book is available from the British Library.

ISBN: 1-905064-99-3

Typeset by Creative, Langbank, Scotland.
Printed and bound in Wales.
Distributed by NBN International, Plymouth, Devon.

# Contents

# Foreword

*Claire Rayner*
*President of The Patients Association*

Patients and their families are rightly entitled to have access to good-quality, independent and reliable information concerning a diverse range of conditions and a wide variety of medications that are available to treat them. Indeed, there is a growing recognition amongst the majority of healthcare professionals that well-informed patients are more likely to adopt a more active role in the management of their illness and will therefore feel more satisfied with the care that they receive. Such an effect has the potential not only to directly benefit the patient and their families, but can also maximise limited healthcare resources within an already over-stretched NHS. However, at present access to this kind of information is limited, despite the fact that as many as one-in-four adults (12 million people in the UK alone) want ready access to this knowledge prior to visiting their doctor.

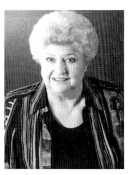

Photograph courtesy of
Amanda Rayner

The importance of patient self-management is a key component of current NHS strategy. Indeed, this has been widely acknowledged in an NHS-led campaign called the Expert Patient Programme (*www.expertpatient.nhs.uk*). This is a self-management course which aims to give people the confidence, skills and knowledge to manage their condition better and take more control of their lives. The Expert Patient Programme defines an Expert Patient as one who has had the condition for long enough to have learnt the language doctors use.

*BESTMEDICINE* aims to meet the information and educational needs of both patients and healthcare professionals alike. The information found in the *BESTMEDICINE* series will assist patients and their families to obtain the level of information they now need to understand and manage their medical condition in partnership with their doctor. However, as *BESTMEDICINE* draws much of its content from medical publications written by doctors for doctors, some readers may find these books rather challenging when they first approach them. Despite this, I strongly believe that the effort that you invest in reading this book will be fully repaid by the increased knowledge they you will gain about this condition. Indeed, the extensive glossary of terms that can be found within each book certainly makes understanding the text a great deal easier, and the Patient Notes section is also very informative and reassuringly written by a doctor for the less scientifically minded reader. *BESTMEDICINE* represents the world's first source of independent, unabridged medical information that will appeal to patients and their families as well as healthcare professionals. This development should be welcomed and applauded, and I would commend these books to you.

**Claire Rayner, November 2004**

Claire Rayner has been involved with the Patients Association for many years and has considerable expertise and experience from a professional background in nursing and journalism and her personal experience as a patient and carer. She is well known as a leading 'Agony Aunt' and as a medical correspondent for many popular magazines. Claire has also published articles in a number of professional journals, as well as over forty medical, nursing and patient advice books.

# An introduction to *BESTMEDICINE*

## The source: information for healthcare professionals

Over the years, it has become increasingly apparent that there is a dearth of drug-related information that is independently compiled and robustly reviewed, and which also acknowledges the challenges faced by healthcare professionals when applying evidence-based medicine whilst practising at the 'front line' of patient care. As such, many healthcare professionals feel a certain ambivalence towards the numerous drug review publications that are currently on offer and, indeed, many do not have confidence in the information that can be found within their pages. In response to the need for a more impartial information resource – one that is independent of the pharmaceutical industry and the health service – we developed a novel publication, which was launched to meet this perceived lack of independent information. This peer-reviewed publication is called *Drugs in Context* and was launched in May 2003 and is the source of much of what you will find in this edition of *BESTMEDICINE*.

## Uniquely independent

*Drugs in Context* is unique in that it reviews the significant clinical and pharmacological evidence underpinning the use of a single drug, in the disease area(s) where it is used and the practice setting where it is most commonly prescribed. Over 50 issues are published each year covering numerous diseases and conditions. The principal goal of *Drugs in Context* is to become the definitive drug and disease management resource for all healthcare professionals. As such, over the coming years, the publication plans to review all of the significant drugs that are currently used in clinical practice.

## Reliable and impartial information for patients too

In addition to the lack of impartial information for the healthcare professional, we also firmly believe that there is a significant and growing number of patients who are not served well in this regard either. Indeed, it is becoming apparent to us that many patients would welcome access to the same sources of information on drugs and diseases that their doctors and other healthcare professionals have access to.

There are numerous sources of information currently available to patients – ranging from leaflets and books to websites and other electronic media. However, despite their best intentions, the rigour and accuracy of many of these resources cannot be relied upon due to significant variation in the quality of the material. Perhaps the major problem facing a patient or a loved one who is hunting for specific information relating to a disease or the drug that has been prescribed by their doctor is that there is simply too much material available, making sifting through it to find a relevant fact akin to looking for a needle in a haystack! More importantly, many of these resources can often (albeit unintentionally) patronise the reader who has made every effort to actively seek out information that can serve to reassure themselves about the concerned illness and about the medication(s) prescribed for it.

## Can knowledge be the 'BESTMEDICINE'?

We firmly believe as healthcare professionals, that an informed patient is more likely to take an active role in the management of their disease or condition and, therefore, will be more likely to benefit from any course of treatment. This means that everyone will benefit – the patient, their family and friends, the healthcare professionals involved in their care, and the NHS and the country as a whole! Indeed, such is the importance of patient education, that the NHS has launched an initiative emphasising the need for patients to assume a more active role in the management of their condition via the acquisition of knowledge and skills related specifically to their disease. This initiative is called the Expert Patients Programme (*www.expertpatients.nhs.uk*).

## Filling the need for quality information

Many of our observations about the lack of quality education have underpinned the principles behind the launch of *BESTMEDICINE*, much of the content of which is drawn directly from the pages of *Drugs in Context*, as written by and for healthcare professionals. *BESTMEDICINE* aims to appeal primarily to the patient, loved-one or carer who wants to improve their knowledge of the disease in question, the evidence for and against the drugs available to treat the disease and the practical challenges faced by healthcare professionals in managing it.

## A whole new language!

We fully acknowledge that a lot of medical terminology used in order to expedite communication amongst the medical community will be new to many of you, some terms may be difficult to pronounce and sometimes surplus to requirements. However, rather than significantly abridge the content and risk excluding something of importance to the reader, we have instead provided you with a comprehensive glossary of terms and what we hope will be helpful additional GP discussion pieces at the end of each section to aid understanding further. We have also provided you with an introduction to the processes underlying drug development and the key concepts in disease management which we hope you will also find informative and which we strongly recommend that you read before tackling the rest of this edition of *BESTMEDICINE*.

## No secrets

By providing the same information to patients and their families as healthcare professionals we believe that *BESTMEDICINE* will help to foster better relationships between patients, their families and doctors and other healthcare professionals and ultimately may even improve treatment outcomes.

This edition is one of a number of unique collections of disease summaries and drug reviews that we will be making widely available over the coming months. You will find details about each issue as it is published at *www.bestmedicine.com*.

We do hope that you find this edition of *BESTMEDICINE* illuminating.

Dr George Kassianos, GP, Bracknell; Editor-in-Chief – *Drugs in Context*, Editor – *BESTMEDICINE*
Dr Jonathan Morrell, GP, Hastings; Medical Editor (Primary Care) – *Drugs in Context*
Dr Michael Schachter, Consultant Physician, St Mary's Hospital Paddington; Clinical Pharmacology Editor – *Drugs in Context*

# Reader's guide

We acknowledge that some of the medical and scientific terminology used throughout *BESTMEDICINE* will be new to you and will address sometimes challenging concepts. However, rather than abridge the content and risk excluding important information, we have included this Reader's Guide to dissect and explain the contents of *BESTMEDICINE* in order to make it more digestible to the less scientifically minded reader. We recommend that you familiarise yourself with the drug development process, summarised below, before embarking on the Drug Reviews. This brief synopsis clarifies and contextualises many of the specialist terms encountered in the Drug Reviews.

Following this Reader's Guide, you will find that *BESTMEDICINE* is made up of two main sections – a Disease Overview and the Drug Reviews – both of which are evidence-based and as such have been highly referenced. All references are listed at the end of a section. Importantly, the manuscript has been 'peer-reviewed', which means that it has undergone rigorous checks for accuracy both by a practising doctor and a specialist in drug pharmacology. The Disease Overview and Drug Reviews are sandwiched between two opinion pieces, an Editorial, written by a recognised expert in the field, and an Improving Practice article, written by a practising GP with a specialist interest in the disease area. It is important to bear in mind that these authors are addressing their professional colleagues, rather than a 'lay' reader, providing you with a fascinating and unique insight into many of the challenges faced by doctors in the day-to-day practice of medicine.

The Disease Overview, Drug Reviews and Improving Practice sections are all followed by a short commentary by Dr Mark Davis entitled Patient Notes. In these sections, Dr Davis reiterates some of the key issues raised in rather more 'user-friendly' language.

As mentioned previously, much of the content of *BESTMEDICINE* has been taken directly from *Drugs in Context,* which is written by and for healthcare professionals. Consequently, some of the language used may be difficult for the less scientifically minded reader. To help with this, in addition to the Patient Notes, we have included a comprehensive glossary of those terms underlined in the text. Terms will not be underlined in tables or figures, but the more difficult words will be defined in the Glossary.

## Disease overview

The disease overview provides a brief synopsis of the disease, its symptoms, diagnosis and a critique of the currently available treatment options.

- The epidemiology, or incidence and distribution of the disease within a population, is discussed, with particular emphasis on UK-specific data.
- The aetiology section describes the specific causes or origins of the

disease, which are usually a result of both genetic and environmental factors. Multifactorial diseases result from more than one causative element. If an individual has a genetic predisposition, they are more susceptible to developing the disease as a result of their genetic make-up.

- The functional changes that accompany a particular syndrome or disease constitute its pathophysiology.

- The management of a disease may be influenced by treatment guidelines, specific directives published by government agencies, professional societies, or by the convening of expert panels. The National Institute for Clinical Excellence (NICE), an independent sector of the NHS comprised of experts in the field of treatment, is one such body.

- The social and economic factors that characterise the influence of the disease, describe its socioeconomic impact. Such factors include the cost to the healthcare provider to treat the disease – in terms of GP consultations, drug costs and the subsequent burden on hospital resources – or the cost to the patient or employer with respect to the number of work days lost as a consequence of ill health.

This edition of *BESTMEDICINE* focuses on one class of antihypertensive drugs. However, to give our readers further information regarding other available treatments, we have also included an overview of other medications currently available. Future editions of *BESTMEDICINE* will look at other drug classes in more detail.

## Drug reviews

☞ The pharmacokinetics of a drug are of interest to healthcare professionals because it is important for them to understand the action of a drug on the body over a period of time.

The drug reviews are not intended to address every available treatment for a particular disease. Rather, we focus on the major drugs currently available in the UK for the treatment of the featured disease and evaluate their performance in clinical trials and their safety in clinical practice. The basic pharmacology of the drug – the branch of science that deals with the origin, nature, chemistry, effects and uses of drugs – is discussed initially.[a] This includes a description of the mechanism of action of the drug, the manner in which it exerts its therapeutic effects, and its pharmacokinetics (or the activity of the drug within the body over a period of time). Pharmacokinetics encompasses the absorption of the drug into or across the tissues of the body, its distribution to specific functional areas, its metabolism – the process by which it is broken down within the body into by-products (metabolites) – and ultimately, its removal or excretion from the body. The most frequently used pharmacokinetic terms that are used in the drug review sections of this issue of *BESTMEDICINE* are explained in Table 1.

---

[a]As this issue of *BESTMEDICINE* deals with one class of blood pressure-lowering drugs (the angiotensin receptor blockers), the pharmacology section is presented as a separate chapter and summarises the basic pharmacological profile of the drug class as a whole.

**Table I.** Key pharmacokinetic terms.

| Term | Definition |
|---|---|
| Agonist | A drug/substance that has affinity for specific cell receptors triggering a biological response. |
| Antagonist | A drug/substance that blocks the action of another by binding to a specific cell receptor without eliciting a biological response. |
| AUC (area under curve) | A plot of the concentration of a drug against the time since initial administration. It is a means of analysing the bioavailability of a drug. |
| Binding affinity | An attractive force between substances that causes them to enter into and remain in chemical contact. |
| Bioavailability | The degree and rate at which a drug is absorbed into a living system or is made available at the site of physiological activity. |
| Clearance | The rate at which the drug is removed from the blood by excretion into the urine through the kidneys. |
| $C_{max}$ | The maximum concentration of the drug recorded in the blood plasma. |
| Cytochrome P450 (CYP) system | A group of enzymes responsible for the metabolism of a number of different drugs and substances within the body. |
| Dose dependency | In which the effect of the drug is proportional to the concentration of drug administered. |
| Enzyme | A protein produced in the body that catalyses chemical reactions without itself being destroyed or altered. The suffix 'ase' is used when designating an enzyme. |
| Excretion | The elimination of a waste product (in faeces or urine) from the body. |
| Half-life ($t_{1/2}$) | The time required for half the original amount of a drug to be eliminated from the body by natural processes. |
| Inhibitor | A substance that reduces the activity of another substance. |
| Ligand | Any substance that binds to another and brings about a biological response. |
| Potency | A measure of the power of a drug to produce the desired effects. |
| Protein binding | The extent to which a drug attaches to proteins, peptides or enzymes within the body. |
| Receptor | A molecular structure, usually (but not always) situated on the cell membrane, which mediates the biological response that is associated with a particular drug/substance. |
| Synergism | A phenomenon in which the combined effects of two drugs are more powerful than when either drug is administered alone. |
| $t_{max}$ | The time taken to reach $C_{max}$. |
| Volume of distribution ($V_D$) | The total amount of drug in the body divided by its concentration in the blood plasma. Used as a measure of the dispersal of the drug within the body once it has been absorbed. |

Whilst the basic pharmacology of a drug is clearly important, the main focus of each drug review is to summarise the drug's performance in controlled clinical trials. Clinical trials examine the effectiveness, or clinical efficacy, of the drug against the disease or condition it was developed to treat, as well as its safety and tolerability – the side-effects associated with the drug and the likelihood that the patient will tolerate treatment. Adherence to drug treatment, or patient compliance, reflects the tendency of patients to comply with the terms of their treatment regimen. Compliance may be affected by treatment-related side-effects or the convenience of drug treatment. The safety of the drug also encompasses its contra-indications – conditions under which the drug should never be prescribed. This may mean avoiding use in special patient populations (e.g. young or elderly patients, or those with co-existing or comorbid conditions, such as liver or kidney disease) or avoiding co-administration with certain other medications.

A brief synopsis of the drug development process is outlined below, in order to clarify and put into context many of the specialist terms encountered throughout the drug reviews.

### The drug development process

Launching a new drug is an extremely costly and time-consuming venture. The entire process can cost an estimated £500 million and can take between 10 and 15 years from the initial identification of a potentially useful therapeutic compound in the laboratory to launching the finished product as a treatment for a particular disease (Figure 1). Much of this time is spent fulfilling strict guidelines set out by regulatory authorities, in order to ensure the safety and quality of the end product.

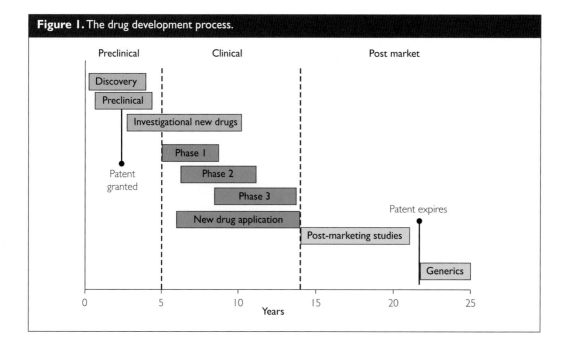

**Figure 1.** The drug development process.

As a consequence of this, a drug can fail at any stage of the development process and its development abandoned. Once identified and registered, the new drug can be protected by a patent for 20 years, after which time other companies are free to manufacture and market identical drugs, called generics. Thus, the pharmaceutical company has a finite period of time before patent expiry to recoup the cost of drug development (of both successful drugs and those drugs that do not make it to the marketplace) and return a profit to their shareholders.

Potential new drugs are identified by the research and development (R&D) department of the pharmaceutical company. After a candidate drug has been selected for development, it enters a rigorous testing procedure with five distinct phases – preclinical, which takes place in the laboratory, and phases 1, 2, 3 and 4, which involve testing in humans. Approval from the regulatory body is essential before the drug can be marketed and is dependent on the satisfactory completion of all phases of testing. In the UK, the Medicines and Healthcare Products Agency (MHRA) and the European Medicines Evaluation Agency (EMEA) regulate the development process and companies must apply to these organisations for marketing authorisation. Within Europe, the Mutual Recognition Procedure means that the approval of a drug in one country (the Reference Member State), forms the basis for its subsequent approval in other European Union member states. This can make the approval process more efficient and may lead to approval being granted in several European countries at once. Once approval has been granted, the drug will be given a licence detailing the specific disease or conditions it is indicated to treat and the patient groups it may be used in. The drug will be assigned either prescription-only medicine (POM) or over-the counter (OTC) status. POMs can only be obtained following consultation with a doctor, who will actively supervise their use.

## Preclinical testing

Preclinical testing is essential before a drug can progress to human clinical trials. It is estimated that only one of every 1000 compounds that enter the preclinical stage continue into human testing (phases 1–4). Preclinical testing, or screening, is for the main-part performed in animals, and every effort is made to use as few animals as possible and to ensure their humane and proper care. Generally, two or more species (one rodent, one non-rodent) are tested, since a drug may affect one species differently from another.

Although a drug will never act in exactly the same way in animals as in humans, animal models are designed to mimic a human disease condition as closely as possible and provide information essential to drug development. _In vitro_ experiments – literally meaning 'in glass' – are performed outside the living system in a laboratory setting. _In vivo_ experiments are performed in the living cell or organism.

It is during the preclinical phase that the pharmacodynamics of the drug will first be examined. These include its mechanism of action, or the way in which it exerts its therapeutic effects. The drug's pharmacokinetics, toxicology (potentially hazardous or poisonous effects) and the formulation of the drug – the manner in which it is taken (e.g. tablet, injection, liquid) – are also assessed at this point in development.

## Phase 1

Phase 1 trials are usually conducted in a small group of 10–80 healthy volunteers and further evaluate the biochemical and physiological effects of the drug – its chemical and biological impact within the body. An appropriate dosage range will be established at this point – the maximum and minimum therapeutic concentrations of the drug which are associated with a tolerable number of side-effects (secondary and usually adverse events unrelated to the beneficial effects of the drug). The mechanism of action and pharmacokinetic effects of the drugs are also further explored in this, the first group of human subjects to receive the drug.

## Phase 2

If no major problems are revealed during phase 1 development, the drug can progress to phase 2 trials which take place in 100–300 patients diagnosed with the disease or condition that the drug is designed to treat. At this stage it is important to determine the effectiveness, or efficacy, of the drug. If the drug is no better than placebo then it will not be granted a licence. The side-effect or adverse event profile of the drug is re-examined at this stage, and is particularly pertinent in these patients, who may react more severely to the drug than healthy volunteers. The likelihood and severity of drug interactions is also of great importance in this patient group. Drug interactions – in which the action of one drug interferes with the action of another – can occur if the patient is taking more than one form of medication for the treatment of a comorbid disease or condition. If multiple drugs are administered together, or concomitantly, then the risk of drug interactions is increased.

## Phase 3

Phase 3 clinical trials involve between 1000 and 3000 patients diagnosed with the relevant disease or condition. The recruitment of patients and the co-ordination and analysis of the trials is costly, so the pharmaceutical company will not embark on this stage unless they are sufficiently convinced of the therapeutic benefits of their drug. Essentially, phase 3 trials are replications of phase 2 trials but on a larger scale. The duration of the trial depends on the type of drug and the length of time required in order to determine the efficacy of the drug. For example, an antibiotic trial will have a shorter duration than the trial of a drug intended to treat long-term conditions, such as Alzheimer's disease. Acute treatment describes a short-term schedule given over a period of days or weeks, and chronic treatment refers to longer-term treatment schedules, lasting over periods of months or years.

Clinical trials may compare the new drug with an existing drug – a comparative trial – or may simply compare the new drug with no active drug treatment at all – a placebo-controlled trial. The participants who receive a comparator treatment or placebo are termed controls. In placebo-controlled trials, patients are given a placebo – an inert substance with no specific pharmacological activity – in place of the active drug. Patients will be unaware that the substance they are taking is placebo, which will be visually identical to the active treatment. This approach rules out any psychological effects of drug treatment – a patient may perceive that their condition has improved simply through the action of taking a tablet. In order to be considered clinically effective, the experimental drug must produce better results than the placebo.

The clinical trial should be designed in such a way as to limit the degree of bias it carries. The blinding of the trial is one means of eliminating bias. Double-blind trials, in which neither the doctor nor the patient knows which is the real drug and which is the placebo or comparator drug, are the most informative. In single-blind trials, only the patient is unaware of what they are taking, and in open-label trials, all participants are aware of treatment allocation. Conducting the trial across a number of clinics or hospitals, either abroad or in the same country (multicentre trials), further eliminates bias, as does randomisation, the random allocation of patients to treatment groups. At the start of the study, the baseline characteristics of the study population are recorded and are used as a starting point for all subsequent comparisons.

Efficacy is commonly measured by means of primary and secondary endpoints. Endpoints mark a recognised stage in the disease process and are used to compare the outcome in different treatment arms of clinical trials. The endpoint of one trial may be a marker of improvement or recovery whereas another trial may use the deterioration of the patient (morbidity) or death (mortality) to signify the end of the trial. Either way, endpoints represent valid criteria by which to compare treatments. On a similar note, surrogate markers are laboratory measurements of biological activity within the body that provide an indirect measure of the effect of treatment on disease state (e.g. blood pressure and cholesterol levels).

Statistical analysis allows the investigator to draw rational conclusions from clinical trials regarding the effectiveness of their drug. If the patient data generated during the course of a clinical trial are statistically significant, then there is a high probability that the given result, be it an improvement or a decline in the health of the patient, is due to a specific effect of drug treatment, rather than a chance occurrence. The data are put through a number of mathematical procedures that ultimately produce a $p$-value. This value reflects the probability that the result occurred by chance. For example, if the $p$-value is less than or equal to 0.05, the result is usually considered to be statistically significant. Such a $p$ value indicates that there is a 95% probability that the result did not occur by chance. The smaller the $p$-value, the more significant the result. When quoting clinical findings,

☛ *Someone is always aware of who is taking what in a clinical trial. Whilst neither a doctor nor a patient may be aware of their treatment in a double-blind trial, there is a secure coding system, known only to the investigator, which contains the various treatment allocations.*

the *p*-value is often given in brackets in order to emphasise the importance of the finding.

Once a drug has progressed through the key stages of development and demonstrated clear efficacy with an acceptable safety profile, the data are collated and the pharmaceutical company will then submit a licence application to the regulatory authorities – a new drug application (NDA).

## Phase 4 (Post-marketing studies)

Phase 4 testing takes place after the drug has been marketed and involves large numbers of patients, sometimes including those groups that may have previously been excluded from clinical trials (e.g. pregnant women and elderly or young patients). These trials are usually open-label, so the patient is aware of what they are taking, without control groups. They provide valuable information regarding the tolerability of the drug, and may reveal any long-term adverse events associated with treatment. Post-marketing surveillance continues throughout the life-span of the drug, and constantly monitors the safety, usage and performance. Doctors are advised to inform the MHRA and the Committee on Safety of Medicines (CSM) of any adverse events they encounter.

# Editorial

*Professor Bryan Williams*
*Professor of Medicine, University of Leicester Medical School, Leicester*

Hypertension is extremely common, affecting approximately 20% of adults, with half of the over-65 year age group affected. The World Health Organization recently identified hypertension as one of the most important preventable causes of death worldwide. Thus, the case for treating hypertension is compelling with the evidence base supporting the effectiveness of treatment the largest in clinical medicine.

It is interesting to reflect on how attitudes and approaches to treatment have evolved over the past 30 years. Initial studies focused on proving that lowering blood pressure would reduce <u>cardiovascular</u> <u>morbidity</u> and <u>mortality</u>. Studies were then refined to focus on different populations and subgroups with varying cardiovascular risk. These subgroups included individuals with diabetes, <u>target-organ damage</u> (e.g. <u>left ventricular hypertrophy</u>, <u>microalbuminuria</u>), hyperlipidaemia, renal disease, older people with <u>isolated systolic hypertension</u>, and different ethnic groups and gender. Such studies have provided us with rich seams of information that have led to the publication of guidelines that have in turn, assisted in the implementation of the evidence base in clinical practice.

However, inadequate implementation of this impressive evidence base persists, and is one of the reasons why we are failing to achieve blood pressure targets in practice. In fact, more people on antihypertensive treatments have poorly controlled blood pressure than are achieving recommended blood pressure targets. This has been confounded further by progressive lowering of targets, as the benefits of treatment in people with lower blood pressures have been realised. As such, the size of the challenge is as great today as it was more than 30 years ago!

How do we improve implementation of this evidence in our clinical practice? What is the best system of care for our patients with hypertension? These areas have been substantially under-researched and yet probably have the greatest potential to improve population-based care for people with hypertension.

It is accepted that lowering blood pressure is very effective at reducing the risk of stroke, heart failure and <u>myocardial infarction</u>. Nevertheless, clinicians have been slow to recognise that achieving blood pressure targets will require more than one drug, with combinations required more often than not. Different combinations will be more effective in certain populations and in those with specific manifestations of target-organ damage. Defining the ideal combination of drugs to achieve optimal blood pressure control and optimal cardiovascular protection is in its infancy, but represents a major shift in emphasis away from <u>monotherapy</u> comparisons that have preoccupied trial designers for so many years.

☛ Remember that the author of this Editorial is addressing his healthcare professional colleagues rather than the 'lay' reader. This provides a fascinating insight into many of the challenges faced by doctors in the day-to-day practice of medicine (see Reader's Guide).

☛ This is a common theme that will be repeated throughout this book – most patients require more than one drug to get their blood pressure controlled.

If we accept that lowering blood pressure reduces <u>cardiovascular</u> risk and that combinations of drugs are likely to be required to achieve recommended blood pressure goals, it is apparent that fixed-dose combinations should also improve concordance with therapy. It is also reasonable to assume that most physicians would welcome guidance on logical drug combinations and in what order to use them. To this end, the British Hypertension Society recently recommended a treatment algorithm based on the 'AB/CD' rule (see Disease Overview and Improving Practice). This algorithm provides us with a much needed treatment template to plan the sequence of care for individual patients that is not restrictive and advises on logical drug combinations. This template could be easily incorporated into practice-based software programmes to provide individualised care plans tailored to individual patients' characteristics and needs. In managing cardiovascular risk, it is also essential to recognise that many patients would also benefit from concomitant treatment with aspirin and <u>statins</u>.

The development of molecular modelling has enabled the pharmaceutical industry to refine its drug targets and produce even more selective agents that block key pathways involved in blood pressure regulation. Such an approach has the potential to provide greater <u>efficacy</u> with fewer adverse effects. Whether these approaches will ultimately translate into improved patient outcome will depend not only on the quality of the individual drug constituents, but also on defining the most appropriate population for each drug combination and the most appropriate method to deliver care, as indicated above. Herein lies the challenge for those of us charged with the responsibility of treating hypertension, which continues to be one of the most important, preventable causes of death worldwide.

# I. Disease overview – Hypertension

Dr Jennifer Moorman and Dr Duncan West
CSF Medical Communications Ltd

## Summary

Hypertension (i.e. blood pressure ≥140/90 mmHg) is a leading cause of death and disability worldwide. It is estimated that over one-third of adults in the UK are hypertensive. Inadequate control of blood pressure is a major risk factor for the development of coronary heart disease (CHD) and stroke. However, despite recent improvements in the diagnosis and treatment of hypertension, it has been estimated that only 9% of hypertensives in the UK attain a target blood pressure of 140/90 mmHg or lower. The benefits of effective blood pressure lowering have been clearly demonstrated. Patients with controlled blood pressure live longer and have a reduced risk of morbidity from stroke, myocardial infarction (MI), heart failure and renal failure. Various guidelines have been published to assist physicians in the management of patients with hypertension. Regular blood pressure monitoring is essential and drug therapy is currently recommended for patients with a sustained systolic blood pressure (SBP) of ≥160 mmHg or a sustained diastolic blood pressure (DBP) of ≥100 mmHg. However, these thresholds are lower for patients with cardiovascular disease (CVD) or diabetes (140–159/90–99 mmHg). These guidelines also enable a patient's prognosis and treatment options to be determined on the basis of their total cardiovascular risk. The pathophysiology of hypertension is complex and poorly understood. A number of physiological mechanisms are involved in the maintenance of blood pressure, although the renin–angiotensin system has been the principal focus in the rational design of antihypertensive agents.

## Introduction

Hypertension (which in the general population means blood pressure ≥140/90 mmHg) remains a major public health problem, being one of the leading causes of death and disability worldwide after smoking and malnutrition, and a major risk factor for CVD.[1–3] Although substantial progress has been made in the diagnosis and treatment of the condition in recent years, blood pressure is normalised in less than one-third of treated hypertensives worldwide, leading to serious long-term health problems for the individuals concerned, to say nothing of the millions of hypertensives who go undiagnosed.[4]

Hypertension is a common condition affecting 600 million people worldwide and resulting in the deaths of 3 million people every year.[5] In the US, 24% of the adult population (43 million people) have hypertension.[6] However, the prevalence in the UK is reported to be higher, with 37% of adults over 16 years of age identified as being hypertensive.[7] The prevalence of hypertension increases markedly with advancing age (Figure 1).[8,9] In the British Women's Heart and Health Study survey of 4286 women aged 60–79 years, 50% were found to be hypertensive.[10] Furthermore, the prevalence of the condition is likely to increase in the coming years with the projected ageing of populations worldwide.

Despite significant progress being made in the diagnosis and treatment of hypertension, blood pressure control worldwide remains largely uncontrolled. The poor control of hypertension appears to be the result of poor detection and awareness of the condition, coupled with inadequate treatment. A key component of this inadequate treatment is

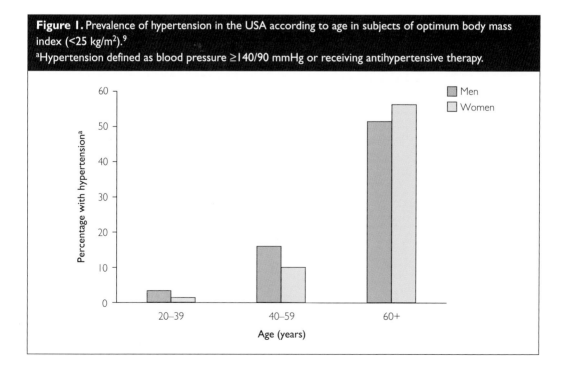

**Figure 1.** Prevalence of hypertension in the USA according to age in subjects of optimum body mass index (<25 kg/m²).[9]
[a]Hypertension defined as blood pressure ≥140/90 mmHg or receiving antihypertensive therapy.

the predominance of <u>monotherapy</u> in clinical practice.[7] Consequently, new hypertension guidelines emphasise the need for combination drug therapy to allow patients to achieve target blood pressure levels.

The rates of hypertension treatment and control increased significantly between the 1994 and 1998 UK health surveys. However, there is further room for improvement in the management of hypertension, both in the UK and other countries, emphasising the importance of auditing the management of patients with CVD.

- Data from the National Health and Nutrition Examination Survey III (NHANES) indicate that only 24.4% of hypertensives in the US aged between 18 and 74 years achieved blood pressure values below the target value of 140/90 mmHg.[8]
- A health survey conducted throughout England in 1998 reported that only 9% of hypertensives attained target blood pressure values of 140/90 mmHg.[7]
- Even in countries where target blood pressure values were set as 160/95 mmHg (e.g. Canada, Australia, Scotland and Spain), control was achieved in only 16, 19, 18 and 20% of patients, respectively.[11]

Awareness of hypertension in the general population also remains poor. A population-based, case-control study conducted in England highlighted poor patient awareness of hypertension through analysis of cases identified from a stroke register (1994–95). Less than 30% of patients (267 stroke, 534 control) were found to have adequate blood pressure control (<140/90 mmHg) and only 56% of the stroke patients were aware of their hypertension.[12] This situation appears to be mirrored in the US: in a study of 636 people from a community in Minnesota, 53% were diagnosed with hypertension, though only 39% were aware of their condition.[13]

There is substantial evidence that uncontrolled hypertension can have profound consequences for the individual. For example, poorly controlled hypertension:

- can contribute to <u>end-organ damage</u> in the heart, brain, eyes and kidneys
- is a major risk factor for the development of CHD and underlying <u>atherosclerosis</u> (Figure 2)[2,9,14]
- increases the risk of stroke.[15]

Although <u>suboptimal</u> control of hypertension is clearly detrimental to patients, significant benefits are gained when blood pressure is sufficiently reduced. Studies have shown that individuals with adequate blood pressure control live longer than those with uncontrolled hypertension.[16] Optimal blood pressure control appears to be particularly crucial in patients with diabetes or <u>chronic renal failure</u>. Moreover, lowering elevated blood pressure reduces <u>morbidity</u> from stroke, MI, <u>congestive heart failure</u> and renal failure, and recent outcomes studies have demonstrated that antihypertensive agents offer clinical benefits beyond their blood pressure lowering <u>efficacy</u>.[8,17–20]

> A health survey conducted in England in 1998 reported that only 9% of hypertensives attained target blood pressure values of 140/90 mmHg.

> Lowering elevated blood pressure reduces morbidity from stroke, MI, congestive heart failure and renal failure.

**Figure 2.** Relationship between systolic (top) and diastolic (bottom) blood pressure and incidence of coronary heart disease (CHD).[14]

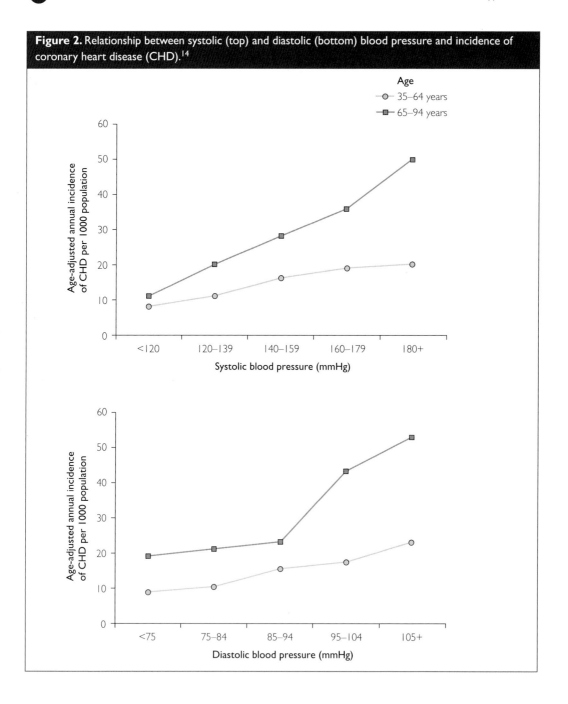

- The Hypertension Optimal Treatment (HOT) study and the UK Prospective Diabetes Study (UKPDS) have demonstrated that intensive blood pressure lowering significantly lowers the risks of cardiovascular events in hypertensive diabetics.[21,22]
- The Multiple Risk Factor Intervention Trial (MRFIT) has provided direct evidence that graded elevations of blood pressure are a strong independent risk factor for end-stage renal disease.[23]

- The Heart Outcomes Prevention Evaluation (HOPE) study has demonstrated a significant improvement in clinical outcomes (reduced fatality and lowered risk of cardiovascular events) in high-risk patients prescribed an angiotensin-converting enzyme (ACE) inhibitor.[17]
- The European Trial on Reduction of Cardiac Events with Perindopril in Stable Coronary Artery Disease (EUROPA) has shown that even in low-risk patients, ACE inhibitor therapy improves clinical outcomes in all at-risk patients with coronary artery disease.[18]
- The Perindopril Protection Against Recurrent Stroke (PROGRESS) study has demonstrated that ACE inhibitor therapy produces a reduction in the risk of stroke in patients with a history of stroke or transient ischaemic attack (TIA).[19]
- The Losartan Intervention For Endpoint Reduction in Hypertension (LIFE) study reported greater reductions in cardiovascular morbidity and mortality with an angiotensin II receptor antagonist compared with β-blocker therapy in patients with left ventricular hypertrophy. Moreover, the difference between the treatment arms was driven largely by a 25% greater reduction in the risk of fatal/non-fatal stroke with the angiotensin II receptor antagonist despite broadly similar blood pressure reductions.[20]

Inadequate compliance with therapy is believed to be one of the major causes of uncontrolled hypertension; between 30 and 60% of patients may be non-compliant with their antihypertensive regimens.[24] The main causes of non-compliance with antihypertensive therapy are thought to be:
- the asymptomatic nature of hypertension
- unacceptable side-effects of therapy
- suboptimal antihypertensive therapy
- lack of communication between doctor and patient.[25]

## Diagnosis

Individuals with severe hypertension may experience dizziness, blurred vision or headaches; however, moderate hypertension is generally asymptomatic and is often detected only during a routine consultation. Nevertheless, undetected hypertension can result in serious long-term damage to the heart, kidneys, eyes and other organs and it is thus vital that blood pressure is assessed regularly, particularly in patients over the age of 60 years.

In recognition of the fact that the relationship between cardiovascular risk and blood pressure begins at very low levels of pressure, new guidelines for the classification and management of hypertension have recently been published by the European Society of Hypertension–European Society of Cardiology (ESH–ESC), Joint National Committee on Prevention, Detection, Evaluation and Treatment of High Blood Pressure (JNC-VII), the World Health Organization–International Society of Hypertension (WHO–ISH) and

It is vital that blood pressure is assessed regularly, particularly in patients over the age of 60 years.

the British Hypertension Society (BHS).[3,26–30] The recently published BHS guidelines emphasise the need to assess and reduce total cardiovascular risk, moving beyond the control of single risk factors, such as hypertension, by multiple interventions, including statin and aspirin therapy where indicated.[29,30] The ESH–ESC and WHO–ISH guidelines classify 'normal' levels of blood pressure as optimal, normal and high–normal (Table 1).[26,28] The classification of blood pressure levels given by the BHS are also equated with those of the ESH–ESC and the WHO–ISH guidelines.[29,30]

The BHS, ESH–ESC and WHO–ISH guidelines all define hypertension as blood pressure of 140/90 mmHg or greater.[26,28–30] The new BHS guidelines recommend the following thresholds and treatment targets:

- start drug therapy in all patients with sustained SBP of 160 mmHg or greater, or sustained DBP of 100 mmHg or greater despite non-pharmacological measures
- drug treatment is also indicated in patients with SBP of 140–159 mmHg or DBP of 90–99 mmHg (grade 1) if target-organ damage is present, if there is evidence of established CVD or diabetes, or the 10-year CVD risk is at least 20%
- for most patients a target of 140 mmHg or lower for SBP and 85 mmHg or lower for DBP is recommended; for patients with diabetes a target of 130/80 mmHg or lower is recommended. Lower targets are also recommended in those at high risk of CVD.[29,30]

**Table 1.** The ESH–ESC, WHO–ISH and BHS classification of blood pressure.[26,28–30]

| Category | SBP (mmHg) | DBP (mmHg) |
|---|---|---|
| Optimal BP | <120 | <80 |
| Normal BP | <130 | <85 |
| High–normal BP | 130–139 | 85–89 |
| Hypertension | | |
|    Grade 1 (mild) | 140–159 | 90–99 |
|    Grade 2 (moderate) | 160–179 | 100–109 |
|    Grade 3 (severe) | ≥180 | ≥110 |
| Isolated systolic hypertension | | |
|    Grade 1 | 140–159 | <90 |
|    Grade 2 | ≥160 | <90 |

When a patient's systolic blood pressure (SBP) and diastolic blood pressure (DBP) fall into different categories, the higher category should apply. BP, blood pressure.

Appropriate lifestyle modification should also be encouraged in patients with mild (grade 1) hypertension who are not treated, and their blood pressures and CVD risk should be reassessed annually.

All adults should have their blood pressure measured at least every 5 years. Those with high–normal values (130–139/85–89 mmHg) and those who have had high readings at any time should have their blood pressure measured annually. Repeated measurements are required in order to distinguish between sustained hypertension and 'white-coat hypertension', a condition in which a patient's blood pressure is elevated in the doctor's surgery or clinic, but is normal at other times. Although the latter group may be at greater risk than normotensive patients, this condition may not warrant a diagnosis or treatment of hypertension.[31] The BHS recommendations for taking blood pressure should be followed (Table 2).[29,30]

> All adults should have their blood pressure measured at least every 5 years.

In addition to follow-up blood pressure measurements, patients with documented hypertension (>140/90 mmHg) should also receive further evaluation to identify:
- known causes of raised blood pressure (e.g. renal disease)
- contributory factors (e.g. obesity, high salt and/or alcohol intake)
- complications of hypertension (e.g. previous stroke or left ventricular hypertrophy [LVH])
- cardiovascular risk factors (e.g. smoking or a family history of CVD).[29,30]

All patients should have a thorough history and physical examination with routine investigations limited to a urine strip test for protein and blood, serum creatinine and electrolytes, blood glucose, serum total cholesterol and high density lipoprotein cholesterol and an

---

**Table 2.** Blood pressure measurement.[29,30]

- Follow British Hypertension Society guidelines on technique.
- Use a device with validated accuracy, that is properly maintained and calibrated.
- Measure sitting blood pressure routinely; standing blood pressure in elderly or diabetic patients.
- Remove tight clothing, support arm at heart level, ensure arm is relaxed and avoid talking during the measurement.
- Use an appropriate size of cuff.
- Lower mercury slowly, by 2 mm/second.
- Read blood pressure to the nearest 2 mmHg.
- Measure diastolic blood pressure as the disappearance of sounds (phase 5).
- Take the mean of two measurements at each visit. More recordings are required if there are marked differences in initial measurements.
- Use the average for several visits when estimating cardiovascular risk in mild hypertension.
- Do not treat on the basis of an isolated reading.

electrocardiogram.[29,30] Further diagnostic procedures such as chest radiograph, urine microscopy and culture, and echocardiography are not required routinely, although an echocardiogram is useful for the diagnosis of LVH.[29,30]

The new ESH–ESC and WHO–ISH guidelines also advocate the stratification of the total cardiovascular risk in each patient into one of four categories – low, medium, high and very high risk. These categories can also be used to determine a patient's prognosis and need for treatment, as well as the speed and intensity with which antihypertensive drug treatment should be introduced (Table 3).[26,28] These guidelines recommend the immediate initiation of drug therapy in patients categorised as very high risk and in those with multiple risk factors.[26,28] The BHS guidelines in use in the UK are summarised in Figure 3.[29,30] These guidelines include assessment of absolute risk of CVD rather than CHD which reflects the importance of stroke prevention as well as CHD prevention. New charts to calculate the 10-year CVD risk are included in the BHS guidelines.[30]

> Guidelines recommend the immediate initiation of drug therapy in patients categorised as very high risk and in those with multiple risk factors.

## Pathophysiology of hypertension

The pathophysiology of hypertension is uncertain, though it is probable that a number of interrelated factors contribute to the condition, with their relative roles differing between individuals.[32] In around 5% of individuals, hypertension is caused by underlying renal or adrenal disease and is termed secondary hypertension. The major causes of secondary hypertension are:

- renal disease (e.g. parenchymal disease, renovascular disease and renin-producing tumours)

**Table 3.** Stratification of total 10-year cardiovascular risk according to grade of hypertension.[26,28]

| Additional risk factors[b] and disease history | Blood pressure (mmHg) and 10-year risk level[a] | | |
|---|---|---|---|
| | Grade 1 (mild) 140–159/90–99 | Grade 2 (moderate) 160–179/100–109 | Grade 3 (severe) ≥180/110 |
| No other risk factors | Low risk | Medium risk | High risk |
| 1 or 2 risk factors | Medium risk | Medium risk | Very high risk |
| 3 or more risk factors, target-organ damage[c] or diabetes | High risk | High risk | Very high risk |
| Associated clinical condition[d] | Very high risk | Very high risk | Very high risk |

[a]Low risk, <15%; medium risk, 15–20%; high risk, 20–30%; very high risk, >30%.
[b]Age (men >55 years, women >65 years), smoking, total cholesterol >6.5 mmol/L, family history of premature cardiovascular disease.
[c]Left ventricular hypertrophy, proteinuria, atherosclerotic plaques, retinal artery narrowing.
[d]Cerebrovascular disease, coronary heart disease or heart failure, renal disease including diabetic nephropathy and renal failure (serum creatinine >177 mmol/L), dissecting aneurysm, symptomatic arterial disease and advanced hypertensive retinopathy.

**Figure 3.** British Hypertension Society guidelines for the management of hypertension.[29]
[a]Unless malignant phase of hypertensive emergency, confirm over 1–2 weeks then treat.
[b]If CV complications, target-organ damage, or diabetes are present, confirm over 3–4 weeks then treat; if absent remeasure weekly and treat if blood pressure persists at this level over 4–12 weeks.
[c]If CV complications, target organ damage, or diabetes are present, confirm over 3–4 weeks then treat; if absent remeasure monthly and treat if this level is maintained and if estimated 10-year CVD risk is ≥20%.
[d]Assessed with risk chart for CVD.
CV, cardiovascular; CVD, cardiovascular disease.

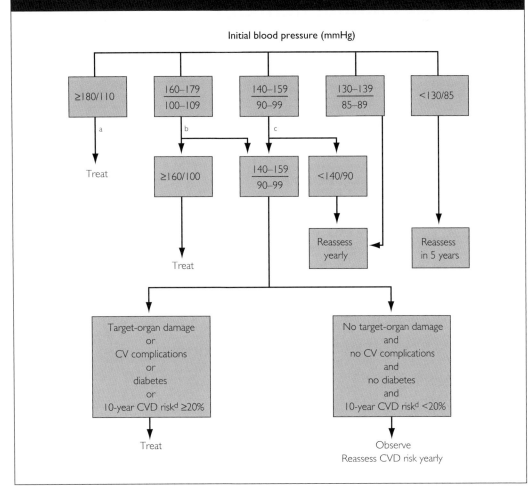

- drugs (e.g. oestrogen contraceptives, corticosteroids, liquorice, carbenoxelone, sympathomimetics and non-steroidal anti-inflammatory drugs)
- endocrine causes (e.g. acromegaly, Cushing's syndrome, primary hyperaldosteronism, congenital hyperplasia, phaeochromocytoma, thyroid disease, hyperparathyroidism)
- coarctation of the aorta
- pregnancy.[33]

In the remaining 95% of hypertensives, no clear identifiable cause can be found and such cases are known as primary or essential hypertension.

A number of physiological mechanisms are involved in the maintenance of normal blood pressure, and a disturbance in such systems may play a role in the development of hypertension. Cardiac output and peripheral resistance are directly involved in blood pressure control, but other important control mechanisms include:

- the renin–angiotensin system
- the autonomic nervous system
- other factors such as bradykinin, endothelin, endothelial-derived relaxing factor (nitric oxide), atrial natriuretic peptide and ouabain.[32]

## Cardiac output and peripheral resistance

In early hypertension, elevation of blood pressure may be caused by raised cardiac output, followed by a compensatory rise in peripheral arteriolar resistance.[32]

## Renin–angiotensin system

This is the most important endocrine system affecting blood pressure control. Angiotensin II is a potent vasoconstrictor that acts via angiotensin II type 1 ($AT_1$) receptors located on arterioles and in the adrenal cortex and increases blood pressure and stimulates the release of aldosterone, producing a further rise in blood pressure resulting from sodium and water retention.[32]

## Kallikrein–kinin system

The kallikrein–kinin system is another important vasoactive pathway. Plasma kallikrein forms the potent peptide vasodilator bradykinin which binds to kinin receptors on nearby endothelial cells. This in turn liberates vasoactive prostaglandins or nitric oxide, which results in vasodilation and increased capillary permeability.[34,35]

## Autonomic nervous system

There is little evidence of a clear role of adrenaline and noradrenaline in the aetiology of hypertension. Nevertheless, drugs that block the sympathetic nervous system lower blood pressure and it is probable that hypertension is caused by an interaction between the autonomic nervous system and the renin–angiotensin system.[32]

Of all these physiological mechanisms, blockade of the renin–angiotensin system has been the focus of the greatest interest in recent years in the rational design of antihypertensive agents, since this system is implicated in the control of blood pressure, water balance and cardiovascular structure and function. Figure 4 shows the pathways for generation of angiotensin II.[32]

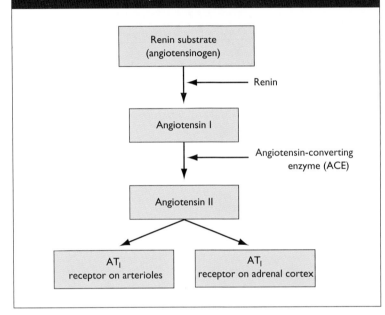

**Figure 4.** The renin–angiotensin system and its effects on blood pressure via angiotensin II type I ($AT_1$) receptors on arterioles and aldosterone release ($AT_1$ receptors on the adrenal cortex).[32] Prevention of the formation of angiotensin II is the target of antihypertensive agents developed over the past decade because of the putative involvement of this hormone in hypertension and cardiovascular disease. The actions of angiotensin II can be prevented by agents that either inhibit its formation (through inhibition of angiotensin-converting enzyme [ACE]) or antagonise its actions at $AT_1$ receptors.

## Risk factors

Although the precise cause of hypertension remains unclear, the following risk factors increase the chance of its development:

- history of hypertension among first-degree relatives
- African race
- male gender
- older age (men >55 years; women >65 years)
- obesity
- high alcohol consumption
- sedentary or inactive lifestyle.[8,32,36]

## The economic cost of hypertension

Hypertension is a highly prevalent condition that incurs substantial direct and indirect healthcare costs each year. Whilst economic data are limited in the UK population, in the US hypertension was reported to cost US$10 billion annually in direct medical expenditures in 1991.[37] Of these costs, a large proportion can be attributed to patients' poor compliance with therapy and switching medications.

The direct costs of switching and discontinuing prescriptions for hypertension in the UK have been calculated using the MediPlus database, which holds information on 156 GP practices.

- The total annual cost associated with switching antihypertensive therapy was estimated at £26.9 million (for 7741 newly diagnosed patients).
- Patients who switched from initial therapy incurred an extra cost of £56 each per year, representing a 20% increase over those continuing on original therapy.[38]
- In the US in 1997, the annual healthcare cost per patient with hypertension was reported as US$341 for those who were compliant with therapy, compared with US$694 for those who were not.[39]

The development of hypertension is associated with an increased risk of CVD and accelerates the progression of <u>diabetic nephropathy</u> and retinopathy. Consequently, the long-term costs associated with the condition can be expected to be considerable. This is illustrated by the findings of a 19-year follow-up study of more than 10,000 patients in Finland. In this study, severely hypertensive men lost 2.6 more years of work than <u>normotensive</u> men, 1.7 years of which were attributable to CVD. The total costs for severe hypertension were US$219,300, with 43% being due to CVD.[40]

## Key points

- Hypertension is a major public health problem and is one of the leading causes of death and disability worldwide.

- Hypertension is poorly controlled because of a lack of detection and awareness of the condition and inadequate treatment.

- Uncontrolled hypertension is a major risk factor for the development of CVD, and can cause long-term damage to the eyes, kidneys and other organs.

- Hypertension is often <u>asymptomatic</u> and may only be detected during routine health checks.

- Hypertension incurs substantial direct and indirect healthcare costs, a large proportion of which can be attributed to poor compliance with therapy.

- The cause of hypertension is known in only a small proportion of cases; in the remainder, it may be caused by a dysregulation in blood pressure control mechanisms.

# References

A list of the published evidence which has been reviewed in compiling the preceding section of *BESTMEDICINE*.

1  Murray CJ, Lopez AD. Evidence-based health policy: lessons from the Global Burden of Disease Study. *Science* 1996; **274**: 740–3.

2  Dustan HP, Roccella EJ, Garrison HH. Controlling hypertension. A research success story. *Arch Intern Med* 1996; **156**: 1926–35.

3  Chobanian AV, Bakris GL, Black HR *et al*. The Seventh Report of the Joint National Committee on Prevention, Detection, Evaluation, and Treatment of High Blood Pressure: the JNC 7 report. *JAMA* 2003; **289**: 2560–72.

4  Waeber B. Achieving blood pressure targets in the management of hypertension. *Blood Press* 2001; **19(Suppl 2)**: 6–12.

5  The World Health Organization. Guidelines set new definitions, update treatment for hypertension. *Bull World Health Organ* 1999; **77**: 293.

6  Burt VL, Whelton P, Roccella EJ *et al*. Prevalence of hypertension in the US adult population. Results from the Third National Health and Nutrition Examination Survey, 1988–1991. *Hypertension* 1995; **25**: 305–13.

7  Primatesta P, Brookes M, Poulter NR. Improved hypertension management and control: results from the health survey for England 1998. *Hypertension* 2001; **38**: 827–32.

8  The sixth report of the Joint National Committee on prevention, detection, evaluation, and treatment of high blood pressure. *Arch Intern Med* 1997; **157**: 2413–46.

9  Brown CD, Higgins M, Donato KA *et al*. Body mass index and the prevalence of hypertension and dyslipidemia. *Obes Res* 2000; **8**: 605–19.

10  Lawlor DA, Bedford C, Taylor M, Ebrahim S. Geographical variation in cardiovascular disease, risk factors, and their control in older women: British Women's Heart and Health Study. *J Epidemiol Community Health* 2003; **57**: 134–40.

11  Marques-Vidal P, Tuomilehto J. Hypertension awareness, treatment and control in the community: is the 'rule of halves' still valid? *J Hum Hypertens* 1997; **11**: 213–20.

12  Du X. Prevalence, treatment, control, and awareness of high blood pressure and the risk of stroke in Northwest England. *Prev Med* 2000; **30**: 288–94.

13  Meissner I, Whisnant JP, Sheps SG *et al*. Detection and control of high blood pressure in the community: do we need a wake-up call? *Hypertension* 1999; **34**: 466–71.

14  Cupples LA, D'Agostino RB, Kiely D. The Framingham Study. *An Epidemiological Investigation of Cardiovascular Disease, Section 34*. Some risk factors related to the annual incidence of cardiovascular disease and death using pooled repeated biennial measurements: Framingham Heart Study, 30-year follow-up. Bethesda, MD: National Heart, Lung and Blood Institute, 1987.

15  Klungel OH, Stricker BH, Paes AH *et al*. Excess stroke among hypertensive men and women attributable to undertreatment of hypertension. *Stroke* 1999; **30**: 1312–18.

16  Havlik RJ, LaCroix AZ, Kleinman JC *et al*. Antihypertensive drug therapy and survival by treatment status in a national survey. *Hypertension* 1989; **13(Suppl 5)**: 128–32.

17  Yusuf S, Sleight P, Pogue J *et al*. Effects of an angiotensin-converting-enzyme inhibitor, ramipril, on cardiovascular events in high-risk patients. The Heart Outcomes Prevention Evaluation Study Investigators. *N Engl J Med* 2000; **342**: 145–53.

18  Fox KM. Efficacy of perindopril in reduction of cardiovascular events among patients with stable coronary artery disease: randomised, double-blind, placebo-controlled, multicentre trial (the EUROPA study). *Lancet* 2003; **362**: 782–8.

19  Randomised trial of a perindopril-based blood-pressure-lowering regimen among 6105 individuals with previous stroke or transient ischaemic attack. *Lancet* 2001; **358**: 1033–41.

20  Lindholm LH, Ibsen H, Dahlof B *et al*. Cardiovascular morbidity in patients with diabetes in the Losartan Intervention For Endpoint reduction in hypertension study (LIFE): a randomised trial against atenolol. *Lancet* 2002; **359**: 1004–10.

21  Tight blood pressure control and risk of macrovascular and microvascular complications in type 2 diabetes: UKPDS 38. UK Prospective Diabetes Study Group. *BMJ* 1998; **317**: 703–13.

22  Hansson L, Zanchetti A, Carruthers SG *et al*. Effects of intensive blood-pressure lowering and low-dose aspirin in patients with hypertension: principal results of the Hypertension Optimal Treatment (HOT) randomised trial. HOT Study Group. *Lancet* 1998; **351**: 1755–62.

23  Klag MJ, Whelton PK, Randall BL *et al*. Blood pressure and end-stage renal disease in men. *N Engl J Med* 1996; **334**: 13–18.

24  Shaw E, Anderson JG, Maloney M, Jay SJ, Fagan D. Factors associated with noncompliance of patients taking antihypertensive medications. *Hosp Pharm* 1995; **30**: 201–7.

25  Rudd P. Compliance with antihypertensive therapy: raising the bar of expectations. *Am J Manag Care* 1998; **4**: 957–66.

26  2003 European Society of Hypertension–European Society of Cardiology guidelines for the management of arterial hypertension. *J Hypertens* 2003; **21**: 1011–53.

27  MacMahon S, Peto R, Cutler J *et al*. Blood pressure, stroke, and coronary heart disease. Part 1, Prolonged differences in blood pressure: prospective observational studies corrected for the regression dilution bias. *Lancet* 1990; **335**: 765–74.

28  1999 World Health Organization–International Society of Hypertension Guidelines for the Management of Hypertension. Guidelines Subcommittee. *J Hypertens* 1999; **17**: 151–83.

29 Williams B, Poulter NR, Brown MJ *et al.* British Hypertension Society guidelines for hypertension management 2004 (BHS-IV): summary. *BMJ* 2004; **328**: 634–40.

30 Williams B, Poulter NR, Brown MJ *et al.* British Hypertension Society guidelines. Guidelines for management of hypertension: report of the fourth working party of the British Hypertension Society, 2004 – BHS IV. *J Hum Hypertens* 2004; **18**: 139–85.

31 Krakoff LR, Phillips RA. White-coat hypertension. *Lancet* 1996; **348**: 1443–4.

32 Beevers G, Lip GY, O'Brien E. ABC of hypertension: The pathophysiology of hypertension. *BMJ* 2001; **322**: 912–16.

33 Adcock BB, Ireland RB. Secondary hypertension: a practical diagnostic approach. *Am Fam Physician* 1997; **55**: 1263–70.

34 Bhoola KD, Figueroa CD, Worthy K. Bioregulation of kinins: kallikreins, kininogens, and kininases. *Pharmacol Rev* 1992; **44**: 1–80.

35 Campbell DJ. The renin–angiotensin and the kallikrein–kinin systems. *Int J Biochem Cell Biol* 2003; **35**: 784–91.

36 Montani JP, Antic V, Yang Z, Dulloo A. Pathways from obesity to hypertension: from the perspective of a vicious triangle. *Int J Obes Relat Metab Disord* 2002; **26(Suppl 2)**: S28–38.

37 Stason WB. Opportunities to improve the cost-effectiveness of treatment for hypertension. *Hypertension* 1991; **18**: 1161–6.

38 Hughes D, McGuire A. The direct costs to the NHS of discontinuing and switching prescriptions for hypertension. *J Hum Hypertens* 1998; **12**: 533–7.

39 Rizzo JA, Simons WR. Variations in compliance among hypertensive patients by drug class: implications for health care costs. *Clin Ther* 1997; **19**: 1446–57.

40 Kiiskinen U, Vartiainen E, Puska P, Aromaa A. Long-term cost and life-expectancy consequences of hypertension. *J Hypertens* 1998; **16**: 1103–12.

# Acknowledgements

Figure 2 is adapted from the Framingham Study, 1987.[14]

Figure 3 is adapted from Williams *et al.*, 2004.[29]

# PATIENT NOTES
*Dr Mark Davis*

## What is hypertension?

Hypertension (or high blood pressure) is one of the main causes of disability and death throughout the world. It causes problems such as strokes, heart attacks, heart failure and kidney damage. Usually these problems develop over many years when either high blood pressure has not been diagnosed or, for various reasons, it has been suboptimally treated. In western societies high blood pressure becomes more common as we get older. For example, studies have shown that 50% of women aged over 60 years are likely to have the condition.

## What are the benefits of reducing blood pressure?

Reducing high blood pressure by making changes to our lifestyles and by using appropriate drug therapy can provide individuals with great health benefits. The Health Development Agency, a government-funded agency concerned with public health, recently announced that by reducing some of the major cardiovascular risk factors – smoking, raised cholesterol and high blood pressure – even by a small amount, we would reduce heart disease deaths by 50%, which equates to about 50,000 deaths per year.

## What are the symptoms of high blood pressure?

High blood pressure usually produces no symptoms until the damage to our organs occurs. This is called 'end organ damage' and may affect the brain, the kidneys, or the peripheral blood vessels in the heart, and can manifest as serious conditions such as a heart attack or stroke. Given the importance of this, it is vitally important that every adult has their blood pressure monitored on a regular basis.

## What causes hypertension?

In about 95% of people with high blood pressure, the cause of their condition is not certain. These people are said to have 'essential hypertension'. This condition is likely to be the result of a number of interrelated problems. For example, lifestyle is a major contributory factor to essential hypertension and includes factors such as obesity, physical inactivity and high alcohol consumption. The remaining 5% of individuals have an

*It is vitally important that every adult has their blood pressure monitored on a regular basis.*

identifiable cause and are said to have 'secondary hypertension'. These individuals often develop high blood pressure at a younger age and are often much harder to treat.

## How is blood pressure measured?

The height of blood pressure is measured in millimetres of mercury (mmHg) and is presented as two numbers. The higher figure (systolic blood pressure) is the pressure in the arteries when the heart contracts. The lower figure (diastolic blood pressure) relates to the pressure when the heart is filling. Blood pressure varies according to the time of day and the level of activity, and therefore it is important that blood pressure measurements are taken at least twice on each of several different days before a decision to treat is made. The individual patient should be made aware of the actual blood pressure reading, and more importantly, whether this is normal, high–normal or raised.

As the number of places where blood pressure can be measured increases, it is vitally important that the person measuring the blood pressure has the skill to interpret the reading. In people with no apparent health problems and normal blood pressure, a repeat measurement every 5 years appears to be sufficient.

More and more people are now being given the opportunity to measure their blood pressure at home using one of the many semi-automatic sphygmomanometers (blood-pressure monitors) that are widely available in pharmacists around the country. When undertaking this home monitoring it is important to use one of the machines that have been shown to be accurate. The British Hypertension Society (BHS) has checked some machines for accuracy and these are listed on their website (*www.hyp.ac.uk/bhs*). However, as a general rule, devices that measure blood pressure at the wrist or finger cannot be relied upon for accurate measurements. Home monitoring is particularly useful when repeated measurements are needed to establish a diagnosis or to decide whether treatment needs to be started or increased. It is important to remember that home blood pressure readings are usually lower than readings taken at a general practice or hospital (so-called 'clinic' readings). As our blood pressure targets are based upon clinical trials that have employed 'clinic' blood pressure readings, home readings need to be increased to be equivalent to these clinic readings. A pragmatic way to do this is to add 10/5 mmHg to the home reading.

## Making a decision to treat – what do the guidelines say?

When the doctor, nurse and patient decide on the available treatment options to manage high blood pressure, this should be

*Blood pressure varies according to the time of day and the level of activity.*

based on the level of risk of an individual. If someone already has evidence of end-organ damage such as a previous heart attack, or has diabetes, then their blood pressure needs to be reduced to the target of 130/80 mmHg, wherever possible. In those with a particularly high blood pressure (i.e. more than 160/100 mmHg), this single risk factor puts the individual at a sufficiently high enough risk to justify the initiation of treatment. In everyone else, the decision to treat depends on the overall level of cardiovascular disease risk of the individual. A calculation of cardiovascular disease risk takes into account factors such as smoking, levels of blood fats (cholesterol) and age (see *www.bestmedicine.com* for an example of a cardiovascular disease risk calculator). The BHS recommends treatment with drug therapy if patients' absolute risk of cardiovascular disease exceeds 20% over a 10-year period. The extent of cardiovascular disease risk is calculated using either charts or a computer programme. The BHS suggests a target of 140/85 mmHg for people with uncomplicated high blood pressure.

## What other factors should be considered when treating high blood pressure?

We know that many people with high blood pressure are unaware that they have the condition. Also of concern is the fact that many people decide to stop, or may never take, the treatment they are prescribed. There are several reasons for this. Understandably people are reluctant to take medication for a condition that usually has no symptoms. In addition, all of the blood-pressure lowering medication that we use can have some side-effects in some patients. When deciding to start treatment, healthcare professionals must ensure that the patient is fully involved in the decision-making process. They should understand what level of risk they face and decide for themselves (with suitable advice) what action needs to be taken. Should weight reduction or increased exercise be required then practical suggestions should be offered to help the patient achieve this. If drug treatment is required each patient should understand what the drug does and what side-effects may occur. This information is described in detail for one class of drugs that reduce blood pressure – the angiotensin II receptor antagonists [or angiotensin receptor blockers] – in the following chapters of this edition of *BESTMEDICINE*. It is also important for the patient to realise at the outset that more than one drug is invariably needed to get their blood pressure under control. However, it is usually possible to get the blood pressure to target levels using a combination of drugs that either cause no, or minimal and acceptable, side-effects.

*The BHS suggests a target of 140/85 mmHg for people with uncomplicated high blood pressure.*

Lifestyle improvements should always be attempted whether or not drug treatment is started. These lifestyle measures are detailed in the BHS guidelines and include dietary changes such as reducing salt, fat and alcohol intake, whilst also increasing fruit and vegetable consumption. Increasing physical activity and reducing excessive weight is also seen as having a beneficial effect on raised blood pressure.

The medical community has moved away from considering risk factors for cardiovascular disease in isolation. As a result of this shift in practice, the doctor or nurse will now measure and discuss all of your risk factors with you, as part of the decision to treat and on an ongoing basis in order to review your progress after treatment has been initiated. As a result of this you may, for example, be found to have a level of cholesterol (blood fats) that further increases your risk of cardiovascular disease. If this is the case, you may be offered further medication to reduce cholesterol levels in your blood, thereby reducing the chances of suffering a condition such as a heart attack. Another important risk factor for cardiovascular disease is type 2 diabetes. Like raised blood pressure, this can cause few symptoms particularly in its early stages. However, the presence of type 2 diabetes can be picked up during your blood pressure review and then treated accordingly.

*Increasing physical activity and reducing excessive weight is also seen as having a beneficial effect on raised blood pressure.*

# 2. Treatment of hypertension – an overview

*Dr Eleanor Bull*
*CSF Medical Communications Ltd*

## Summary

The treatment of hypertension is usually initiated with single drug therapy, with the subsequent addition of further drugs until adequate control of blood pressure is achieved. Any treatment approach should be tailored towards the individual patient and should take into account age, race and concomitant disease status. The major blood pressure-lowering drugs are divided into five major groups: diuretics; β-adrenoceptor antagonists (β-blockers); angiotensin-converting enzyme (ACE) inhibitors; angiotensin II receptor antagonists (alternatively called angiotensin receptor blockers); and calcium-channel blockers. Mechanistically, these drugs differ considerably; for example, diuretics lower blood pressure by preventing the urinary loss of sodium, whilst ACE inhibitors block the formation of angiotensin II, a potent vasoconstricting agent. Whilst all of these agents effectively lower blood pressure, some drugs are better suited to individual patients than others (e.g. certain β-blockers are contra-indicated in patients with asthma). Thus, selection of the appropriate drug therapy determines not only treatment success but also influences patient safety.

*This section provides an overview of the different classes of blood pressure-lowering drugs that are widely used to control blood pressure. The Drug Review chapters in this edition of BESTMEDICINE focuses solely on one class of drugs – the angiotensin II receptor antagonists (alternatively called angiotensin receptor blockers).*

## Introduction

In general hypertensive patient populations, no one class of agent has been shown to be any more effective at lowering blood pressure than another, with single drug therapy reducing blood pressure by, on average, by 7–8%.[1] There is considerable inter-individual variability in the response to single antihypertensive drugs, which may reflect the marked heterogeneity that exists in the pathogenesis of hypertension. The choice of antihypertensive therapy is influenced by many factors, including the previous experiences of the patient with blood pressure-lowering agents, drug costs, the risk profile of the patient (e.g. target-organ damage, cardiovascular or renal disease, or diabetes) and the patient's age, race and personal preferences (Table 1).[1,2]

*There is considerable inter-individual variability in the response to single antihypertensive drugs.*

**Table 1.** Indications and contra-indications for the major classes of antihypertensive drugs.[1]

| Drug class | Examples | Compelling indications | Possible indications | Caution | Compelling contra-indications |
|---|---|---|---|---|---|
| ACE inhibitors | Captopril, enalapril, lisinopril, perindopril | Heart failure, left ventricular dysfunction, post MI, established CHD, type I diabetic nephropathy, secondary stroke prevention | Chronic renal disease, type II diabetic nephropathy, proteinuric renal disease | Renal impairment, peripheral vascular disease | Pregnancy, renovascular disease |
| β-blockers | Atenolol, bisoprolol, metoprolol, nebivolol | MI, angina | Heart failure | Heart failure, peripheral vascular disease, diabetes (except with CHD) | Asthma, COPD, heart block |
| Calcium-channel blockers (dihydropyridine) | Amlodipine, lacidipine, lercanidipine, nifedipine | Elderly, isolated systolic hypertension | Elderly, angina | – | – |
| Calcium-channel blockers (rate-limiting) | Diltiazem, verapamil | Angina | MI | Combination with β-blockers | Heart block, heart failure |
| Thiazide/thiazide-like diuretics | Bendroflumethiazide, hydrochlorthiazide | Elderly, isolated systolic hypertension, heart failure, stroke prevention | – | – | Gout |

CHD, coronary heart disease; COPD, chronic obstructive pulmonary disease; MI, myocardial infarction.

## Diuretics

In simplistic terms, <u>diuretics</u> are agents that promote the <u>excretion</u> of urine via their effects on kidney function. <u>Monotherapy</u> with diuretics controls blood pressure in a large percentage of patients with essential hypertension, as well as reducing <u>cardiovascular</u> <u>morbidity</u> and <u>mortality</u>.[3]

Diuretics fall into one of three main groups:

- <u>thiazide</u> and thiazide-like (e.g. bendroflumethiazide [bendrofluazide], chlortalidone, hydrochlorthiazide, indapamide)
- <u>potassium-sparing</u> (e.g. amoloride, triamterene, spironolactone)
- loop (furosemide, bumetanide, torasemide).

Thiazide and thiazide-like diuretics lower blood pressure by a complex series of mechanisms. The principal mechanism involves urinary loss of sodium as a result of the blockade of renal re-<u>absorption</u> of sodium at the beginning of the <u>distal convoluted tubule</u>.[1] Thiazide diuretics differ from thiazide-like diuretics mechanistically, in terms of their <u>ion channel</u>-blocking activity, duration of action and <u>carbonic anhydrase inhibitory</u> activity.[1] However, the clinical implications of this have yet to be confirmed.

When used in the management of hypertension, a low dose of a thiazide diuretic (e.g. bendroflumethiazide, 2.5 mg/day) produces a maximal or near-maximal blood pressure-lowering effect, with very little <u>biochemical disturbance</u>. Higher doses may be associated with marked changes in plasma potassium and <u>uric acid</u> levels, impaired glucose tolerance, and small increases in blood levels of <u>low density lipoprotein cholesterol (LDL-C)</u> and <u>triglycerides</u>. Moreover, these higher doses offer little advantage in terms of improved blood pressure control compared with lower doses.[1,4] Consequently, patients may be at increased risk of <u>hypokalaemia</u> when treated with higher doses of thiazide diuretics, although potassium supplements are rarely required when thiazides are used in the routine management of hypertension.[4] Thiazide diuretics act within 1–2 hours of oral administration and most have a duration of action that persists for 12–24 hours. They are usually administered early in the day so that <u>diuresis</u> does not interfere with the patient's sleep.[4] The use of thiazide and thiazide-like diuretics has been associated with erectile dysfunction in some patients.[1] Furthermore, patients with gout and those undergoing treatment with lithium are not generally suitable for treatment with these agents.[1]

In contrast to the thiazides, the potassium-sparing diuretics act by blocking <u>sodium–potassium exchange</u> in the <u>renal distal tubules</u> of the kidney.[5] Potassium-sparing diuretics do not feature heavily in the routine management of hypertension, although they may be used to limit potassium loss in patients treated with thiazide/thiazide-like diuretics.[1]

The <u>loop diuretics</u> (e.g. furosemide, bumetanide) inhibit the re-absorption of sodium and chloride from the ascending limb of the <u>loop of Henle</u> in the renal tubule and are most frequently used in the treatment of <u>pulmonary oedema</u> due to left ventricular failure and in patients with <u>chronic</u> heart failure.[4] As with the potassium-sparing

> <u>Diuretics</u> fall into one of three main groups: <u>thiazide</u> and thiazide-like, <u>potassium-sparing</u> and loop.

> A low dose of a thiazide (e.g. bendroflumethiazide, 2.5 mg/day) produces a maximal or near-maximal blood pressure-lowering effect, with very little biochemical disturbance.

diuretics, these agents have no place in the routine management of blood pressure.[1] However, a loop diuretic may be used to lower blood pressure in hypertensive patients who are resistant to thiazide therapy, although generally, the sustained duration of action of thiazides makes them the preferred therapy option.[1,4]

## β-blockers

Originally developed for the treatment of angina, β-blockers (e.g. atenolol, bisoprolol, metoprolol, nebivolol) were subsequently found to lower blood pressure and now represent one of the most widely used class of antihypertensive agents.[1] In addition to their blood pressure-lowering effects, β-blockers have also been shown to reduce the morbidity and mortality associated with myocardial infarction (MI), congestive heart failure[a] and angina.[6]

In general terms, β-blockers prevent the binding of catecholamines (e.g. adrenaline and noradrenaline) to the β-adrenoceptors in the heart, peripheral vasculature, bronchi, pancreas and liver. Despite their longevity, the mode of action of β-blockers in lowering blood pressure remains controversial, although it is known that they reduce cardiac output, limit renin release from the kidney and alter baroceptor reflex sensitivity, as well as blocking peripheral β-adrenoceptors.[4]

Individual β-blockers differ in terms of their receptor selectivity, gastrointestinal absorption, lipid solubility, brain penetration, concentration within the cardiac tissue and renal clearance.[7] Since age, race, cigarette smoking and concomitant drug therapy can also influence the pharmacokinetics of β-blockers, the importance of tailoring specific drug therapy to the individual patient is indisputable.[7] For example, the water soluble β-blockers (e.g. atenolol, celiprolol, nadolol) are less likely to enter the brain, and may therefore cause less sleep disturbance and nightmares.[4] However, these drugs are excreted by the kidneys and thus, may not be appropriate in patients with renal impairment.[4]

Intrinsic sympathomimetic activity (or partial agonist activity), which describes the tendency of β-blockers to stimulate as well as to block adrenergic receptors, is a further distinguishing feature of individual β-blockers. Oxprenolol, pindolol, acebutolol and celiprolol show intrinsic sympathomimetic activity and subsequently, tend to cause less bradycardia and less coldness of the extremities than other β-blockers.[4] Labetalol, celiprolol, carvedilol and nebivolol have additional mild vasodilatory properties that cannot simply be ascribed to β-adrenoceptor antagonism, although the therapeutic benefits of this effect are unconfirmed.

The non-selective blockade of bronchial β-adrenoceptors and the resultant bronchoconstriction, represents a significant danger to patients with respiratory disease (e.g. asthma) and restricts the widespread use of β-blockers in such patients. If there is no alternative, patients with

> Individual β-blockers differ in terms of their receptor selectivity, gastrointestinal absorption, lipid solubility, brain penetration, concentration within the cardiac tissue and renal clearance.

---

[a]The use of β-blockers should be avoided in patients with worsening unstable heart failure and heart failure which is stable and uncorrected.

asthma or bronchospasm may be cautiously treated with a cardioselective β-blocker, that by definition, has limited bronchiolar effects (e.g. atenolol, bisoprolol, metoprolol, nebivolol).[4] However, no β-blocker is completely cardiospecific. Common side-effects associated with β-blockers include lethargy, aches in the limbs on exercise, impaired concentration and memory, erectile dysfunction, vivid dreams and exacerbation of the symptoms of peripheral vascular disease and Raynaud's syndrome.[1] β-blockers may also cause adverse metabolic effects, including impairment of blood glucose control and worsening of dyslipidaemia (reduced high density lipoprotein cholesterol [HDL-C] and raised triglycerides), and may increase the likelihood of new-onset diabetes.[1] Their adverse events on insulin resistance have restricted the use of β-blockers in at-risk patients. Despite this, large controlled trials (e.g. the UK Prospective Diabetes Study [UKPDS]) have shown β-blockers to be highly effective in reducing the risk of cardiovascular events and death in post-MI patients with diabetes.[8]

## Angiotensin-converting enzyme (ACE) inhibitors

The ACE inhibitors (e.g. captopril, enalapril, lisinopril, perindopril) block the conversion of angiotensin I to angiotensin II by competitively inhibiting ACE. Angiotensin II is a potent vasoconstrictor of blood vessels and stimulates the adrenal cortex to release aldosterone, which further increases blood pressure by increasing the retention of sodium and water by the kidney.[9] By reducing levels of angiotensin II, ACE inhibitors promote vasodilatation and ultimately reduce blood pressure.

One of the most common adverse events associated with the regular use of ACE inhibitors is a dry persistent cough, reported in 10–20% of users.[1] Although this is not life-threatening, it is responsible for many cases of premature treatment discontinuation.[10] The mechanisms underlying ACE inhibitor-induced cough are probably linked to the suppression of kininase II activity, which may be followed by an accumulation of kinins, substance P and prostaglandins.[10]

Angioedema is another well-recognised and potentially life-threatening side-effect of ACE inhibitor treatment, although it is much less common than cough, affecting 0.1–0.2% of patients.[11] The incidence of angioedema can be up to three-fold higher amongst black patient populations, although the reasons behind this are unclear.[11,12] Other adverse events associated with ACE inhibitors include rash, hypotension, renal impairment, pancreatitis, and upper respiratory-tract symptoms such as sinusitis, rhinitis and sore throat.[4] Gastrointestinal effects associated with ACE inhibitors include nausea, vomiting, dyspepsia, diarrhoea and constipation.[4]

The use of ACE inhibitors is contra-indicated in patients with hypersensitivity to ACE inhibitors and in patients with known or suspected renovascular disease.[4] ACE inhibitors may be used with caution in those patients:

● in whom the renin–angiotensin system is already activated (i.e. patients receiving high doses of diuretics, patients on a low-sodium

> One of the most common adverse events associated with the regular use of ACE inhibitors is a dry persistent cough, reported in 10–20% of users.

☞ The related drugs –
the angiotensin
receptor antagonists
are covered in detail
in the following
chapters of this book.

diet, patients on dialysis, dehydrated patients or those with heart failure[1,4]

● with peripheral vascular disease or generalised atherosclerosis, owing to the risk of clinically silent renovascular disease[4]

● with severe or symptomatic aortic stenosis, owing to a risk of hypotension[4]

● with collagen vascular disease, owing to the risk of agranulocytosis[4]

● with a history of idiopathic or hereditary angioedema[4]

● of child-bearing potential, owing to a risk of foetal malformation.[1]

## Calcium-channel blockers

The calcium-channel blockers (e.g. amlodipine, lercanidipine, nifedipine, verapamil) act by selectively inhibiting the cellular influx of calcium ions via L-type calcium channels found in cardiac myocytes and in the smooth muscle of arteries, veins and non-vascular smooth muscle cells.[13] Thus, these drugs may reduce myocardial contractility, depress the formation and propagation of electrical impulses within the heart, and reduce coronary or systemic vascular tone, ultimately leading to vasodilatation and the lowering of blood pressure.[4] Calcium-channel blockers are widely used in the treatment of both hypertension and angina. The antihypertensive effects of the calcium-channel blockers occur independently of fluid volume status, concomitant drug therapy and comorbid conditions, making them a valuable class of blood pressure-lowering agents.[14]

The majority of the controversy surrounding the calcium-channel blockers has centred on whether these drugs increase the risk of cardiovascular events and mortality.[15] The development of sustained-release, long-acting formulations (e.g. extended-release verapamil) may have raised the profile of the calcium-channel blockers by eliminating the major fluctuations in blood pressure and heart rate associated with short-acting agents (e.g. short-acting nifedipine).[15] Large clinical studies, including the Antihypertensive and Lipid Lowering Treatment to Prevent Heart Attack Trial (ALLHAT) and Controlled Onset Verapamil Investigation of Cardiovascular Endpoints (CONVINCE) have further confirmed the cardiovascular safety of these agents.[16,17]

The
calcium-channel
blockers are
heterogeneous in
terms of their
chemistry,
pharmacology and
clinical effects, and
also vary widely in
their preferred
site of action.

The calcium-channel blockers are heterogeneous in terms of their chemistry, pharmacology and clinical effects, and also vary widely in their preferred site of action. Particular differences exist between verapamil, diltiazem and the dihydropyridine calcium-channel blockers (i.e. amlodipine, felodipine, isradipine, lacidipine, lercanidipine, nicardipine, nifedipine, nimodipine and nisoldipine).[18] The dihydropyridine calcium-channel blockers are more selective at blocking L-type calcium channels in vascular smooth muscle cells, and thereby induce vascular relaxation with a fall in vascular resistance and arterial pressure.[1]

'Rate-limiting' calcium-channel blockers (e.g. diltiazem, verapamil) block calcium channels in cardiac myocytes, thereby reducing cardiac output.[1] These agents cause less peripheral oedema than the dihydropyridine derivatives but are negatively inotropic and negatively chronotropic and should therefore be avoided in patients with compromised left ventricular function.[4]

Calcium-channel blockers are generally well tolerated. The most common adverse events associated with their use include flushing, headache, hypotension and dose-dependent peripheral oedema.[1,15] Verapamil is frequently associated with constipation. Bradycardia and heart block, resulting from the slowing of sinoatrial and atrioventricular nodal conduction particularly affect patients treated with the non-dihydropyridine calcium-channel blockers.[15]

Calcium-channel blockers are generally well tolerated. The most common adverse events associated with their use include flushing, headache, hypotension and peripheral oedema.

## Key points

- Thiazide and thiazide-like diuretics, which block the renal re-absorption of sodium at the distal convoluted tubule, control blood pressure at low doses in a large percentage of patients with hypertension.

- High doses of thiazide diuretics may be associated with marked reductions in plasma potassium and significant changes in metabolic parameters.

- β-blockers – agents that prevent the binding of catecholamines to β-adrenoceptors in the heart, vasculature and pulmonary system – vary considerably in terms of their receptor selectivity, pharmacokinetics, vasodilatory effects and intrinsic sympathomimetic activity.

- In view of their non-selective action on pulmonary β-adrenoceptors, certain β-blockers are contra-indicated in patients with asthma. Other relatively cardiospecific β-blockers (e.g. atenolol, nebivolol) may be used with extreme caution in these patients.

- ACE inhibitors reduce blood pressure by blocking the enzymatic conversion of angiotensin I to angiotensin II – a potent vasoconstrictor.

- Up to 20% of patients treated with ACE inhibitors may experience a dry, persistent cough. More seriously, a very small proportion of patients may develop angioedema.

- The calcium-channel blockers selectively inhibit the cellular influx of calcium ions, thereby reducing vascular tone and lowering blood pressure.

- Concerns regarding the potentiation of cardiovascular events by calcium-channel blockers have been largely dismissed by controlled studies of long-acting agents, performed in large patient populations.

# References

A list of the published evidence which has been reviewed in compiling the preceding section of *BESTMEDICINE*.

1 Williams B, Poulter N, Brown M *et al.* Guidelines for management of hypertension: report of the fourth working party of the British Hypertension Society, 2004-BHS IV. *J Hum Hypertens* 2004; **18**: 139–85.

2 Guidelines Committee. 2003 European Society of Hypertension–European Society of Cardiology guidelines for the management of arterial hypertension. *J Hypertens* 2003; **21**: 1011–53.

3 Reyes A. Diuretics in the therapy of hypertension. *J Hum Hypertens* 2002; **16**: S78–83.

4 *British National Formulary (BNF) 48*. London: British Medical Association and Royal Pharmaceutical Society of Great Britain. September, 2004.

5 Wright J. Choosing a first-line drug in the management of elevated blood pressure: what is the evidence? 1: Thiazide diuretics. *CMAJ* 2000; **163**: 57–60.

6 Ritter JM. Nebivolol: endothelium-mediated vasodilating effect. *J Cardiovasc Pharmacol* 2001; **38(Suppl 3)**: S13–16.

7 Frishman W, Alwarshetty M. Beta-adrenergic blockers in systemic hypertension: pharmacokinetic considerations related to the current guidelines. *Clin Pharmacokinet* 2002; **41**: 505–16.

8 Cruickshank J. Beta-blockers and diabetes: the bad guys come good. *Cardiovasc Drugs Ther* 2002; **16**: 457–70.

9 Wright J. Choosing a first-line drug in the management of elevated blood pressure: what is the evidence? 3: Angiotensin-converting-enzyme inhibitors. *CMAJ* 2000; **163**: 293–6.

10 Overlack A. ACE inhibitor-induced cough and bronchospasm. Incidence, mechanisms and management. *Drug Saf* 1996; **15**: 72–8.

11 Vleeming W, van Amsterdam J, Stricker B, de Wildt D. ACE inhibitor-induced angioedema. Incidence, prevention and management. *Drug Saf* 1998; **18**: 171–88.

12 Sica D, Black H. Current concepts of pharmacotherapy in hypertension: ACE inhibitor-related angioedema: can angiotensin-receptor blockers be safely used? *J Clin Hypertens* 2002; **4**: 375–80.

13 Muntwyler J, Follath F. Calcium channel blockers in treatment of hypertension. *Prog Cardiovasc Dis* 2001; **44**: 207–16.

14 Messerli F. Calcium antagonists in hypertension: from hemodynamics to outcomes. *Am J Hypertens* 2002; **15**: S94–7.

15 Eisenberg M, Brox A, Bestawros A. Calcium channel blockers: an update. *Am J Med* 2004; **116**: 35–43.

16 Black H, Elliott W, Grandits G *et al.* Principal results of the Controlled Onset Verapamil Investigation of Cardiovascular End Points (CONVINCE) trial. *JAMA* 2003; **289**: 2073–82.

17 Major outcomes in high-risk hypertensive patients randomized to angiotensin-converting enzyme inhibitor or calcium channel blocker *vs* diuretic: The Antihypertensive and Lipid-Lowering Treatment to Prevent Heart Attack Trial (ALLHAT). *JAMA* 2002; **288**: 2981–97.

18 Israili Z. The use of calcium antagonists in the therapy of hypertension in the elderly. *Am J Ther* 2003; **10**: 383–95.

# 3. Pharmacology of the angiotensin II receptor antagonists

*Dr Eleanor Bull*
*CSF Medical Communications Ltd*

## Chemistry

A number of angiotensin II receptor antagonists are commercially available (candesartan [Amias®], eprosartan [Teveten®], irbesartan [Aprovel®], losartan [Cozaar®], olmesartan [Olmetec®], telmisartan [Micardis®] and valsartan [Diovan®]), which show considerable heterogeneity in terms of their chemical structures (Figure 1). Olmesartan, losartan and candesartan are all administered as prodrugs, and are converted to their active forms following administration, whereas the other angiotensin II receptor antagonists are administered in their active forms. Losartan was the first angiotensin II receptor antagonist to be licensed in the UK. Telmisartan was developed from the active metabolite of losartan by the substitution of a lipophilic benzimidazole group for an imidazole moiety. Valsartan was formed by

☛ *This section is a condensed summary of the pharmacological data presented in the original issue of* Drugs in Context *from which each individual drug review is derived.*

**Figure 1.** The chemical structures of angiotensin II receptor antagonists.

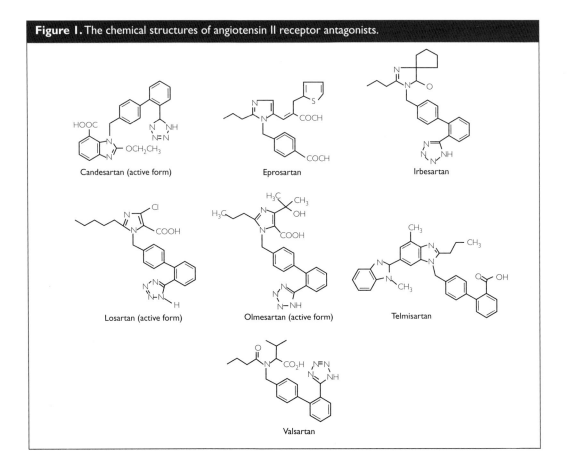

Candesartan (active form)

Eprosartan

Irbesartan

Losartan (active form)

Olmesartan (active form)

Telmisartan

Valsartan

replacement of the heterocyclic imidazole group of losartan with a non-planar, acetylated amino acid. Eprosartan is a non-biphenyl, non-tetrazole angiotensin II receptor antagonist that is chemically distinct from other drugs of the class.

## Mechanism of action

The angiotensin II receptor antagonists share a common mechanism of action in that they all act selectively on angiotensin II (AT$_1$) receptors – found in vascular smooth muscle, the adrenal glands, kidneys and heart – and displace angiotensin II from its binding site. By interrupting the renin–angiotensin cascade, as shown in Figure 2, these drugs prevent a number of the physiological actions of angiotensin II, including arteriolar vasoconstriction and aldosterone-mediated sodium and water retention.[1] Ultimately, this manifests clinically as a significant reduction in blood pressure. Unlike the angiotensin-converting enzyme (ACE) inhibitors (e.g. enalapril [Innovace®], perindopril [Coversyl®], lisinopril [Zestril®]), the angiotensin II receptor antagonists inhibit angiotensin II activity without disrupting bradykinin metabolism, and are thus not expected to potentiate bradykinin-mediated adverse events such as cough.

> All of the angiotensin II receptor antagonists act selectively on angiotensin II (AT$_1$) receptors to displace angiotensin II from its binding site.

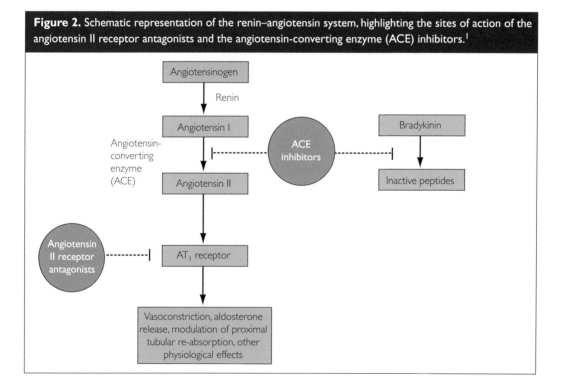

**Figure 2.** Schematic representation of the renin–angiotensin system, highlighting the sites of action of the angiotensin II receptor antagonists and the angiotensin-converting enzyme (ACE) inhibitors.[1]

## Selectivity and potency

The structural heterogeneity within the angiotensin II receptor antagonist drug class also leads to differences in the affinity of the different drugs for the $AT_1$ receptor, giving rise to differences in potency and pharmacokinetic parameters. Thus, there are notable variations in the time of onset, duration of action and potency of the individual drugs.[2] Some of these differences are explored in more detail in the individual drug reviews in this edition of *BESTMEDICINE.*

One characteristic that is likely to influence the clinical efficacy of an angiotensin II receptor antagonist is its ability to bind competitively or non-competitively to the $AT_1$ receptor. Levels of circulating angiotensin II can increase over time with continuous blockade of angiotensin II receptors by angiotensin II receptor antagonists.[3] As a consequence, the pharmacological effects of competitive antagonists, such as eprosartan and losartan, may be overcome by elevated levels of angiotensin II, leading to a shortening in their duration of action. By definition, the therapeutic activity of non-competitive antagonists, such as olmesartan, telmisartan, irbesartan and valsartan, is unaffected by increased levels of angiotensin II, resulting in a long terminal half-life, and a prolonged duration of action.[4]

> The therapeutic activity of non-competitive antagonists is unaffected by increased levels of angiotensin II, resulting in a long terminal half-life, and a prolonged duration of action.

## Effect on sympathetic outflow

In contrast to many of the other $AT_1$ receptor antagonists, eprosartan also exerts an inhibitory action on sympathetic nerve activity by blocking presynaptic $AT_1$ receptors, thus inhibiting the release of the neurotransmitter, noradrenaline. Although the clinical relevance of this is still under investigation, reducing noradrenaline release would be expected to have beneficial effects on blood pressure control. Arterial compliance is reduced by increased sympathetic activity, which can lead to a selective increase in systolic blood pressure.[5] Thus, by blocking sympathetic activity and inhibiting the effects of angiotensin II, eprosartan may improve blood pressure via a dual mechanism.[6]

# Pharmacokinetics

The pharmacokinetic properties of the individual angiotensin II receptor antagonists are summarised in Table 1.[7–20] The pharmacokinetic profiles of all angiotensin II receptor antagonists are unaffected by co-administration with food, which further simplifies their dosage regimens. For all compounds, the predominant route of elimination is biliary, though a varying proportion of an oral dose is excreted in the urine.

> ☞ The pharmacokinetics of a drug are of interest to healthcare professionals because it is important for them to understand the action of a drug on the body over a period of time.

**Table 1.** The pharmacokinetic parameters of the different angiotensin II receptor antagonists.[7–20]

| Drug | Active metabolite | $t_{max}$ (hours) | Protein binding (%) | Half-life (hours) | Bioavailability (%) | Volume of distribution (L) | Metabolism |
|---|---|---|---|---|---|---|---|
| Candesartan | Prodrug | 4 | >99 | 9–12 | 14 | 9 | CYP 2C9 |
| Eprosartan | No | 1–3 | 98 | 5–9 | 13 | 13 | Not CYP |
| Irbesartan | No | 1.5–2 | 96 | 11–15 | 60–80 | 53–93 | CYP 2C9 |
| Losartan | Prodrug | 1 | >99 | 2 | 33 | 34 | CYP 2C9 CYP 3A4 |
| Olmesartan | Prodrug | 2 | 99.7 | 13 | 27 | 16–29 | Not CYP |
| Telmisartan | No | 0.5–1 | 99.5 | 24 | 43 | 500 | Not CYP |
| Valsartan | No | 2 | 94–97 | 7 | 23 | 17 | Not CYP |

CYP, cytochrome P450; $t_{max}$, time to reach maximum drug plasma concentration.

### Special patient populations

Although the pharmacokinetic properties of some angiotensin II receptor antagonists may fluctuate when administered to elderly patients, there is generally no need for dosage adjustment in this patient population, although patients aged over 75 years may require slightly modified regimens (Table 2).[8,10,11,13,15,17,19] For patients with renal and hepatic impairment, the starting and maximum dose of angiotensin II receptor antagonist depends on the particular drug (Table 2).

**Table 2.** Angiotensin II receptor antagonists: recommended dosage adjustments in special patient populations.[8,10,11,13,15,17,19]

| Drug | Recommended dosage regimen (mg/day) | Dosage adjustment in special patient populations |
|---|---|---|
| Candesartan | Initial: 8<br>Maximum: 16 | **Renal impairment:** Restrict initial dose to 4 mg/day<br>**Hepatic impairment (mild-to-moderate):** Restrict initial dose to 2 mg/day |
| Eprosartan | Initial: 600<br>Maximum: 800 | **Elderly:** In patients over 75 years of age, restrict initial dose to 300 mg/day<br>**Renal impairment:** In patients with creatinine clearance <60 mL/minute, restrict initial dose to 300 mg/day<br>**Hepatic impairment (mild-to-moderate):** Restrict initial dose to 300 mg/day |
| Irbesartan | Initial: 150<br>Maximum: 300 | **Elderly:** In patients over 75 years of age, restrict initial dose to 75 mg/day |
| Losartan | Initial: 50<br>Maximum: 100 | **Elderly:** In patients over 75 years of age, restrict initial dose to 25 mg/day<br>**Renal impairment:** In patients with creatinine clearance <20 mL/minute, restrict initial dose to 25 mg/day<br>**Hepatic impairment:** Consider a lower dose |
| Olmesartan | Initial: 10<br>Maximum: 40 | **Elderly:** In patients over 75 years of age, restrict maximum dose to 20 mg/day<br>**Renal impairment:** In patients with creatinine clearance 20–60 mL/minute, restrict maximum dose to 20 mg/day. Not recommended in patient with creatinine clearance <20 mL/minute.<br>**Hepatic impairment:** Not recommended |
| Telmisartan | Initial: 40<br>Maximum: 50 | **Hepatic impairment (mild-to-moderate):** Restrict maximum dose to 40 mg/day |
| Valsartan | Initial: 80<br>Maximum: 160 | **Elderly:** In patients over 75 years of age, restrict initial dose to 40 mg/day<br>**Renal impairment (moderate-to-severe):** In patients with creatinine clearance 20–60 mL/minute, restrict initial dose to 40 mg/day.<br>**Hepatic impairment (mild-to-moderate):** Restrict initial dose to 40 mg/day and maximum dose to 80 mg/day. Not recommended in patients with severe hepatic impairment. |

# References

A list of the published evidence which has been reviewed in compiling the preceding section of *BESTMEDICINE.*

1   Plosker G, Foster R. Eprosartan: a review of its use in the management of hypertension. *Drugs* 2000; **60**: 177–201.

2   Israili Z. Clinical pharmacokinetics of angiotensin II (AT1) receptor blockers in hypertension. *J Hum Hypertens* 2000; **14**: S73–86.

3   Norwood D, Branch E, Smith B, Honeywell M. Olmesartan medoxomil for hypertension: a clinical review. *Drug Forecast* 2002; **27**: 611–18.

4   McConnaughey M, McConnaughey J, Ingenito A. Practical considerations of the pharmacology of angiotensin receptor blockers. *J Clin Pharmacol* 1999; **39**: 547–59.

5   Brooks D, Ruffolo R. Pharmacological mechanism of angiotensin II receptor antagonists: implications for the treatment of elevated systolic blood pressure. *J Hypertens Suppl* 1999; **17**: S27–32.

6   Hedner T. Management of hypertension: the advent of a new angiotensin II receptor antagonist. *J Hypertens Suppl* 1999; **17**: S21–5.

7   Easthope S, Jarvis B. Candesartan cilexetil: an update of its use in essential hypertension. *Drugs* 2002; **62**: 1253–87.

8   Takeda UK Ltd. Amias® (candesartan). *Summary of product characteristics.* High Wycombe, UK, 2004.

9   McClellan K, Balfour J. Eprosartan. *Drugs* 1998; **55**: 713–18.

10  Solvay Healthcare Limited. Teveten® (eprosartan). *Summary of product characteristics.* Southampton, UK, 2004.

11  Bristol-Myers Squibb Pharmaceuticals Ltd. Aprovel® (irbesartan). *Summary of product characteristics.* Hounslow, UK, 2004.

12  Gillis J, Markham A. Irbesartan. A review of its pharmacodynamic and pharmacokinetic properties and therapeutic use in the management of hypertension. *Drugs* 1997; **54**: 885–902.

13  Merck Sharp & Dohme Limited. Cozaar® (losartan). *Summary of product characteristics.* Hoddesdon, UK, 2003.

14  Lo M, Goldberg M, McCrea J *et al.* Pharmacokinetics of losartan, an angiotensin II receptor antagonist, and its active metabolite EXP3174 in humans. *Clin Pharmacol Ther* 1995; **58**: 641–9.

15  Sankyo Pharma UK Limited. Olmetec® (olmesartan). *Summary of product characteristics.* Amersham, UK, 2004.

16  Schwocho L, Masonson H. Pharmacokinetics of CS-866, a new angiotensin II receptor blocker, in healthy subjects. *J Clin Pharmacol* 2001; **41**: 515–27.

17  Boehringer Ingelheim Limited. Micardis® (telmisartan). *Summary of product characteristics.* Bracknell, UK, 2004.

18  Sharpe M, Jarvis B, Goa K. Telmisartan: a review of its use in hypertension. *Drugs* 2001; **61**: 1501–29.

19  Novartis Pharmaceuticals UK Ltd. Diovan® (valsartan). *Summary of product characteristics.* Camberley, UK, 2004.

20  Markham A, Goa K. Valsartan. A review of its pharmacology and therapeutic use in essential hypertension. *Drugs* 1997; **54**: 299–311.

# 4. Drug review – Candesartan (Amias®)

Dr Richard Clark
CSF Medical Communications Ltd

## Summary

Candesartan is a member of the angiotensin II receptor antagonist group of antihypertensives. It is both potent and selective, and is administered as the prodrug, candesartan cilexetil, which is rapidly converted to the active form. Candesartan has a greater or equivalent efficacy to other antihypertensive agents including the angiotensin-converting enzyme (ACE) inhibitors, calcium-channel blockers, thiazide diuretics and other angiotensin II receptor antagonists. Furthermore, candesartan has an overall incidence of adverse events that is similar to placebo, and also appears to be better tolerated than either ACE inhibitors or calcium-channel blockers.

## Introduction

The renin–angiotensin system plays a pivotal role in the control of blood pressure, and as such, is implicated in the development of hypertension. Angiotensin II is the key effector peptide in this system, and plays an important role in regulating arterial blood pressure and cardiovascular homeostasis. The development of ACE inhibitors represented a major advance in the treatment of hypertension. Whilst ACE inhibitors block the conversion of angiotensin I to angiotensin II, other pathways that generate angiotensin II are unaffected by this inhibition. Furthermore, as the ACE inhibitor target enzyme is not very specific, ACE inhibitor treatment can cause an accumulation of bradykinin – a vasodilator but also an inflammatory mediator that can lead to side-effects such as cough.

Angiotensin II receptor antagonists have several theoretical advantages over ACE inhibitors as they specifically bind to type 1 angiotensin II ($AT_1$) receptors and block the binding of angiotensin II. This specificity for $AT_1$ receptors translates into a more favourable side-effect profile.

This section focuses on the clinical efficacy, tolerability and safety of candesartan, a non-peptide angiotensin II receptor antagonist used in the treatment of hypertension. The accumulated evidence supporting the use of candesartan within this indication will be discussed in the context of data obtained from studies with other antihypertensive medications.

# Clinical efficacy and tolerability

## *Placebo-controlled and dose-ranging studies*

☞ *Dose-ranging studies are particularly important to ensure that the optimum dose of a drug can be determined in order that benefit can be realised with the least risk of side-effects.*

Several randomised, <u>double-blind</u>, <u>placebo-controlled</u> clinical trials have been conducted covering the 2–64 mg/day dose range[a] for candesartan, with one trial comparing once- and twice-daily dosing regimens.[1–5] The observations made in these studies are presented in Table 1. In summary, all candesartan doses were shown to be more effective than placebo in terms of controlling <u>systolic (SBP)</u> and <u>diastolic blood pressure (DBP)</u>. Moreover, the incidence of adverse events was similar in patients receiving placebo or candesartan. The incidence and severity of adverse events did not appear to be related to the dose of candesartan over this dose range. Finally, there was no significant advantage for a twice-daily over a once-daily dosing regimen.[4]

*Candesartan, 8 or 16 mg once daily, are the optimal maintenance doses for the majority of patients.*

The results of six randomised, double-blind, placebo-controlled, dose–response studies have been pooled.[6] A total of 1482 patients with mild-to-moderate hypertension were treated with candesartan, 2, 4, 8 or 16 mg, or placebo, once-daily for at least 4 weeks, and blood pressure was measured 24 hours after the last dose (<u>trough</u> blood pressure). Candesartan, 2, 4, 8 and 16 mg doses resulted in placebo-corrected mean reductions in trough DBP of 2.5, 4.5, 6.0 and 8.0 mmHg, respectively, and approximately 5, 7, 10 and 12 mmHg, respectively, in trough SBP. Thus, a clinically significant and dose-dependent antihypertensive effect was observed for candesartan, 4–16 mg once daily, and it appears that candesartan, 8 or 16 mg once daily, are the optimal maintenance doses for the majority of patients.

## *Candesartan vs other angiotensin II receptor antagonists*

The antihypertensive effects of candesartan and losartan have been compared directly in several randomised, double-blind trials, and these are summarised in Table 2.[3,7–10] Two of these studies have compared candesartan and losartan at doses licensed in the UK (i.e. candesartan up to 16 mg/day, and losartan up to 100 mg/day),[3,7] whilst other US-based trials evaluated doses up to the maximum levels approved in the US (candesartan, 32 mg/day, and losartan, 100 mg/day).

The antihypertensive <u>efficacy</u> of candesartan, 8 or 16 mg/day, was compared with that of losartan, 50 mg/day, in 337 patients over 8 weeks.[3] This study demonstrated that candesartan, 16 mg, reduced trough DBP by 3.7 mmHg more than losartan, 50 mg ($p=0.013$; Figure 1). At a dose of 8 mg/day, candesartan reduced DBP by 8.9 mmHg compared with approximate 6 mmHg reductions observed in patients receiving losartan, 50 mg (no <u>p-value</u> reported). However, a second randomised, double-blind, parallel-group study did not find a statistically significant difference in terms of trough DBP reductions between candesartan, 8–16 mg/day, and losartan, 50–100 mg/day.[7]

---

[a]The licensed dose range of candesartan in the UK is 2–16 mg/day.

**Table 1.** Summary of double-blind, randomised trials comparing candesartan with placebo in patients with hypertension.[1–5]

| Drug regimen | Patients | Outcomes |
|---|---|---|
| Candesartan, 8–16 mg once daily, losartan, 50–100 mg once daily, or placebo 8-week, randomised, double-blind, forced-titration study[1] | n=268 DBP 95–110 mmHg | • Significant reductions in ambulatory SBP and DBP were observed at 4 and 8 weeks in patients receiving candesartan or losartan compared with those on placebo ($p<0.05$). <br> • 24-hour ambulatory SBP was reduced by a greater extent with candesartan than with losartan treatment (−13.4 vs −9.3 mmHg, respectively; $p<0.01$). However, there was no difference in 24-hour ambulatory DBP between the two active treatments ($p>0.05$). <br> • There were no significant differences between candesartan, losartan and placebo groups with regard to the frequency of adverse events (43, 45 and 46%, respectively; $p>0.05$). |
| Candesartan, 2–32 mg once daily, or placebo 8-week, randomised, double-blind, study[2] | n=365 DBP 95–114 mmHg | • All doses of candesartan reduced trough DBP and SBP by a greater extent than placebo ($p<0.005$ and parallel-group $p<0.001$, respectively). <br> • A dose–response relationship was apparent ($p\leq0.0001$), with greater reductions of SBP and DBP at higher doses of candesartan. <br> • There was no apparent increase in adverse events with increasing dose of candesartan. The majority of adverse events were mild-to-moderate intensity and resolved without discontinuing treatment. |
| Candesartan, 8 or 16 mg once daily, losartan, 50 mg once daily, or placebo 8-week, randomised, double-blind, parallel-group study[3] | n=337 DBP 95–114 mmHg | • Candesartan, 8 and 16 mg, reduced trough DBP by 8.9 and 10.3 mmHg, respectively, compared with those receiving placebo (both $p<0.001$ vs placebo). <br> • Candesartan, 16 mg, reduced trough DBP by 3.7 mmHg more than losartan, 50 mg ($p=0.013$). <br> • The frequency of adverse events was similar in the candesartan, losartan and placebo groups. |

DBP, diastolic blood pressure; SBP, systolic blood pressure.

| Drug regimen | Patients | Outcomes |
|---|---|---|
| Placebo or candesartan, 8 mg once daily, for 4 weeks, then either candesartan, 16 mg once daily, or candesartan, 8 mg twice daily 8-week, randomised, double-blind, parallel-group, forced-titration study[4] | n=277 DBP 95–109 mmHg | • Candesartan, 16 mg once daily, and 8 mg twice daily, reduced trough DBP by 9.4 and 10.3 mmHg, respectively (both $p<0.001$ vs baseline). Trough SBP was reduced by 11.1 and 12.6 mmHg, respectively (both $p<0.001$ vs baseline).<br>• No significant difference was observed between the once- and twice-daily dosing regimens with regard to trough DBP or SBP ($p>0.05$).<br>• Both candesartan regimens were superior to placebo in reducing trough SBP and DBP (both $p<0.05$).<br>• No significant between-group differences were observed in terms of the incidence or severity of adverse events (no $p$-value reported). |
| Placebo or candesartan dose titration from 8 mg to 16, 32 and 64 mg once daily, at 2-weekly intervals[5] 8-week, randomised, double-blind, forced-titration study | n=133 DBP 95–114 mmHg | • Treatment with all doses of candesartan were superior to placebo in reducing trough SBP and DBP ($p<0.001$ and $p<0.01$, respectively).<br>• A dose–response relationship was observed for candesartan up to 32 mg but an additional clinically meaningful effect on blood pressure was noted with the 64 mg dose.<br>• The incidence and intensity of adverse events were similar in the placebo and candesartan groups, and there were no dose-related adverse events over the candesartan, 8–64 mg range. |

**Table 1.** Continued

DBP, diastolic blood pressure; SBP, systolic blood pressure.

Candesartan, 8–16 mg/day, and losartan, 50–100 mg/day, reduced DBP by 13.1 (95% confidence interval [CI] 12.4–13.8) and 12.4 (95% CI 11.7–13.0) mmHg, respectively. However, the same study reported that candesartan was superior compared with losartan in reducing SBP at the aforementioned doses. Thus, it appears that candesartan, 8–16 mg/day, has a greater systolic, but not diastolic, antihypertensive efficacy than losartan, 50–100 mg/day, but the 16 mg daily dose of candesartan is superior to losartan, 50 mg/day.

When the broader dose range of candesartan available in the US was used in clinical studies (16–32 mg/day), candesartan appears to be a

**Table 2.** Summary of double-blind, randomised trials comparing candesartan with losartan in patients with hypertension.[3,7–10]

| Drug regimen | Patients | Outcomes |
| --- | --- | --- |
| Candesartan, 8 or 16 mg once daily, losartan 50 mg once daily, or placebo<br>8-week, randomised, double-blind, parallel-group study[3] | n=337<br>DBP 95–114 mmHg | • Candesartan, 8 and 16 mg, reduced trough DBP by 8.9 and 10.3 mmHg, respectively, compared with those receiving placebo (both p<0.001 vs placebo).<br>• Candesartan, 16 mg, reduced trough DBP by 3.7 mmHg more than losartan, 50 mg (p=0.013).<br>• The frequency of adverse events was similar in the candesartan, losartan and placebo groups. |
| Candesartan, 8–16 mg/day, losartan, 50–100 mg/day, or losartan, 50 mg/day, ± HCTZ, 12.5 mg/day<br>12-week, randomised, double-blind parallel-group study[7] | n=1161<br>DBP 95–115 mmHg | • Greater reductions in trough SBP from baseline were observed in patients receiving candesartan than in those receiving losartan monotherapy (15.8 mmHg [95% CI 14.7–16.9] vs 14.4 mmHg [95% CI 13.3–15.5], respectively).<br>• The difference in reductions in trough DBP from baseline between candesartan and losartan monotherapy was not significant (13.1 mmHg [95% CI 12.4–13.8] vs 12.4 mmHg [95% CI 11.7–13.0], respectively).<br>• The incidence of adverse events and patient withdrawals were similar in all treatment groups. |
| Candesartan, 16–32 mg/day, losartan, 50–100 mg/day<br>8-week, randomised, double-blind, parallel-group study[8] | n=332<br>DBP 95–114 mmHg | • Candesartan reduced trough DBP more than losartan (11.0 vs 8.9 mmHg, respectively; p=0.016).<br>• Candesartan reduced peak DBP more than losartan (12.6 vs 9.6 mmHg, respectively; p=0.005).<br>• The differences between reductions in trough SBP and peak SBP for candesartan and losartan treatments did not reach statistical significance (11.9 vs 10.0 and 16.5 vs 14.4 mmHg, respectively; p=0.25 and p=0.24, respectively).<br>• 58 and 64% of patients given candesartan and losartan, respectively, experienced adverse effects (no p-value reported). |

[a]Trough DBP at week 8 <90 mmHg, or a decrease from baseline of at least 10 mmHg.
[b]Trough DBP at week 8 <90 mmHg.
CI, confidence interval; DBP, diastolic blood pressure; HCTZ, hydrochlorothiazide; SBP, systolic blood pressure.

## Table 2. Continued

| Drug regimen | Patients | Outcomes |
| --- | --- | --- |
| Candesartan, 16–32 mg/day, losartan, 50–100 mg/day 8-week, randomised, double-blind, parallel-group, forced-titration study[9] | n=654 DBP 95–114 mmHg | • Candesartan lowered trough SBP and DBP more than losartan treatment (13.3 vs 9.8 and 10.9 vs 8.7 mmHg, respectively; $p<0.001$ for both comparisons). • Candesartan also reduced peak SBP and DBP more than losartan treatment (15.2 vs 12.6 and 11.6 vs 10.1 mmHg, respectively; $p<0.05$ for both comparisons). • A greater proportion of patients were classed as responders[a] or controlled[b] in the candesartan than in the losartan group (62.4 vs 54.0% and 56.0 vs 46.9%, respectively; $p=0.033$ and $p=0.023$, respectively). • Of those receiving candesartan and losartan, 45 and 47%, respectively, experienced treatment-emergent adverse events, and both treatments were generally well tolerated. |
| Candesartan, 16–32 mg/day, losartan, 50–100 mg/day 8-week, randomised, double-blind, parallel-group, forced-titration study[10] | n=611 DBP 95–114 mmHg | • Candesartan lowered trough SBP and DBP more than losartan treatment (13.4 vs 10.1 and 10.5 vs 9.1 mmHg, respectively; both $p<0.05$). • Candesartan also reduced peak SBP and DBP more than losartan treatment (15.5 vs 12.0 and 12.9 vs 9.5 mmHg, respectively; both $p<0.005$). • Numerically, more patients were classed as responders[a] or controlled[b] in the candesartan than the losartan group, though these differences were not significant (58.8 vs 52.1% and 49.0 vs 44.6%, respectively; $p>0.05$). • The most common adverse events in the candesartan group were headache (7.2%), respiratory infection (3.9%) and sinusitis (3.9%). The most common adverse events in the losartan group were respiratory infection (7.9%), headache (5.9%) and rhinitis (3.6%). |

[a]Trough DBP at week 8 <90 mmHg, or a decrease from baseline of at least 10 mmHg.
[b]Trough DBP at week 8 <90 mmHg.
CI, confidence interval; DBP, diastolic blood pressure; HCTZ, hydrochlorothiazide; SBP, systolic blood pressure.

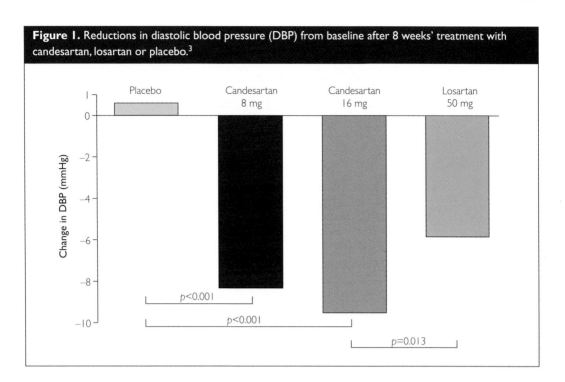

**Figure 1.** Reductions in diastolic blood pressure (DBP) from baseline after 8 weeks' treatment with candesartan, losartan or placebo.[3]

more effective antihypertensive agent than losartan both with respect to trough, peak, or 48-hour post-dose DBP (Table 2).[8–10]

Various meta-analyses have compared the efficacy of angiotensin II receptor antagonists and have generated conflicting results. For example, Conlin et al. did not find a significant difference in terms of antihypertensive efficacy between losartan and the other agents in this class of drugs, though this did not review data available after 1998 and few studies were direct comparisons.[11] Another review encompassing new drug application data from the Food and Drug Administration (FDA) in the US found that the reductions in trough DBP were markedly greater with candesartan than with losartan, valsartan or irbesartan (no p-values reported).[12] However, the results of direct comparisons in the form of double-blind trials are preferable even to well-executed meta-analyses, and thus we await further head-to-head trials before drawing firm conclusions. On the balance of data, it would appear to be fair to conclude that candesartan is at least as effective an antihypertensive agent as losartan.[12]

Candesartan is at least as effective an antihypertensive agent as losartan.

## Candesartan vs ACE inhibitors

Several trials have performed head-to-head comparisons between candesartan and ACE inhibitors such as enalapril, lisinopril and perindopril. Data from these studies are summarised in Table 3.[13–19] Treatment with candesartan has certain distinct advantages over enalapril. Although both agents appear to be generally well tolerated, a number of studies have shown that the overall burden of adverse events is lower for candesartan treatment, in particular a lower incidence of dry

**Table 3.** Summary of double-blind, randomised trials comparing candesartan with angiotensin-converting enzyme (ACE) inhibitors in patients with hypertension.[13–19]

| Drug regimen | Patients | Outcomes |
| --- | --- | --- |
| Candesartan, 8–16 mg/day, or enalapril, 10–20 mg/day 8-week, randomised, double-blind, parallel-group, forced-titration study[13] | n=395 DBP 95–114 mmHg | • Ambulatory SBP and DBP (measured 22–24 hours post-dose from baseline to 8 weeks' treatment) were lower in patients receiving candesartan than enalapril (13.5 vs 9.9 and 8.7 vs 5.8 mmHg, respectively; $p<0.008$ and $p<0.032$, respectively).<br>• Ambulatory SBP and DBP (measured 24–36 hours post-dose from baseline to 8 weeks' treatment) showed greater reductions in patients receiving candesartan than enalapril (11.4 vs 7.2 and 8.0 vs 4.5 mmHg, respectively; $p<0.002$ and $p<0.001$, respectively). |
| Candesartan, 4–8 mg/day, or enalapril, 10–20 mg/day, or placebo 8-week, randomised, double-blind, parallel-group study[14] | n=227 DBP 95–109 mmHg | • Similar reductions in SBP and DBP were obtained in the candesartan and enalapril groups (13 vs 14 and 10 vs 10 mmHg, respectively; $p>0.05$).<br>• The response rate[a] in the candesartan and enalapril groups (60 vs 63%, respectively) and normalisation rates[b] (61 vs 63%, respectively) were not significantly different (no p-value given).<br>• The incidence of adverse events was lower in the candesartan than the enalapril group and similar to that in the placebo group (11, 24 and 16%, respectively). |
| Candesartan, 8–16 mg/day, or enalapril, 10–20 mg/day, or HCTZ, 12.5–25 mg/day 12-week, randomised, double-blind, parallel-group study[15] | n=227 women DBP 95–115 mmHg | • Candesartan treatment lowered SBP/DBP by 17/11 and 19/11 mmHg after 6 and 12 weeks' treatment, respectively.<br>• This reduction was greater ($p<0.01$) than treatment with either enalapril (12/8 and 13/9 mmHg) or HCTZ (12/7 and 13/8 mmHg) after 6 and 12 weeks' treatment, respectively.<br>• The proportion of patients receiving candesartan, enalapril or HCTZ whose blood pressure was controlled[b] was 60, 51 and 43%, respectively; $p<0.01$ for candesartan vs HCTZ.<br>• Though the incidence of patients reporting at least one adverse event was similar in the candesartan, enalapril and HCTZ groups (60, 67 and 64%, respectively), patients experienced less dry cough ($p<0.001$) with candesartan than enalapril. |

[a]Reduction in trough DBP from baseline of at least 10 mmHg. [b]Trough DBP ≤90 mmHg.
[c]Reduction in trough DBP from baseline of at least 10 mmHg and/or trough DBP ≤90 mmHg.
DBP, diastolic blood pressure; HCTZ, hydrochlorothiazide; SBP, systolic blood pressure.

## Table 3. Continued

| Drug regimen | Patients | Outcomes |
|---|---|---|
| Candesartan, 4–12 mg/day, or lisinopril, 10–20 mg/day 24-week, randomised, prospective, crossover study[16] | n=73 DBP >90 mmHg or SBP >150 mmHg | • SBP and DBP were similar for candesartan and lisinopril treatments with regard to systolic or diastolic clinic BP or 24-hour ambulatory blood pressure (no p-values reported). • Patients with the greatest morning surge in blood pressure had greater decreases in clinic SBP/DBP with candesartan than lisinopril ($p<0.05$). |
| Candesartan/HCTZ 8/12.5 mg/day, or lisinopril/HCTZ 10/12.5 mg/day 26-week, randomised, double-blind, parallel-group study[17] | n=353 DBP 95–115 mmHg | • Trough SBP and DBP were not significantly different between the candesartan and lisinopril groups (mean difference 2.1 and 0.5 mmHg, both $p=0.20$). • No significant differences were found between the candesartan and lisinopril groups for proportion of responders[c] (54.4 vs 62.1%, respectively; $p=0.094$) and the number of controlled patients[b] (45.1 vs 44.8%, respectively; $p>0.2$). • Candesartan/HCTZ was better tolerated than lisinopril/HCTZ, with fewer patients experiencing at least one adverse event than in the lisinopril group (68.9 vs 79.5, respectively; $p=0.02$). |
| Candesartan, 16 mg/day, lisinopril, 20 mg/day, or its combination (candesartan, 16 mg/day, plus lisinopril, 20 mg/day) 24-week, randomised, double-blind, parallel-group study[18] | n=199 type 2 diabetics with urinary albumin: creatine ratio of 2.5–25 mg/mmol DBP 90–110 mmHg | • There were no significant differences between candesartan and lisinopril treatments for reductions in SBP (9.5 vs 9.7 mmHg, respectively; $p>0.2$), DBP (12.4 vs 15.7 mmHg, respectively; $p=0.18$) or urinary albumin:creatine ratio (30 vs 46%, respectively; $p=0.058$). • At 24 weeks, combination treatment was more effective in reducing microalbuminuria than candesartan but not lisinopril monotherapy (50, 24 and 39%, respectively; $p=0.04$ vs candesartan and $p>0.2$ vs lisinopril). • All treatments were generally well tolerated. |
| Candesartan, 16 mg/day, or perindopril, 4 mg/day 12-month, randomised, double-blind, parallel-group study[19] | n=96 type 2 diabetics DBP >90 and <105 mmHg | • Candesartan reduced DBP to a lesser degree than perindopril (8 vs 11 mmHg, respectively; $p<0.05$). • There was no significant difference between candesartan and perindopril treatments in SBP reductions (12 vs 13 mmHg, respectively; $p>0.05$). |

[a]Reduction in trough DBP from baseline of at least 10 mmHg. [b]Trough DBP ≤90 mmHg.
[c]Reduction in trough DBP from baseline of at least 10 mmHg and/or trough DBP ≤90 mmHg.
DBP, diastolic blood pressure; HCTZ, hydrochlorothiazide; SBP, systolic blood pressure.

cough.[14,15] Furthermore, candesartan has been shown to have an equivalent, or greater, antihypertensive efficacy to enalapril, both with regard to SBP and DBP reductions, response and normalisation rates.[13–16] However, the practical relevance of this comparison may be questionable, given the significantly longer duration of action of candesartan compared with enalapril. No significant differences in antihypertensive efficacy have been observed between candesartan and lisinopril, or between candesartan–hydrochlorothiazide (HCTZ) and lisinopril–HCTZ combinations,[16–18] with the exception of a reported superiority for candesartan in controlling the morning surge of blood pressure in a subgroup of patients in one trial.[16] Candesartan is also associated with fewer adverse effects than lisinopril when both are given in combination with HCTZ. One trial of 96 patients with type 2 diabetes showed that perindopril was more effective than candesartan in lowering DBP but not SBP, but few data were presented to allow a proper comparison of these agents' relative tolerability profiles. Thus, it is difficult to draw direct conclusions on the relative efficacy/tolerability of these two agents.

In summary, candesartan is at least as effective as a variety of ACE inhibitors for the treatment of hypertension and appears to be better tolerated.

### Candesartan vs calcium-channel blockers

Candesartan has been compared directly with calcium-channel blockers, such as amlodipine and felodipine, in randomised, double-blind or open-label trials. Data from these studies are summarised in Table 4.[20–22] Candesartan was shown to be at least as effective as amlodipine or felodipine in reducing SBP and DBP in patients with mild systemic or systolic hypertension, and was also better tolerated, with a lower incidence of peripheral oedema.[20–22] Furthermore, candesartan also appears to be effective and well tolerated in patients with moderate-to-severe hypertension when combined with amlodipine and/or HCTZ, or in elderly patients with systolic hypertension.[21,22]

### Comparison or combination with HCTZ

Candesartan and the diuretic, HCTZ, reduce blood pressure by a similar magnitude in obese patients, but candesartan, and not HCTZ, has the added benefit of increasing insulin sensitivity in this population (Table 5).[23] Thus, candesartan appears to be a more appropriate treatment than HCTZ for obese patients with hypertension. In addition, a combination of candesartan plus HCTZ was shown to be more effective than HCTZ monotherapy and placebo in treating patients with mild-to-moderate hypertension (DBP 90–110 mmHg), or in those with severe hypertension (DBP >110 mmHg; Table 5).[24,25]

A combination of candesartan, 4–16 mg, plus HCTZ, 12.5–25 mg, effectively reduces blood pressure in the majority of patients, and those treated with these combinations exhibit greater reductions in blood pressure than when either agent is used as monotherapy.[26] The antihypertensive effect of candesartan–HCTZ has also been compared

> Candesartan is at least as effective as a variety of ACE inhibitors for the treatment of hypertension and appears to be better tolerated.

> Candesartan is at least as effective as amlodipine or felodipine in reducing SBP and DBP, and is better tolerated.

**Table 4.** Summary of clinical trials of comparisons and combinations of candesartan with calcium-channel blockers.[20–22]

| Drug regimen | Patients | Outcomes |
|---|---|---|
| Candesartan, 16–32 mg/day, or amlodipine, 5–10 mg/day 8-week, randomised, double-blind, parallel-group, forced-titration study[20] | n=251 DBP 90–99 mmHg | • Candesartan treatment was at least as effective as amlodipine, with trough SBP/DBP reductions of 15.2/10.2 vs 15.4/11.3 mmHg, respectively (p>0.05).<br>• Peripheral oedema occurred less frequently in patients receiving candesartan than amlodipine (8.9 vs 22.1%, respectively; p=0.005).<br>• The number of patients discontinuing treatment due to adverse events in the candesartan and amlodipine groups was 3.3 and 9.4%, respectively; no p-value reported). |
| Candesartan, 8–16 mg/day, plus amlodipine, 5 mg/day, then HCTZ, 25 mg/day, as required 12-week, open-label study[21] | n=185 DBP >100 mmHg | • After 12 weeks, 19% of patients were receiving candesartan, 8 mg, 15% candesartan, 16 mg, 29% candesartan, 16 mg, plus amlodipine, and 18% candesartan, 16 mg, plus amlodipine and HCTZ.<br>• Overall, DBP was reduced by 19.8 mmHg, from 107.8 at baseline to 88.0 mmHg and SBP was reduced by 32.9 mmHg, from 174.4 at baseline to 141.5 mmHg.<br>• Candesartan is an effective antihypertensive agent as monotherapy, or when combined with amlodipine or HCTZ.<br>• All agents were generally well tolerated, either as monotherapy or in combination. |
| Candesartan, 16 mg; felodipine, 5 mg; candesartan, 16 mg, plus felodipine, 5 mg; or placebo 4-month, randomised, double-blind, four-way crossover study[22] | n=31 elderly patients with systolic hypertension SBP ≥160 mmHg | • Candesartan and felodipine lowered ambulatory blood pressure (SBP/DBP) by a similar extent (12.2/7.5 vs 11.9/5.7 mmHg, respectively).<br>• Combination treatment lowered ambulatory blood pressure (SBP/DBP) by 21.0/11.2 mmHg, a reduction greater than that for either monotherapy (p<0.005).<br>• The combination of candesartan and felodipine had an additive effect on blood pressure reductions, and combination and monotherapies were both generally well tolerated. |

DBP, diastolic blood pressure; HCTZ, hydrochlorothiazide; SBP, systolic blood pressure.

**Table 5.** Summary of randomised, double-blind clinical trials of candesartan and HCTZ.[23–25]

| Drug regimen | Patients | Outcomes |
|---|---|---|
| Candesartan, 8–16 mg/day, or HCTZ, 25–50 mg/day 12-week, randomised, double-blind, parallel-group study[23] | n=127 obese patients (BMI 30–40 kg/m$^2$) DBP ≥95 and ≤115 mmHg | • Trough SBP and DBP were both reduced from baseline by a similar extent with candesartan and HCTZ ($p<0.001$). <br> • Patients receiving candesartan showed beneficial increases in insulin sensitivity, as indicated by a reduction in the IRI (−23.2 at baseline to −17.6 at 12 weeks, $p<0.01$). <br> • In contrast, HCTZ was associated with an increase in the IRI (−19.2 to −21.4, $p<0.02$). <br> • Candesartan appears to be a more appropriate treatment for hypertension in obese patients with hypertension. |
| Candesartan, 16 mg/day, for 4 weeks, then 8 weeks' double-blind treatment with either candesartan, 16 mg/day, plus placebo, or candesartan, 16 mg/day, plus HCTZ, 12.5 mg 12-week, randomised, double-blind, parallel-group study[24] | n=328 DBP 90–110 mmHg | • Treatment with the candesartan–HCTZ combination was more effective in reducing SBP/DBP than candesartan plus placebo (−12.0 vs −7.5 and −7.5 vs −5.5 mmHg, respectively; $p=0.010$ and $p=0.037$, respectively). <br> • There was a similar pattern and low frequency of adverse events in both treatment groups. |
| Candesartan, 8–16 mg/day, plus HCTZ, 12.5 mg/day, or placebo, plus HCTZ, 12.5 mg/day 4-week, randomised, double-blind, study[25] | n=217 DBP ≥110 mmHg | • Candesartan–HCTZ was more effective than placebo–HCTZ in reducing trough DBP (−9.1 vs −3.1, respectively; $p=0.0001$). <br> • Similarly, trough SBP was reduced by a greater extent with candesartan–HCTZ than with placebo–HCTZ (−11.3 vs −4.1, respectively; $p=0.0009$). <br> • More patients treated with candesartan than placebo responded to treatment (53 vs 29%) and achieved DBP of under 90 mmHg (32 vs 15%) (no $p$-values reported). <br> • Candesartan–HCTZ was equally well tolerated as placebo–HCTZ. |

BMI, body-mass index; DBP, diastolic blood pressure; HCTZ, hydrochlorothiazide; IRI, insulin resistance index; SBP, systolic blood pressure.

with that of losartan–HCTZ and lisinopril–HCTZ (see preceding sections of this review). In summary, these trials have demonstrated that candesartan–HCTZ has superior efficacy to the losartan–HCTZ combination and is at least as effective as lisinopril in combination with HCTZ.[7,17] In addition, candesartan–HCTZ was better tolerated than lisinopril–HCTZ.[17] Candesartan, 16 mg, plus HCTZ, 12.5 mg, is the recommended dosage of this fixed combination both in Europe and in the US, and a fixed-dose combination tablet is available (in some countries) for patients in whom adequate blood pressure control is not achieved with the maximum dose of candesartan as monotherapy.[26] Candesartan, 32 mg, plus HCTZ, 12.5 mg, combination tablets are also available in the USA for patients whose blood pressure is not adequately controlled by candesartan, 32 mg/day.[26]

## Switching studies

The efficacy and tolerability profile of candesartan has been investigated in patients previously treated with ACE inhibitors, β-blockers, calcium-channel blockers or thiazide diuretics, and who failed to tolerate these drugs.[27] Such patients (n=968), with mild-to-moderate hypertension (DBPs and SBPs of 95 and 180 mmHg, or less, respectively), were enrolled into an 8-week, randomised, open-label, parallel-group trial. Patients received candesartan, 8 or 16 mg/day, for 4 weeks, at which time the dose of candesartan could be doubled, as appropriate, in patients in the candesartan 8 mg treatment arm. (Note: patients who were previously treated with β-blockers had to progressively reduce their β-blocker dose before receiving candesartan treatment in order to avoid an increase in blood pressure resulting from abrupt cessation of treatment.) Clinic SBPs and DBPs were reduced from baseline after 8-weeks' treatment (in both treatment groups) by 12.1 and 5.8 mmHg, respectively ($p<0.01$). Reductions in blood pressure occurred regardless of the previous type of antihypertensive medication that the patient had failed to tolerate. Furthermore, the number of adverse events dropped from 1125 at baseline to 129 and 46 after 4 and 8 weeks' treatment, respectively. In conclusion, candesartan is an effective and well-tolerated alternative to other classes of antihypertensive agents, when, despite their efficacy, they are not well tolerated.[27]

> Candesartan is an effective and well-tolerated alternative to other classes of antihypertensive agents, when, despite their efficacy, they are not well tolerated.

## Add-on therapy

The efficacy of candesartan as an add-on therapy has been assessed in large numbers of patients (n=6465) with untreated hypertension or with hypertension not controlled by other antihypertensive medications (SBP and/or DBP of 140–179 and 90–109 mmHg, respectively).[28] In patients with raised DBP (n=5446), candesartan, 16–32 mg/day, was effective as monotherapy, reducing SBP/DBP by 18.7/13.1 mmHg, respectively ($p<0.05$ vs baseline; Figure 2). Candesartan was also effective when added to pre-existing antihypertensive therapy (Figure 2). Similar reductions were also obtained for patients with isolated systolic hypertension (n=1014), whether candesartan was administered as monotherapy (reducing SBP/DBP by 17.0/4.4 mmHg, respectively; $p<0.05$ vs baseline), or as an add-on treatment. A separate publication, also based on data from this trial, focused specifically on the effects of candesartan on isolated systolic hypertension.[29] The additional benefits of candesartan as add-on therapy were apparent regardless of the age, gender or race of patients with systolic or diastolic hypertension.[28,29]

**Figure 2.** Effect of candesartan, 16–32 mg/day, as monotherapy or as add-on treatment to other antihypertensive agents on systolic (top) and diastolic blood pressure (bottom).[28] All treatments showed improvements from baseline ($p$<0.05). Patients initially received candesartan, 16 mg/day either as monotherapy or as add-on therapy to pre-exisiting background therapy. If blood pressure was uncontrolled after 2 or 4 weeks' treatment then the dose of candesartan was doubled to 32 mg/day. No dosage information was available for the add-on therapies because a variety of different agents within each class were used. ACE, angiotensin-converting enzyme; BP, blood pressure.

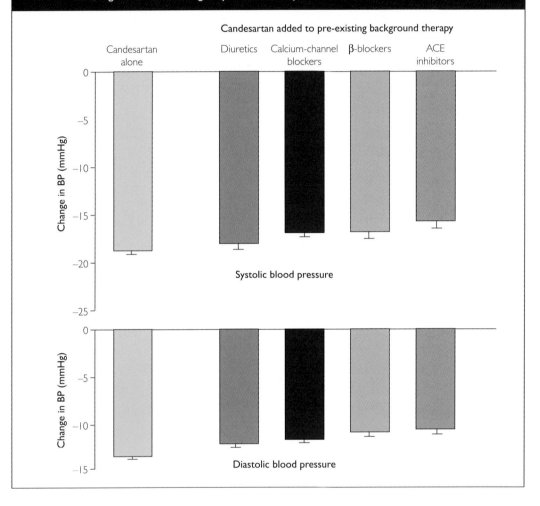

It has been postulated that combining an ACE inhibitor with an angiotensin II receptor antagonist may lead to a more complete blockade of the renin–angiotensin–aldosterone pathway than that achieved by either agent alone. Clinically, this may translate as greater control of blood pressure than with the equivalent monotherapeutic treatment strategies. Two identically designed randomised, multicentre studies have directly compared whether the addition of candesartan treatment to existing treatment with the ACE inhibitor, lisinopril, is more effective in terms of blood-pressure lowering than an increase in the dose of lisinopril.[30] Patients (n=1096) uncontrolled on lisinopril, 20 mg/day, were randomised to 8 weeks' treatment with high-dose lisinopril (40 mg/day) or to 2 weeks' treatment with candesartan, 16 mg/day, followed by 6 weeks of high-dose candesartan (32 mg/day). Pooled data from both studies demonstrated that blood pressure was reduced by a slightly greater extent in the lisinopril plus candesartan group than in those who received high-dose lisinopril (between group difference of –3.1/–1.7 mmHg; $p$=0.05 in favour of candesartan plus lisinopril). Effective blood pressure control (i.e. <140/90 mmHg) was achieved by 42.7 and 36.9% in the lisinopril plus candesartan group and the high-dose lisinopril group, respectively (difference not significant). Both treatment regimens were well tolerated, with a similar frequency of adverse events in both arms. However, patients unable to tolerate lisinopril, 20 mg/day, would have been excluded from this analysis and this probably accounts for the equivalent incidence of adverse events in both groups. Moreover, hyperkalaemia – a potential concern when administering both agents in combination – was only very rarely reported in these studies. Thus, in conclusion, in patients whose blood pressure control is not controlled by lisinopril monotherapy, adding candesartan to their existing treatment regimen is an alternative to increasing the dose of lisinopril. However, further studies are required to evaluate whether a true additive effect is derived from combining these two distinct classes of agents. Moreover, greater benefit in terms of blood-pressure lowering may be derived from combining either agent with an agent that has a completely distinct mechanism of action (e.g. a diuretic or calcium-channel blocker).[31]

## Long-term studies

The long-term treatment of patients for hypertension with candesartan has been investigated in two open-label trials (study 1, n=388; study 2, n=244 patients).[32] Patients with mild-to-moderate hypertension (DBP 95–109 mmHg) enrolled in these studies were administered a flexible dosing regimen of candesartan, 4–16 mg/day. Candesartan was shown to lower SBP and DBP effectively with its antihypertensive effects maintained over the long term (≤12 months). By the end of treatment, 81.1% of patients were classed as responders (reduction in clinic DBP to <90 mmHg and/or a ≥10 mmHg reduction), and 73.8% had a normalised DBP (<90 mmHg). Candesartan appeared to be well tolerated in this long-term trial, with only 5% of patients discontinuing treatment as a result of adverse events. The majority of adverse events that did occur became apparent within the first 3 months of treatment and their incidence decreased steadily thereafter. Thus, candesartan maintains its antihypertensive effects and good tolerability profile with long-term administration.

## Elderly patients

The efficacy and tolerability of candesartan treatment has been investigated extensively in elderly hypertensive patient populations.[33–35] Candesartan has been compared with HCTZ in patients over 75 years of age, in a 24-week, randomised, double-blind trial.[33] Candesartan, 8–16 mg/day, and HCTZ, 12.5 mg/day, reduced clinic DBP by a similar extent (12.0 and 11.4 mmHg, respectively; $p>0.05$), although candesartan was better tolerated, with a lower incidence of hypokalaemia and hyperuricaemia.[33]

Patients over 65 years of age with a DBP of 95–114 mmHg (n=193) were randomised to double-blind treatment with candesartan, 8 mg, or placebo for 6 weeks.[34] After 6 weeks the dose of candesartan was doubled, if required, and was continued for the remaining 6 weeks of the study. Approximately 48% of patients had their dose of candesartan increased from 8 to 16 mg/day. At the end of the trial trough SBP and DBPs were reduced by 13.6 and 7.5 mmHg, respectively (both $p<0.001$ *vs* placebo). The proportion of patients whose hypertension was controlled (DBP ≤90 mmHg) was higher in the candesartan than in the placebo group (41.7 *vs* 16.8%, respectively; $p<0.001$). Likewise, more patients were classified as responders (DBP ≤90 mmHg and/or a reduction in DBP ≤10 mmHg) in the candesartan than in the placebo group (46.9 *vs* 21.1%, respectively; $p<0.001$). Furthermore, there was no evidence of first-dose hypotension, a well-recognised complication of ACE-inhibitor treatment that is of particular concern in the elderly. Thus, in summary, the antihypertensive action of candesartan does not appear to be unduly influenced by patients' age.[34]

The Study on Cognition and Prognosis in the Elderly (SCOPE) has evaluated whether candesartan treatment in 4964 patients aged between 70–89 years with mild-to-moderate hypertension (SBP: 160–179 mmHg; DBP 90–99 mmHg) would lead to reductions in cardiovascular events, cognitive decline or dementia.[35] Patients entering this prospective, randomised, double-blind, parallel-group trial had their previous antihypertensive medication (where treated) standardised to HCTZ, 12.5 mg/day, which continued throughout the trial. Patients were then randomised to receive candesartan, 8 mg, or placebo. The dose of candesartan was doubled, if necessary, after 1 month. Open-label active antihypertensive therapy could be added, as required, for patients in either group, though addition of an ACE inhibitor or another angiotensin II receptor antagonist was not permitted. Active antihypertensive therapy was used in 84% of the placebo group. The mean follow-up period was 3.7 years.

Patients in both the candesartan and the control groups had their SBPs and DBPs reduced from baseline (21.7/10.8 and 18.5/9.2 mmHg, respectively; both $p<0.001$ *vs* baseline). The mean difference between the two groups was 3.2/1.6 mmHg in favour of the candesartan group (both $p<0.001$ for the candesartan *vs* control group).

There was no significant difference between the candesartan and the control groups in terms of the number of first cardiovascular events (26.7 and 30.0 events per 1000 patient-years, respectively; a risk reduction of 10.9% ($p=0.19$). The event rate and relative risks for cardiovascular and total mortality endpoints are shown in Figure 3. With the exception of non-fatal stroke, candesartan did not have a significant effect on overall morbidity or mortality relative to the control group. In terms of non-fatal stroke, candesartan treatment was associated with a

---

The antihypertensive action of candesartan does not appear to be unduly influenced by patients' age.

In terms of non-fatal stroke, candesartan treatment was associated with a relative risk reduction of 27.8% compared with the control group ($p=0.04$).

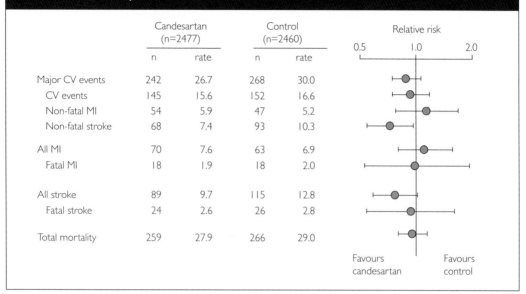

**Figure 3.** Effects of candesartan, 8–16 mg/day, vs placebo control (both groups received additional open-label antihypertensive agents as required) on cardiovascular mortality and morbidity (number of patients [n] and events per 1000 patient-years [rate]). Relative risks are expressed with 95% confidence intervals.[35] CV, cardiovascular; MI, myocardial infarction.

| | Candesartan (n=2477) | | Control (n=2460) | | Relative risk |
|---|---|---|---|---|---|
| | n | rate | n | rate | |
| Major CV events | 242 | 26.7 | 268 | 30.0 | |
| CV events | 145 | 15.6 | 152 | 16.6 | |
| Non-fatal MI | 54 | 5.9 | 47 | 5.2 | |
| Non-fatal stroke | 68 | 7.4 | 93 | 10.3 | |
| All MI | 70 | 7.6 | 63 | 6.9 | |
| Fatal MI | 18 | 1.9 | 18 | 2.0 | |
| All stroke | 89 | 9.7 | 115 | 12.8 | |
| Fatal stroke | 24 | 2.6 | 26 | 2.8 | |
| Total mortality | 259 | 27.9 | 266 | 29.0 | |

relative risk reduction of 27.8% compared with the control group (*p*=0.04). Cognitive function, as determined by the Mini Mental State Examination (MMSE) was not significantly different between the candesartan and control groups (–0.5 and –0.6 points, respectively; *p*=0.2), whilst there was no significant difference between the candesartan and control groups in the incidence of dementia (62 *vs* 57, respectively; *p*>0.2). Both treatment regimens were well tolerated, with 15 and 17% of patients in the candesartan and placebo groups, respectively, withdrawing due to adverse events.

A *post hoc* analysis of the SCOPE study specifically evaluated the clinical outcomes of patients who did not receive any add-on antihypertensive therapy after treatment randomisation. Therefore, this analysis is more reflective of a direct placebo-controlled evaluation of the effects of candesartan treatment.[36] A total of 2098 patients from the entire SCOPE study population did not receive any additional antihypertensive treatment after initial randomisation to candesartan or placebo. Specifically, 1253 of these patients received candesartan, 8–16 mg/day, whilst 845 received placebo. Blood pressure was reduced by 21.8/11.0 mmHg in the candesartan group and by 17.2/8.4 mmHg in the placebo group. The difference in adjusted blood pressure reductions between the two treatment groups (4.7/2.6 mmHg) was significant in favour of candesartan (*p*<0.001, for both SBP and DBP). Moreover, this analysis revealed that candesartan treatment was associated with significantly greater improvements in clinical outcomes relative to placebo. Thus, major cardiovascular events were reduced by 32% with candesartan treatment (*p*=0.013 *vs* placebo), cardiovascular

Candesartan treatment appears to be an appropriate antihypertensive agent for elderly patients with mild hypertension and can reduce major cardiovascular outcomes.

mortality was reduced by 29% (*p*=0.049 *vs* placebo) and total mortality was reduced by 27% (*p*=0.018 *vs* placebo). Cognitive function was maintained in both treatment groups, with no significant differences apparent between the candesartan and placebo groups. There were also no significant differences between the two treatment groups in terms of significant cognitive decline or the number of cases of dementia. Thus, candesartan treatment appears to be an appropriate antihypertensive agent for elderly patients with mild hypertension and can reduce major cardiovascular outcomes in this patient population.

A further *post hoc* analysis of data from the SCOPE study evaluated the effects of candesartan treatment upon the risk of stroke in elderly patients with isolated systolic hypertension.[37] This analysis was conducted because isolated systolic hypertension is the most common form of hypertension in the elderly, whilst stroke is the primary cardiovascular complication within this population. A total of 1518 patients in the SCOPE study were considered to have isolated systolic hypertension (i.e. SBP >160 mmHg and DBP <90 mmHg). Over the course of the study, blood pressure in these patients was significantly reduced by 22/6 mmHg in the candesartan group and by 20/5 mmHg in the placebo group. Despite this very small difference in blood pressure reduction between the two treatment groups, candesartan treatment was associated with a significant relative risk reduction in the incidence of fatal and non-fatal stroke of 42% (*p*=0.05 *vs* placebo). This difference was maintained when the data were adjusted to reflect the higher cardiovascular risk that was apparent in the candesartan group at baseline (*p*=0.049 *vs* placebo). Thus, given the minor difference in blood pressure between the two treatment groups, the favourable effects of candesartan treatment on the incidence of stroke in this patient population may be related to effects other than simple blood-pressure lowering *per se*. However, no significant differences between the two treatment groups were reported in other cardiovascular endpoints or in all-cause mortality. Given the low number of strokes that were revealed in both treatment groups in this analysis, further prospectively conducted studies are warranted in this and other patient populations to investigate the potential of candesartan treatment in reducing the risk of stroke further.

A further substudy of the SCOPE trial demonstrated significant improvements for several health-related quality-of-life measures in the candesartan treatment group compared with the control group. These included the Psychological General Well-being Index (PGWB) anxiety, PGWB well being and EuroQoL Health Utility Index current health (*p*=0.01, *p*=0.04 and *p*=0.008, respectively).[38]

## Heart failure

Whilst it is beyond the scope of this edition of *BESTMEDICINE* to review the effects of candesartan beyond its current license in the treatment of hypertension, a number of important clinical trials have evaluated whether there are any mortality and morbidity benefits associated with candesartan treatment in patients with chronic heart failure.[39] Three distinct patient populations were studied: those with left-ventricular ejection fraction (LVEF) of 40% or less who were or were not receiving ACE inhibitors, and patients with LVEF of greater than 40%. Overall, 7601 patients were randomly assigned candesartan (4 or 8 mg/day, titrating up to 32 mg/day) or placebo, and were followed-up for 2 years.[39–42]

The overall mortality rates for the candesartan and placebo groups were 23 and 25%, respectively (covariate adjusted hazard ratio of 0.90 [95% CI 0.82–0.99]; $p=0.032$). This reduction in mortality was driven by a reduction in cardiovascular deaths (Figure 4). In addition,

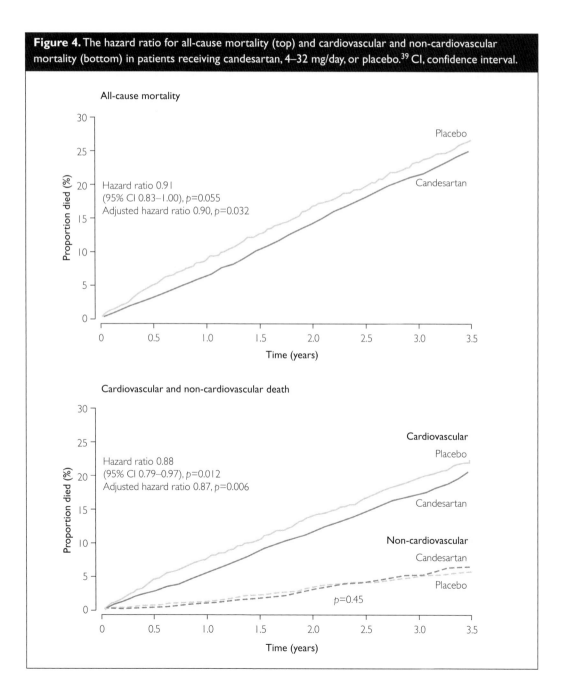

**Figure 4.** The hazard ratio for all-cause mortality (top) and cardiovascular and non-cardiovascular mortality (bottom) in patients receiving candesartan, 4–32 mg/day, or placebo.[39] CI, confidence interval.

fewer hospital admissions for <u>chronic</u> heart failure were reported in the candesartan group compared with those receiving <u>placebo</u> (20 *vs* 24%, respectively; $p<0.0001$). Moreover, candesartan reduced <u>cardiovascular</u> deaths and hospital admissions for heart failure, regardless of LVEF or treatment at <u>baseline</u>. Candesartan was generally well tolerated, but was associated with a greater incidence of discontinuation than placebo as a result of <u>hypotension</u>, hyperkalaemia and increases in <u>serum creatine</u>.[39]

## Safety and tolerability

Given the long-term nature of antihypertensive treatment, the tolerability, rather than the <u>efficacy</u> of antihypertensive agents, is often a limiting factor in their selection.[43] The <u>safety and tolerability</u> of candesartan has been assessed in a <u>pooled analysis</u> of randomised, <u>double-blind</u>, <u>placebo-controlled</u> studies conducted in patients with mild-to-moderate hypertension.[44] The most common <u>adverse events</u> that occurred in at least 2% of patients who received candesartan were headache (10.4%), upper respiratory tract infection (5.1%), back pain (3.2%) and dizziness (2.5%). With the exception of back pain, which occurred more frequently in the candesartan than the placebo group (3.2 *vs* 0.9%, respectively; no <u>*p*-value</u> reported), there were no significant differences in the incidence of adverse events between the candesartan and placebo groups. Importantly, within this same population, there was no evidence of a dose-dependent increase in adverse events. Thus, the proportions of patients with at least one adverse event after receiving placebo or candesartan, 4, 8 or 16 mg, were 33.5, 27.6, 36.2 and 34.8%, respectively).

An analysis of pooled data from double-blind phase 2 or phase 3 studies showed no consistent and/or clinically significant changes in laboratory parameters amongst patients treated with candesartan.[44] A similar proportion of patients in the candesartan and placebo groups experienced changes in laboratory values (7.0 *vs* 5.9%, respectively). Occasional incidences of raised liver <u>enzyme</u> activity (e.g. <u>alanine aminotransferase</u>) were usually transient despite continued candesartan treatment.[44]

## Key points

- Candesartan is administered orally as a <u>prodrug</u>, which is converted to its active form during <u>absorption</u> from the gastrointestinal tract.

- Candesartan binds specifically and tightly to $AT_1$ receptors, causing a long-lasting suppression of the <u>renin–angiotensin system</u> and pronounced antihypertensive action over a 24-hour period.

- Linear and predictable <u>pharmacokinetics</u> across the approved dose range of candesartan translates into a predictable relationship between the dose of candesartan and its antihypertensive <u>efficacy</u>.

- Candesartan may be a more effective antihypertensive agent than losartan, though further direct comparisons are required to confirm this. However, at present, it would be reasonable to conclude that candesartan is at least as effective as losartan.

- Candesartan is at least as effective as a variety of ACE inhibitors in reducing SBP or DBP, with fewer adverse effects, in particular, fewer instances of dry cough.

- Candesartan is at least as effective as the <u>calcium-channel blockers</u>, amlodipine and felodipine, and is better tolerated, with a lower incidence of <u>peripheral oedema</u>.

- The combination of candesartan with HCTZ results in greater reductions in blood pressure than when either agent is used as <u>monotherapy</u>, and the combination is generally well tolerated.

- Candesartan is also effective when added to pre-existing antihypertensive therapy, regardless of patients' age, gender and race.

- Candesartan treatment may reduce the risk of non-fatal stoke, <u>cardiovascular</u> deaths and hospital admissions for heart failure, and increases health-related quality of life.

- The most common <u>adverse events</u> associated with candesartan use are headache, upper respiratory tract infection, back pain and dizziness. In general, candesartan has an adverse event profile that is similar to <u>placebo</u>.

# References

A list of the published evidence which has been reviewed in compiling the preceding section of *BESTMEDICINE*.

1  Lacourciere Y, Asmar R. A comparison of the efficacy and duration of action of candesartan cilexetil and losartan as assessed by clinic and ambulatory blood pressure after a missed dose, in truly hypertensive patients: a placebo-controlled, forced titration study. Candesartan/Losartan study investigators. *Am J Hypertens* 1999; **12**: 1181–7.

2  Reif M, White WB, Fagan TC *et al*. Effects of candesartan cilexetil in patients with systemic hypertension. Candesartan Cilexetil Study Investigators. *Am J Cardiol* 1998; **82**: 961–5.

3  Andersson OK, Neldam S. A comparison of the antihypertensive effects of candesartan cilexetil and losartan in patients with mild to moderate hypertension. *J Hum Hypertens* 1997; **11(Suppl 2)**: S63–4.

4  Zuschke CA, Keys I, Munger MA *et al*. Candesartan cilexetil: comparison of once-daily versus twice-daily administration for systemic hypertension. Candesartan Cilexetil Study Investigators. *Clin Ther* 1999; **21**: 464–74.

5  Bell TP, DeQuattro V, Lasseter KC *et al*. Effective dose range of candesartan cilexetil for systemic hypertension. Candesartan Cilexetil Study Investigators. *Am J Cardiol* 1999; **83**: 272–5.

6  Elmfeldt D, George M, Hubner R, Olofsson B. Candesartan cilexetil, a new generation angiotensin II antagonist, provides dose dependent antihypertensive effect. *J Hum Hypertens* 1997; **11(Suppl 2)**: S49–53.

7  Manolis AJ, Grossman E, Jelakovic B *et al*. Effects of losartan and candesartan monotherapy and losartan/hydrochlorothiazide combination therapy in patients with mild to moderate hypertension. Losartan Trial Investigators. *Clin Ther* 2000; **22**: 1186–203.

8  Gradman AH, Lewin A, Bowling BT *et al*. Comparative effects of candesartan cilexetil and losartan in patients with systemic hypertension. Candesartan Versus Losartan Efficacy Comparison (CANDLE) Study Group. *Heart Dis* 1999; **1**: 52–7.

9  Bakris G, Gradman A, Reif M *et al*. Antihypertensive efficacy of candesartan in comparison to losartan: the CLAIM study. *J Clin Hypertens (Greenwich)* 2001; **3**: 16–21.

10  Vidt DG, White WB, Ridley E *et al*. A forced titration study of antihypertensive efficacy of candesartan cilexetil in comparison to losartan: CLAIM Study II. *J Hum Hypertens* 2001; **15**: 475–80.

11  Conlin PR, Spence JD, Williams B *et al*. Angiotensin II antagonists for hypertension: are there differences in efficacy? *Am J Hypertens* 2000; **13**: 418–26.

12  Hansson L. The relationship between dose and antihypertensive effect for different AT1-receptor blockers. *Blood Press Suppl* 2001; **3**: 33–9.

13  Himmelmann A, Keinanen-Kiukaanniemi S, Wester A *et al*. The effect duration of candesartan cilexetil once daily, in comparison with enalapril once daily, in patients with mild to moderate hypertension. *Blood Press* 2001; **10**: 43–51.

14  Zanchetti A, Omboni S. Comparison of candesartan versus enalapril in essential hypertension. Italian Candesartan Study Group. *Am J Hypertens* 2001; **14**: 129–34.

15  Malmqvist K, Kahan T, Dahl M. Angiotensin II type 1 (AT1) receptor blockade in hypertensive women: benefits of candesartan cilexetil versus enalapril or hydrochlorothiazide. *Am J Hypertens* 2000; **13**: 504–11.

16  Eguchi K, Kario K, Shimada K. Comparison of candesartan with lisinopril on ambulatory blood pressure and morning surge in patients with systemic hypertension. *Am J Cardiol* 2003; **92**: 621–4.

17  McInnes GT, O'Kane KP, Istad H, Keinanen-Kiukaanniemi S, Van Mierlo HF. Comparison of the AT1-receptor blocker, candesartan cilexetil, and the ACE inhibitor, lisinopril, in fixed combination with low dose hydrochlorothiazide in hypertensive patients. *J Hum Hypertens* 2000; **14**: 263–9.

18  Mogensen CE, Neldam S, Tikkanen I *et al*. Randomised controlled trial of dual blockade of renin-angiotensin system in patients with hypertension, microalbuminuria, and non-insulin dependent diabetes: the candesartan and lisinopril microalbuminuria (CALM) study. *BMJ* 2000; **321**: 1440–4.

19  Derosa G, Cicero AF, Ciccarelli L, Fogari R. A randomized, double-blind, controlled, parallel-group comparison of perindopril and candesartan in hypertensive patients with type 2 diabetes mellitus. *Clin Ther* 2003; **25**: 2006–21.

20  Kloner RA, Weinberger M, Pool JL *et al*. Comparative effects of candesartan cilexetil and amlodipine in patients with mild systemic hypertension. Comparison of Candesartan and Amlodipine for Safety, Tolerability and Efficacy (CASTLE) Study Investigators. *Am J Cardiol* 2001; **87**: 727–31.

21  MacGregor GA, Viskoper JR, Antonios TF, He FJ. Efficacy of candesartan cilexetil alone or in combination with amlodipine and hydrochlorothiazide in moderate-to-severe hypertension. UK and Israel Candesartan Investigators. *Hypertension* 2000; **36**: 454–60.

22  Morgan T, Anderson A. A comparison of candesartan, felodipine, and their combination in the treatment of elderly patients with systolic hypertension. *Am J Hypertens* 2002; **15**: 544–9.

23  Grassi G, Seravalle G, Dell'Oro R *et al.* Comparative effects of candesartan and hydrochlorothiazide on blood pressure, insulin sensitivity, and sympathetic drive in obese hypertensive individuals: results of the CROSS study. *J Hypertens* 2003; **21**: 1761–9.

24  Campbell M, Sonkodi S, Soucek M, Wiecek A. A candesartan cilexetil/hydrochlorothiazide combination tablet provides effective blood pressure control in hypertensive patients inadequately controlled on monotherapy. *Clin Exp Hypertens* 2001; **23**: 345–55.

25  Oparil S. Candesartan cilexetil in combination with low-dose hydrochlorothiazide is effective in severe hypertension. *Am J Cardiol* 1999; **84**: 35S–41S.

26  Melian EB, Jarvis B. Candesartan cilexetil plus hydrochlorothiazide combination: a review of its use in hypertension. *Drugs* 2002; **62**: 787–816.

27  Porcellati C, Omboni S. Switching from ACE inhibitors, beta-blockers, calcium antagonists or diuretics to candesartan improves efficacy and tolerability. *Blood Press* 2002; **11**: 310–19.

28  Weir MR, Weber MA, Neutel JM *et al.* Efficacy of candesartan cilexetil as add-on therapy in hypertensive patients uncontrolled on background therapy: a clinical experience trial. ACTION Study Investigators. *Am J Hypertens* 2001; **14**: 567–72.

29  Neutel JM, Weir MR, Moser M *et al.* The effects of candesartan cilexetil in isolated systolic hypertension: a clinical experience trial. *J Clin Hypertens (Greenwich)* 2000; **2**: 181–6.

30  Izzo JL, Weinberg MS, Hainer JW, Kerkering J, Tou CK. Antihypertensive efficacy of candesartan-lisinopril in combination *vs.* up-titration of lisinopril: the AMAZE trials. *J Clin Hypertens (Greenwich)* 2004; **6**: 48–93.

31  Morgan T, Anderson A, Bertram D, MacInnis RJ. Effect of candesartan and lisinopril alone and in combination on blood pressure and microalbuminuria. *J Renin Angiotensin Aldosterone Syst* 2004; **5**: 64–71.

32  Sever P, Holzgreve H. Long-term efficacy and tolerability of candesartan cilexetil in patients with mild to moderate hypertension. *J Hum Hypertens* 1997; **11(Suppl 2)**: S69–73.

33  Neldam S, Forsen B. Antihypertensive treatment in elderly patients aged 75 years or over: a 24-week study of the tolerability of candesartan cilexetil in relation to hydrochlorothiazide. *Drugs Aging* 2001; **18**: 225–32.

34  McInnes GT, O'Kane KP, Jonker J, Roth J. The efficacy and tolerability of candesartan cilexetil in an elderly hypertensive population. *J Hum Hypertens* 1997; **11(Suppl 2)**: S75–80.

35  Lithell H, Hansson L, Skoog I *et al.* The Study on Cognition and Prognosis in the Elderly (SCOPE): principal results of a randomized double-blind intervention trial. *J Hypertens* 2003; **21**: 875–86.

36  Lithell H, Hansson L, Skoog I *et al.* The Study on COgnition and Prognosis in the Elderly (SCOPE); outcomes in patients not receiving add-on therapy after randomization. *J Hypertens* 2004; **22**: 1605–12.

37  Papademetriou V, Farsang C, Elmfeldt D *et al.* Stroke prevention with the angiotensin II type 1-receptor blocker candesartan in elderly patients with isolated systolic hypertension: the Study on Cognition and Prognosis in the Elderly (SCOPE). *J Am Coll Cardiol* 2004; **44**: 1175–80.

38  Degl'Innocenti A, Elmfeldt D, Hofman A *et al.* Health-related quality of life during treatment of elderly patients with hypertension: results from the Study on Cognition and Prognosis in the Elderly (SCOPE). *J Hum Hypertens* 2004; **18**: 239–45.

39  Pfeffer MA, Swedberg K, Granger CB *et al.* Effects of candesartan on mortality and morbidity in patients with chronic heart failure: the CHARM-Overall programme. *Lancet* 2003; **362**: 759–66.

40  Yusuf S, Pfeffer MA, Swedberg K *et al.* Effects of candesartan in patients with chronic heart failure and preserved left-ventricular ejection fraction: the CHARM-Preserved Trial. *Lancet* 2003; **362**: 777–81.

41  Granger CB, McMurray JJ, Yusuf S *et al.* Effects of candesartan in patients with chronic heart failure and reduced left-ventricular systolic function intolerant to angiotensin-converting-enzyme inhibitors: the CHARM-Alternative trial. *Lancet* 2003; **362**: 772–6.

42  McMurray JJ, Ostergren J, Swedberg K *et al.* Effects of candesartan in patients with chronic heart failure and reduced left-ventricular systolic function taking angiotensin-converting-enzyme inhibitors: the CHARM-Added trial. *Lancet* 2003; **362**: 767–71.

43  Andersson OK. Tolerability of a modern antihypertensive agent: candesartan cilexetil. *Basic Res Cardiol* 1998; **93(Suppl 2)**: 54–8.

44  Belcher G, Hubner R, George M, Elmfeldt D, Lunde H. Candesartan cilexetil: safety and tolerability in healthy volunteers and patients with hypertension. *J Hum Hypertens* 1997; **11(Suppl 2)**: S85–9.

## Acknowledgements

Figure 2 is adapted from Andersson and Neldam, 1997.[3]

Figure 3 is adapted from Weir *et al.*, 2001.[28]

Figure 4 is adapted from Lithell *et al.*, 2003.[35]

Figure 5 is adapted from Pfeffer *et al.*, 2003.[39]

# 5. Drug review – Eprosartan (Teveten®)

*Dr Eleanor Bull*
*CSF Medical Communications Ltd*

## Summary

Eprosartan is a potent <u>angiotensin II receptor antagonist</u> currently indicated for the treatment of essential hypertension. By directly blocking the action of angiotensin II on the angiotensin II type 1 ($AT_1$) receptor, eprosartan inhibits <u>vasoconstriction</u> and <u>aldosterone</u> release whilst avoiding the persistent cough that commonly occurs with the <u>angiotensin-converting enzyme (ACE) inhibitors</u>. In contrast to many of the other angiotensin II receptor antagonists, eprosartan also exerts an inhibitory effect on <u>sympathetic neurotransmission</u> and may thus improve arterial compliance. In a clinical setting, eprosartan is significantly better than <u>placebo</u> and at least as effective as the ACE inhibitor, enalapril, at reducing <u>systolic blood pressure (SBP)</u> and <u>diastolic blood pressure (DBP)</u> in patients with hypertension of varying severity. Eprosartan has a low potential for drug–<u>drug interactions</u> and is well tolerated in all patient groups examined, including the elderly and black patient subpopulations. The <u>adverse event</u> profile of eprosartan is similar to that of placebo and doses can be <u>titrated</u> upwards without worsening of adverse events.

## Introduction

The <u>renin–angiotensin system</u> is a complex of <u>enzymes</u>, proteins and peptides that are involved in blood pressure regulation and fluid and <u>electrolyte</u> balance.[1] The final effector substance of the renin–angiotensin system, angiotensin II is a potent vasoconstrictor and acts via $AT_1$ receptors to increase blood pressure and stimulate aldosterone release.[2] The ACE inhibitors (e.g. enalapril, perindopril) are effective antihypertensive agents, although their use is associated with the development of a persistent, non-productive cough in 5–20% of patients.[3,4] This, and other effects – including <u>angioedema</u> – are thought to pertain to a non-selective action on other <u>vasoactive pathways</u>, including the <u>bradykinin</u> system.[3]

The angiotensin II receptor antagonists (e.g. candesartan, eprosartan, irbesartan, losartan, olmisartan, telmisartan, valsartan) offer an alternative approach to the management of hypertension. By directly targeting the $AT_1$ receptor, these agents inhibit angiotensin II activity without disrupting bradykinin metabolism, thus reducing the likelihood of a number of potential side-effects, including cough. This mechanism of action also avoids blocking the potentially beneficial effects of $AT_2$ receptor activation on the vasculature and guards against the production of angiotensin II by ACE-independent pathways.[4,5] The early angiotensin II receptor antagonists (e.g. saralasin) were limited by their partial agonist activity, short duration of action and lack of significant activity after oral administration.[6] The more recent, non-peptide angiotensin II receptor antagonists offer improved selectivity, nanomolar affinity for the $AT_1$ receptor and also lack any agonist activity.[4]

First introduced in the UK in 2000, eprosartan is a potent and selective angiotensin II receptor antagonist indicated for the treatment of essential hypertension. This article reviews the efficacy and tolerability of eprosartan in controlled clinical trials in the context of other available treatments for hypertension. Although there is evidence to suggest that eprosartan may have potential for the management of heart failure, this is beyond the scope of this review and will not be discussed herein.[7–9]

> Eprosartan elicited a dose-dependent decrease in DBP and SBP and a dose-related increase in the number of patients responding to therapy.

## Clinical efficacy

### Placebo-controlled studies

A placebo-controlled, dose-ranging study was conducted in 364 patients with essential hypertension (sitting DBP ≥95 and ≤114 mmHg).[10] Eprosartan was administered at doses of 400–1200 mg once daily for an 8-week period. Overall, eprosartan elicited a dose-dependent decrease in sitting DBP and SBP compared with placebo (Table 1). There was a dose-related increase in the number of patients responding to therapy at study endpoint (response defined as DBP <90 mmHg, or <100 mmHg with a 10 mmHg reduction from baseline). Responses ranged between

**Table 1.** Effect of once-daily eprosartan treatment on sitting diastolic (DBP) and systolic blood pressure (SBP) (trough) at study endpoint.[10]

| | Eprosartan regimen (mg/day) | | | |
| --- | --- | --- | --- | --- |
| | 400 | 600 | 800 | 1200 |
| DBP (mmHg) | | | | |
| Difference from placebo | −1.9 | −3.2 | −2.7 | −4.3 |
| p-value | 0.12 | 0.01 | 0.03 | 0.001 |
| SBP (mmHg) | | | | |
| Difference from placebo | −4.1 | −7.5 | −4.9 | −9.5 |
| p-value | 0.05 | <0.001 | 0.02 | <0.001 |

27.8–43.7% for patients receiving 400–1200 mg eprosartan, compared with 23.6% in placebo-treated patients.

The relative efficacy of two eprosartan treatment regimens – 400–800 mg once daily, or 200–400 mg twice daily – was compared in a placebo-controlled study in 243 patients with mild-to-moderate hypertension.[11] The dose of eprosartan was titrated upwards over a 9-week period and those patients achieving a sitting DBP of below 90 mmHg continued with fixed-dose treatment for a further 4 weeks. At the study endpoint, the baseline change in DBP was –9 mmHg following once-daily eprosartan dosing, –9 mmHg following two daily doses and –4 mmHg following placebo ($p<0.0001$ vs placebo for both eprosartan regimens). Sitting SBP was also significantly reduced following both treatment regimens compared with placebo (–15, –10 and –4 mmHg, for twice daily, once daily and placebo, respectively, $p<0.005$ vs placebo for both eprosartan regimens). Both eprosartan treatment regimens were well tolerated and showed a similar adverse event profile to that of placebo. This study demonstrates that there is no advantage to administering the same total dose of eprosartan twice-daily over once-daily administration.

A double-blind, multicentre study in 200 patients with essential hypertension – diagnosed as sitting DBP greater than 95 mmHg and less than 114 mmHg on two consecutive visits – examined the antihypertensive effect of eprosartan administered at 600 or 1200 mg daily.[12] The baseline SBP and DBP values were 153 and 100 mmHg, respectively. After an 8-week treatment period, the 24-hour change in blood pressure (SBP/DBP) from baseline was 0.2/0.1 mmHg following placebo, –7.9/–5.4 mmHg following 600 mg eprosartan ($p<0.0001$ vs placebo) and –7.4/–5.0 mmHg following 1200 mg[a] eprosartan ($p<0.0001$ vs placebo). Trough ambulatory blood pressure was reduced by –6.3/–4.1 for 600 mg and –7.7/–5.5 for 1200 mg eprosartan with no differences between the active treatment groups, advocating the 600 mg dose over the 1200 mg dose (Figure 1).

An 8-week study conducted in the US, examined the effect of eprosartan, 600 mg once daily, in 243 patients with mild-to-moderate hypertension (sitting DBP 94–114 mmHg).[13] All blood pressure measurements were taken 24 hours ± 90 minutes after dosing. After 8 weeks of eprosartan treatment, sitting DBP was reduced by 7.6 mmHg, compared with 1.9 mmHg following placebo ($p<0.0001$). Following a similar trend, sitting SBP was reduced by 6.1 mmHg in eprosartan-treated patients, yet increased by 0.8 mmHg in those patients receiving placebo ($p<0.0001$). The response rate – characterised as sitting DBP of less than 90 mmHg or a decrease of at least 10 mmHg – was 42% following eprosartan treatment compared with 21% following placebo ($p=0.0003$). Eprosartan had no effect on sitting or standing heart rate and the adverse events reported were similar for eprosartan and placebo groups, and were mild-to-moderate in severity.

> There is no advantage to administering the same total dose of eprosartan twice-daily over once-daily administration.

---

[a]Dose not licensed in the UK.

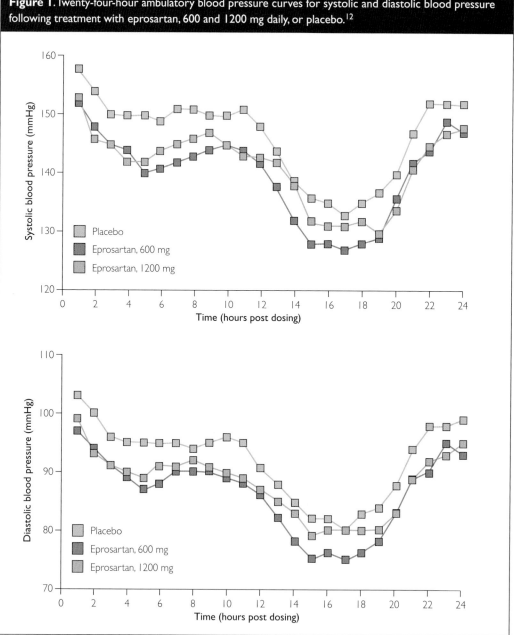

**Figure 1.** Twenty-four-hour ambulatory blood pressure curves for systolic and diastolic blood pressure following treatment with eprosartan, 600 and 1200 mg daily, or placebo.[12]

## Comparative clinical trials

### Eprosartan vs enalapril

A summary of the clinical trials comparing the blood pressure lowering effects of eprosartan with those of the ACE inhibitor, enalapril, is presented in Table 2.[14–18] In general, eprosartan was at least as effective as enalapril at lowering blood pressure and in some instances, the

**Table 2.** Summary of the controlled clinical trials comparing eprosartan with enalapril for the treatment of hypertension.[14–18] Changes in blood pressure reflect those measured at study endpoint.

| Study | Study design | Treatment regimens | Baseline SBP/DBP (mmHg) | Change from baseline in SBP/DBP (mmHg) | Response rate at study endpoint |
|---|---|---|---|---|---|
| Sega et al., 1999[14] | Double-blind 10 weeks n=118 Patients with severe hypertension | Eprosartan 600–800 mg daily | 180/117 | –29*/–20 | 69.5%* |
| | | Enalapril 20–40 mg daily | 178/117 | –21/–16 | 54.2% |
| Elliott et al., 1999[15] | Double-blind 26 weeks n=528 | Eprosartan 200–300 mg twice daily | 156/101 | –16/–13 | 81.7%* |
| | | Enalapril 5–20 mg once daily | 156/101 | –15/–12 | 73.4% |
| Argenziano et al.,1999[16] | Double-blind 26 weeks Elderly patient subgroup n=37 | Eprosartan 200–300 mg twice daily | 165/101 | –19/–14 | 55% |
| | | Enalapril 5–20 mg once daily | 165/100 | –15/–12 | 48% |
| Levine et al., 1999[17] | Double-blind 26 weeks n=40 Black patient subgroup | Eprosartan 200–300 mg twice daily | 156/101 | –19/–11 | 66.7%* |
| | | Enalapril 5–20 mg once daily | 156/102 | –11/–10 | 42.1% |
| Ruilope et al., 2001[18] | Double-blind 12 weeks n=323 Elderly patients | Eprosartan 600–800 mg once daily | 176/98 | –18/–9 | Systolic – 41% Diastolic – 64% |
| | | Enalapril 5–20 mg once daily | 175/98 | –17/–10 | Systolic – 39% Diastolic – 68% |

*p<0.05, eprosartan vs enalapril. DBP, diastolic blood pressure; SBP, systolic blood pressure.

reduction in SBP was more pronounced following eprosartan treatment. The response rate to drug treatment tended to be superior for eprosartan compared with enalapril, usually to a significant degree.

The largest comparative trial conducted to date is that of Elliott and colleagues on behalf of the Eprosartan Study Group.[15] This 26-week international multicentre study included 528 patients with essential hypertension and also prompted further subgroup analyses in elderly and

The response rate to drug treatment tended to be superior for eprosartan over enalapril, usually to a significant degree.

black patient subpopulations.[16,17,19] The dose of eprosartan was <u>titrated</u> upwards to 200–300 mg twice daily over a 12-week period, after which time the option of <u>hydrochlorothiazide add-on therapy</u>, 12.5–25 mg daily, was available if needed. Overall, eprosartan treatment was associated with a significantly superior response rate compared with enalapril (defined as sitting DBP ≤90 mmHg or ≤10 mmHg reduction from <u>baseline</u>). The superior response profile of eprosartan was apparent both at the end of the titration period (70.3 *vs* 62.6% for eprosartan and enalapril, respectively, *p*<0.05) and at the study endpoint (81.7 *vs* 73.4%, *p*=0.018).

A subgroup analysis investigated the impact of both drugs on <u>neurohormone</u> levels, <u>serum lipid profiles</u> and <u>electrocardiogram (ECG)</u> parameters in a representative sample of the patient population from the aforementioned study.[19] Consistent with their respective mechanisms of action, both eprosartan and enalapril increased <u>plasma renin activity</u> but did not affect plasma <u>aldosterone</u> levels. At the study endpoint, <u>angiotensin II</u> levels taken from 100 patients were significantly reduced in the eprosartan group (6.9 *vs* 3.1 ng/mL for eprosartan and enalapril respectively, *p*<0.05). Neither eprosartan nor enalapril altered serum lipid or <u>electrolyte</u> levels and no alteration in ECG parameters was reported in either treatment group.

The antihypertensive effect of eprosartan in 118 patients with severe hypertension (sitting DBP >115 mmHg and <125 mmHg) was compared with that of enalapril over a period of 10 weeks.[14] After an initial titration period, patients received a maximum daily dose of either eprosartan, 600–800 mg daily, or enalapril, 20–40 mg daily. In addition, hydrochlorothiazide was available to all patients if blood pressure remained uncontrolled on maximum doses of eprosartan and enalapril. The proportion of patients requiring additional <u>diuretic</u> treatment was similar for eprosartan and enalapril (39 and 37.3%, respectively). As shown in Table 2, the mean change in sitting DBP at study endpoint was –20.1 mmHg following eprosartan compared with –16.2 mmHg following enalapril, although this did not reach significance. In terms of improvements in SBP, eprosartan was superior to enalapril for both sitting and standing measurements, with eprosartan-treated patients experiencing a mean decrease in sitting SBP of 29.1 mmHg compared with 21.1 mmHg following enalapril treatment (*p*=0.025). The response rate, defined as sitting DBP of less than 90 mmHg or a reduction from baseline of at least 15 mmHg, was 69.5% for eprosartan and 54.2% for enalapril (*p*=0.07). These data suggest that eprosartan may be more effective than enalapril in reducing SBP, at least in patients with severe hypertension.

> Eprosartan may be more effective than enalapril in reducing SBP, at least in patients with severe hypertension.

## Eprosartan in combination with hydrochlorothiazide

For those patients who do not respond well to <u>monotherapy</u> for hypertension, further reductions in blood pressure can be achieved through the combination of two different classes of antihypertensive, for example, an angiotensin II receptor antagonist and a thiazide diuretic. For this reason, eprosartan is frequently co-administered with hydrochlorothiazide.

The efficacy of an eprosartan and hydrochlorothiazide combination
was evaluated in a randomised, double-blind study in 494 patients with
mild-to-moderate hypertension.[20] Patients received either eprosartan,
600 mg daily, alone or in combination with hydrochlorothiazide,
12.5 mg daily, for a total of 8 weeks with a 4-week follow-up period.
Whilst both treatment groups experienced reductions from baseline in
DBP, greater reductions were observed in those patients receiving
eprosartan and hydrochlorothiazide in combination ($p=0.001$; Figure 2).
This finding was echoed by a correspondingly higher response rate in the
combination group, defined as the percentage of patients with a sitting
DBP of less than 100 mmHg, having decreased from baseline by at least
10 mmHg (73.2 *vs* 57.1% for combination and monotherapy,
respectively; $p=0.004$).

An open-label study of 706 patients with mild-to-moderate
hypertension examined the effect of eprosartan, 400–800 mg once daily,
alone or in combination with hydrochlorothiazide (12.5–25 mg).[21]
The study involved a 3–15-week dose-titration period, followed by
12–24 months of maintenance therapy and 5–7 days follow-up. In
total, 83.3% patients completed 12 months and 44.4% completed
24 months of maintenance therapy. Overall, eprosartan – either alone or
in combination with hydrochlorothiazide – was well tolerated,
irrespective of dose, with mild side-effects. Improvements in blood
pressure were maintained throughout the treatment period and high
density lipoprotein cholesterol (HDL-C), triglyceride and glucose
levels were unaffected in the majority of patients. Thus, an
eprosartan–hydrochlorothiazide combination is well tolerated in both
the short and long term, with negligible adverse events.[22]

> An eprosartan–
> hydrochlorothiazide
> combination is well
> tolerated in both
> the short and long-
> term, with negligible
> adverse events.

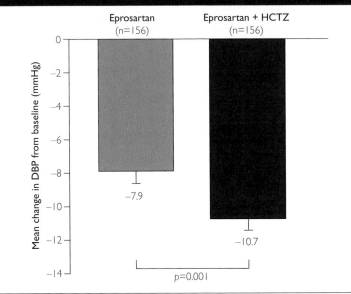

**Figure 2.** Mean change from baseline in sitting diastolic blood pressure
(DBP) at study endpoint in patients receiving eprosartan, 600 mg, or
eprosartan, 600 mg, plus hydrochlorothiazide (HCTZ), 12.5 mg.[20]

## Special patient populations

### Type 2 diabetes

A double-blind, placebo-controlled study of 119 patients with type 2 diabetes and mild essential hypertension (DBP 91–104 mmHg) has evaluated the relative antihypertensive efficacy of eprosartan and telmisartan, and also determined whether either agent had any effect upon glucose homeostasis or plasma lipid profiles.[23] Patients were randomised to 12 months' treatment with either eprosartan 600 mg, telmisartan, 40 mg, or placebo, all given once daily. Both active treatments reduced seated trough SBP compared with baseline (mean reductions: –8 and –7 mmHg for telmisartan and eprosartan, respectively; $p<0.01$ for both $vs$ baseline). Likewise, seated trough DBP was also significantly reduced by both agents, though the DBP-lowering effect was more profound in those who received telmisartan (–8 and –4 mmHg for telmisartan and eprosartan, respectively; $p<0.05$ for this comparison). Interestingly, the plasma lipid profile was significantly improved with telmisartan, but not with eprosartan. Thus, improvements relative to baseline were observed in terms of total cholesterol ($p<0.01$), low density lipoprotein cholesterol (LDL-C; $p<0.01$) and triglyceride levels ($p<0.05$) after telmisartan treatment. Neither agent had any effect on body mass index or glucose metabolism. Thus, whilst eprosartan effectively reduced both SBP and DBP in this mildly hypertensive diabetic patient population, this study demonstrates that telmisartan provides more profound reductions in DBP, with the additional benefit of favourable modifications to the atherogenic lipid profile. Further placebo- and comparator-controlled studies of eprosartan in diabetic patient populations are, however, required to establish its role in this patient population more fully.

### Elderly

Blood pressure and the incidence of hypertension tends to rise progressively with age and thus the elderly represent a major treatment population.[24] Furthermore, elevated blood pressure in this population in particular, is a significant risk factor for the development of cardiovascular complications.[4] Clinical data suggest that eprosartan is well tolerated and effective in older patients.[16,18]

A subgroup analysis of a large comparative trial examined the effect of both eprosartan and enalapril in hypertensive patients over 65 years of age.[15,16] Both eprosartan, 200–300 mg twice daily and enalapril, 5–20 mg daily, were well tolerated over a 26-week period in this patient population and the sub-group analysis closely mirrored the results of the original study. These findings were echoed by a double-blind study in 334 elderly patients (over 65 years of age) with essential hypertension.[18] Patients received either eprosartan, 600–800 mg daily, or enalapril, 5–20 mg daily, for a period of 12 weeks. Both eprosartan and enalapril reduced sitting SBP and DBP from baseline levels by a comparable extent. Adverse events considered to be related to the study medication were mild or moderate in intensity and reported by 6.4% of patients receiving eprosartan compared with 14.7% of those receiving enalapril, reflecting improved tolerability following eprosartan treatment.

More recently a double-blind, randomised, placebo-controlled study prospectively evaluated the antihypertensive efficacy of eprosartan in an elderly patient population with isolated systolic hypertension.[25] Isolated systolic hypertension is the most common form of essential hypertension in the elderly, and thus, it is important to evaluate the antihypertensive efficacy of eprosartan in this patient population. Patients (n=283) had a mean sitting SBP of 170 mmHg at baseline, and were randomised to a 6-week double-blind treatment phase (after an initial 3–5-week placebo run-in phase) during which time they received either placebo or eprosartan, which was titrated according to antihypertensive effect from 600 to 1200 mg/day over 6 weeks. Thereafter, patients were maintained on their optimum monotherapy dose for 3 weeks. Finally, for the remaining 4 weeks of the double-blind treatment phase, patients who did not respond adequately to eprosartan monotherapy (mean sitting SBP ≥145 mmHg) received 4 weeks' single-blind combination therapy with hydrochlorothiazide (12.5 mg/day). Those who responded to eprosartan monotherapy were considered to have completed the study at this point.

After the dose-titration phase, eprosartan monotherapy elicited significant reductions in sitting SBP compared with placebo (−16.1 vs −8.4 mmHg; p<0.00001), with 57.4% of patients considered to be responders to eprosartan monotherapy compared with only 32% of patients receiving placebo (p<0.0001). In those patients who did not respond to eprosartan monotherapy, the addition of hydrochlorothiazide led to a significant decrease in sitting SBP compared with the placebo arm (−21.7 vs −14.4 mmHg; p<0.0002). Both eprosartan monotherapy and eprosartan–hydrochlorothiazide combination therapy also provided significant reductions in standing SBP. Retrospective analyses also demonstrated greater reductions in pulse pressure with eprosartan monotherapy compared with placebo (−16.9 mmHg vs −9.1 mmHg; no p-value reported). There were no effects of age, gender or race upon blood pressure-lowering response, though Caucasian patients tended to respond better to treatment than black patients. Eprosartan was well tolerated in this study with dizziness and asthenia the most commonly reported adverse events. Thus, this study demonstrates that eprosartan in doses up to 1200 mg/day, either alone or in combination with hydrochlorothiazide, was effective and well tolerated in elderly patients with isolated systolic hypertension.

> Eprosartan in doses up to 1200 mg/day, either alone or in combination with hydrochlorothiazide, was effective and well-tolerated in elderly patients with isolated systolic hypertension.

## Ethnic groups

Hypertension is more prevalent in black than Caucasian populations and these patients are relatively resistant to ACE inhibitors, perhaps as a result of an inherently low renin status.[26,27]

In a subgroup analysis of a large comparative trial, the antihypertensive effects of eprosartan were compared with those of enalapril in 40 Afro-Caribbean patients with essential hypertension (Table 2).[15,17] Patients received eprosartan 200–300 mg daily, or enalapril, 5–20 mg daily, with the option for additional hydrochlorothiazide therapy (12.5–25 mg) after week 12 if DBP after the titration period was greater than 90 mmHg. After 26 weeks of treatment, sitting DBP was significantly reduced from baseline by a similar extent in both treatment groups (–10.5 and –9.6 mmHg for eprosartan and enalapril-treated patients, respectively). The incidence of cough also showed a similar trend to that observed in the original study, with eprosartan treatment associated with lower cough rates than enalapril, although this did not reach statistical significance. These data demonstrate that eprosartan is as effective and well tolerated in a black patient subpopulation as in the total population of the original study.[15]

## Safety and tolerability

Hypertension may be associated with few if any symptoms and so any side-effects associated with drug treatment will impact highly on patients' perception of therapy and their compliance with therapy and may affect eventual outcomes.[28] Thus, the minimisation of treatment-related side-effects is paramount to the success of any antihypertensive drug. Eprosartan is well tolerated, both in clinical trials and clinical practice, with a side-effect profile similar to that of placebo.[29] The adverse events most commonly reported following eprosartan treatment (Table 3) are mild-to-moderate in severity and do not usually merit treatment discontinuation. Data accumulated from 17 phase 2b and phase 3 clinical studies involving 2709 patients with hypertension, confirm that the adverse event profile of eprosartan is comparable with

**Table 3.** Adverse events reported during placebo-controlled clinical trials in at least 1% of patients receiving eprosartan.[29] Studies of 8–13 weeks' duration, doses ranged from 200–400 mg twice daily or 400–1200 mg daily.

| Adverse event | Incidence of adverse event (%) | |
| --- | --- | --- |
| | Placebo (n=352) | Eprosartan (n=1202) |
| Viral infection | 1 | 2 |
| Injury | 1 | 2 |
| Fatigue | 1 | 2 |
| Abdominal pain | 1 | 2 |
| Hypertriglyceridaemia | 0 | 1 |
| Arthralgia | 1 | 2 |
| Depression | 0 | 1 |
| Upper respiratory tract disorders | 5 | 8 |
| Rhinitis | 3 | 4 |
| Pharyngitis | 3 | 4 |
| Coughing | 3 | 4 |
| Urinary tract infection | 0 | 1 |

that of placebo.[28] The mean duration of eprosartan treatment was 268 days, with 36% of patients receiving treatment for longer than 1 year. The severity of side-effects was not altered by the duration of drug treatment or the size or the frequency of the dose. Age, sex and ethnic origin also had no bearing on tolerability.

The side-effect profile of eprosartan is generally superior to that of the alternative antihypertensive agents, specifically in terms of the incidence of ACE inhibitor-induced cough or the headache and oedema that has been associated with sustained-release nifedipine.[28] Eprosartan is well tolerated when co-administered with the thiazide diuretic, hydrochlorothiazide, an initiative commonly used to boost the overall antihypertensive effect.[22]

## Incidence of cough

ACE inhibitors are known to produce, in approximately 5–20% of patients taking them, a persistent, dry cough that may impact on patients' quality of life and concordance with a dosage regimen. The incidence of cough following eprosartan has been evaluated in a number of clinical settings and one such study estimated that patients treated with enalapril were 3.45-times more likely to experience treatment-related cough than those receiving eprosartan ($p=0.018$).[15]

A 26-week double-blind study incorporating 529 patients with moderate hypertension, compared the cough-inducing properties of an eprosartan or enalapril treatment regimen.[30] Patients received eprosartan (maximum dose 300 mg twice daily) or enalapril (up to 20 mg daily) for 12 weeks with the optional addition of hydrochlorothiazide treatment for the remaining 14 weeks of the trial. At the study endpoint, twice as many enalapril- than eprosartan-treated patients showed symptoms of cough (7.6 vs 3.2% for enalapril and eprosartan, respectively; $p=0.099$). This difference was more pronounced at the monotherapy endpoint (12 weeks) and reached 9.9 and 2.1% for enalapril and eprosartan, respectively ($p=0.001$).

A similar pattern was reported in a 6-week study which assessed incidence of cough and quality of life following treatment with eprosartan, 300 mg twice daily, enalapril, 20 mg once daily, or placebo, in 136 patients with hypertension and a history of ACE inhibitor-induced cough.[31] Although the percentage of patients experiencing cough was significantly higher following enalapril (23 vs 5% for enalapril, eprosartan and placebo, respectively; $p=0.02$), this figure did not reach significance when adjusted for multiple comparisons. Furthermore, no treatment-dependent differences in quality of life were reported.

## Effect on uric acid excretion

Thiazide diuretics are known to impair uric acid excretion, which in some cases may result in hyperuricaemia and gouty arthritis. In contrast, the angiotensin II receptor antagonist, losartan, has a marked uricosuric effect which may lead to the development of uric acid nephropathy.[32] Consequently, the effect of eprosartan on uric acid excretion has been examined.

At the study endpoint, twice as many enalapril- than eprosartan-treated patients showed symptoms of cough.

A <u>double-blind</u>, <u>placebo-controlled</u> study in 57 mild-to-moderately hypertensive patients reported no differences from <u>baseline</u> values in the <u>excretion</u> of <u>uric acid</u> or <u>serum uric acid</u> concentrations after single or repeated doses of eprosartan, 50–1200 mg daily.[32] This was confirmed in a comparative 4-week study of eprosartan, 600 mg daily, or losartan, 50 mg daily, in 60 patients with mild-to-moderate essential hypertension. Uric acid excretion was unchanged over a 24-hour period following eprosartan, in contrast to marked increases associated with losartan treatment (–0.3 mmol *vs* 0.7 mmol for eprosartan and losartan, respectively, $p<0.03$).[33]

# Key points

● Eprosartan is a non-peptide <u>angiotensin II receptor antagonist</u> which displays a high affinity for the $AT_1$ receptor subtype.

● In addition to blocking the effects of angiotensin II on the vasculature, eprosartan also inhibits the sympathetically mediated impairment of <u>arterial compliance</u>.

● Eprosartan has a <u>renal</u> protective action by completely reversing the pressor effects, <u>aldosterone</u> secretion and renal <u>vasoconstriction</u> induced by angiotensin II.

● In contrast to the other angiotensin II receptor antagonists, eprosartan is not metabolised by <u>hepatic</u> cytochrome P450 <u>enzymes</u> and therefore has a low potential for <u>drug interactions</u>.

● Eprosartan is at least as effective as the ACE inhibitor, enalapril, in reducing blood pressure in patients with mild, moderate and severe hypertension.

● The antihypertensive effect of eprosartan <u>monotherapy</u> is enhanced when given in combination with the <u>thiazide</u> <u>diuretic</u>, hydrochlorothiazide.

● Initial data suggest that eprosartan is effective in reducing blood pressure in mildly hypertensive diabetic patients, though it is not as effective as telmisartan in this patient population.

● Eprosartan is effective and well tolerated in elderly (including those with <u>isolated systolic hypertension</u>) and ethnic subpopulations with no need for dosage adjustment.

● The selective blockade of the $AT_1$ receptor by eprosartan avoids some of the disadvantages which can be associated with the ACE inhibitors – including persistent cough – and confers a good tolerability profile.

# References

A list of the published evidence which has been reviewed in compiling the preceding section of *BESTMEDICINE.*

1 Oparil S, Haber E. The renin–angiotensin system. *N Engl J Med* 1974; **291**: 389–401.

2 Beevers G, Lip G, O'Brien E. ABC of hypertension: the pathophysiology of hypertension. *BMJ* 2001; **322**: 912–16.

3 Hedner T. Management of hypertension: the advent of a new angiotensin II receptor antagonist. *J Hypertens Suppl* 1999; **17**: S21–5.

4 Brooks DP, Ruffolo RR. Pharmacological mechanism of angiotensin II receptor antagonists: implications for the treatment of elevated systolic blood pressure. *J Hypertens Suppl* 1999; **17**: S27–32.

5 Brooks DP, Ohlstein EH, Ruffolo RR. Pharmacology of eprosartan, an angiotensin II receptor antagonist: exploring hypotheses from clinical data. *Am Heart J* 1999; **138**: 246–51.

6 Edwards RM, Aiyar N, Ohlstein EH *et al.* Pharmacological characterization of the nonpeptide angiotensin II receptor antagonist, SK&F 108566. *J Pharmacol Exp Ther* 1992; **260**: 175–81.

7 Hollenberg N. Potential of the angiotensin II receptor 1 blocker eprosartan in the management of patients with hypertension or heart failure. *Curr Hypertens Rep* 2001; **3**: S25–8.

8 Gremmler B, Kunert M, Schleiting H, Ulbricht L. Improvement of cardiac output in patients with severe heart failure by use of ACE-inhibitors combined with the AT1-antagonist eprosartan. *Eur J Heart Fail* 2000; **2**: 183–7.

9 Murdoch DR, McDonagh TA, Farmer R *et al.* ADEPT: Addition of the AT1 receptor antagonist eprosartan to ACE inhibitor therapy in chronic heart failure trial: hemodynamic and neurohormonal effects. *Am Heart J* 2001; **141**: 800–7.

10 Shusterman NH. Safety and efficacy of eprosartan, a new angiotensin II receptor blocker. *Am Heart J* 1999; **138**: 238–45.

11 Hedner T, Himmelmann A. The efficacy and tolerance of one or two daily doses of eprosartan in essential hypertension. The Eprosartan Multinational Study Group. *J Hypertens* 1999; **17**: 129–36.

12 White WB, Anwar YA, Mansoor GA, Sica DA. Evaluation of the 24-hour blood pressure effects of eprosartan in patients with systemic hypertension. *Am J Hypertens* 2001; **14**: 1248–55.

13 Gradman AH, Gray J, Maggiacomo F, Punzi H, White WB. Assessment of once-daily eprosartan, an angiotensin II antagonist, in patients with systemic hypertension. Eprosartan Study Group. *Clin Ther* 1999; **21**: 442–53.

14 Sega R. Efficacy and safety of eprosartan in severe hypertension. Eprosartan Multinational Study Group. *Blood Press* 1999; **8**: 114–21.

15 Elliott WJ. Double-blind comparison of eprosartan and enalapril on cough and blood pressure in unselected hypertensive patients. Eprosartan Study Group. *J Hum Hypertens* 1999; **13**: 413–17.

16 Argenziano L, Trimarco B. Effect of eprosartan and enalapril in the treatment of elderly hypertensive patients: subgroup analysis of a 26-week, double-blind, multicentre study. Eprosartan Multinational Study Group. *Curr Med Res Opin* 1999; **15**: 9–14.

17 Levine B. Effect of eprosartan and enalapril in the treatment of black hypertensive patients: subgroup analysis of a 26-week, double-blind, multicentre study. Eprosartan Multinational Study Group. *Curr Med Res Opin* 1999; **15**: 25–32.

18 Ruilope L, Jager B, Prichard B. Eprosartan versus enalapril in elderly patients with hypertension: a double-blind, randomized trial. *Blood Press* 2001; **10**: 223–9.

19 Gavras I, Gavras H. Effects of eprosartan versus enalapril in hypertensive patients on the renin–angiotensin-aldosterone system and safety parameters: results from a 26-week, double-blind, multicentre study. Eprosartan Multinational Study Group. *Curr Med Res Opin* 1999; **15**: 15–24.

20 Sachse A, Verboom CN, Jager B. Efficacy of eprosartan in combination with HCTZ in patients with essential hypertension. *J Hum Hypertens* 2002; **16**: 169–76.

21 Levine B. Eprosartan provides safe and effective long-term maintenance of blood pressure control in patients with mild to moderate essential hypertension. *Curr Med Res Opin* 2001; **17**: 8–17.

22 Bohm M, Sachse A. Safety and tolerability of eprosartan in combination with hydrochlorothiazide. *Drug Saf* 2002; **25**: 599–611.

23 Derosa G, Ragonesi PD, Mugellini A, Ciccarelli L, Fogari R. Effects of telmisartan compared with eprosartan on blood pressure control, glucose metabolism and lipid profile in hypertensive, type 2 diabetic patients: a randomized, double-blind, placebo-controlled 12-month study. *Hypertens Res* 2004; **27**: 457–64.

24 Wilking S, Belanger A, Kannel W, D'Agostino R, Steel K. Determinants of isolated systolic hypertension. *JAMA* 1988; **260**: 3451–5.

25 Punzi HA, Punzi CF. Once-daily eprosartan mesylate in the treatment of elderly patients with isolated systolic hypertension: data from a 13-week double-blind, placebo-controlled, parallel, multicenter study. *J Hum Hypertens* 2004; **18**: 655–61.

26 Lackland D, Keil J. Epidemiology of hypertension in African Americans. *Semin Nephrol* 1996; **15**: 63–70.

27 Sagnella G. Why is plasma renin activity lower in populations of African origin? *J Hum Hypertens* 2001; **15**: 17–25.

28 Gavras I, Gavras H. Safety and tolerability of eprosartan. *Pharmacotherapy* 1999; **19**: S102–7.

29 Solvay Healthcare Limited. Teveten® (eprosartan). *Summary of product characteristics.* High Wycombe, UK, 2004.

30 Breeze E, Rake EC, Donoghue MD, Fletcher AE. Comparison of quality of life and cough on eprosartan and enalapril in people with moderate hypertension. *J Hum Hypertens* 2001; **15**: 857–62.

31 Rake EC, Breeze E, Fletcher AE. Quality of life and cough on antihypertensive treatment: a randomised trial of eprosartan, enalapril and placebo. *J Hum Hypertens* 2001; **15**: 863–7.

32 Ilson BE, Martin DE, Boike SC, Jorkasky DK. The effects of eprosartan, an angiotensin II AT1 receptor antagonist, on uric acid excretion in patients with mild to moderate essential hypertension. *J Clin Pharmacol* 1998; **38**: 437–41.

33 Puig J, Mateos F, Buno A *et al.* Effect of eprosartan and losartan on uric acid metabolism in patients with essential hypertension. *J Hypertens* 1999; **17**: 1033–9.

## Acknowledgements

Figure 1 is adapted from White *et al.*, 2001.[12]
Figure 2 is adapted from Sachse *et al.*, 2002.[20]

# 6. Drug review – Irbesartan (Aprovel®)

*Dr Jennifer Moorman and Dr Scott Chambers*
*CSF Medical Communications Ltd*

## Summary

Irbesartan is a potent and selective <u>angiotensin II receptor antagonist</u>, which is licensed in the UK for the treatment of essential hypertension and for the management of <u>renal</u> disease in patients with hypertension and <u>type 2 diabetes mellitus</u>. Clinical trials have demonstrated that irbesartan provides effective control of blood pressure over a 24-hour period, and offers equivalent blood-pressure lowering <u>efficacy</u> to other antihypertensive agents from different drug classes including the <u>angiotensin-converting enzyme (ACE) inhibitor</u> enalapril, the <u>β-blocker</u> atenolol, and the calcium-channel blocker amlodipine. In addition, clinical evidence suggests that irbesartan offers greater control of blood pressure than other angiotensin II receptor antagonists, including losartan and valsartan. Irbesartan can be combined with the <u>diuretic,</u> hydrochlorothiazide, to offer greater control of blood pressure in patients who fail to respond to <u>monotherapy</u> with either agent. Irbesartan also has important renoprotective effects in patients with hypertension and diabetes, as demonstrated by two large-scale, longer-term clinical trials. Treatment with irbesartan is generally well tolerated, whether it is used as monotherapy or in combination with hydrochlorothiazide. In controlled clinical trials, the overall incidence of <u>adverse events</u> associated with irbesartan was similar to <u>placebo</u>. Importantly, the incidence of cough was lower with irbesartan than with enalapril, whilst there was also a lower incidence of ankle oedema compared with amlodipine.

## Introduction

Effective pharmacotherapy for hypertension has been available for the last 50 years, with each new class of drug introduced being associated with a reduction in the frequency and severity of adverse events. In recent years, the search for effective and well-tolerated antihypertensive

The non-specific effects of ACE inhibitors are responsible for some of their limiting side-effects such as cough and angioedema, which cannot be tolerated by up to 20% of patients.

agents has focused on blockade of the renin–angiotensin system, since this system has been implicated in the pathogenesis of essential hypertension, renovascular hypertension and congestive heart failure.[1] Angiotensin II is the most active peptide in this system, acting as a powerful vasoconstrictor, facilitating sympathetic neurotransmission and promoting salt and water retention through stimulation of type I angiotensin II ($AT_1$) receptors.[2]

ACE inhibitors interfere with the renin–angiotensin system by direct blockade of ACE, thus reducing the circulating concentrations of angiotensin II. Although such agents are effective treatments for both hypertension and congestive heart failure, their use is associated with a range of problems. In particular, ACE inhibitors do not block the production of angiotensin II completely because it can be generated by non-ACE pathways. Furthermore, ACE is a relatively non-specific enzyme that has substrates in addition to angiotensin II – including bradykinin and other tachykinins – and thus inhibition of ACE can result in accumulation of these substrates.[3] The non-specific effects of ACE inhibitors are responsible for some of their limiting side-effects, such as cough and angioedema, which cannot be tolerated by up to 20% of patients.[4]

Angiotensin II receptor antagonists are the most recently introduced class of antihypertensive agents and were developed to overcome the deficiencies of ACE inhibitors. These agents block the effects of angiotensin II by specifically antagonising its actions at the $AT_1$ receptor.[2] Early clinical evidence suggests that angiotensin II receptor antagonists can provide equivalent blood pressure control to ACE inhibitors, but with better tolerability.[5,6] Losartan was the first agent in this class to become available for clinical use, though six other agents – irbesartan, valsartan, candesartan, telmisartan, eprosartan and olmesartan – are now available. These agents differ in the degree of angiotensin II inhibition, which may translate to clinical differences in efficacy and safety.[7–9] This review summarises the evidence for the clinical efficacy, and safety and tolerability of irbesartan in the treatment of hypertension and other conditions.

## Clinical efficacy in hypertension

### Dose–response studies

There appears to be a clear dose–response relationship for irbesartan at doses of 75–300 mg/day, in terms of both reductions in blood pressure and the percentage of patients who achieve a therapeutic response (seated diastolic blood pressure [DBP] <90 mmHg or reduction from baseline of ≥10 mmHg).[10] These observations are based on pooled data from eight multicentre, randomised, placebo-controlled, double-blind, parallel-group studies involving 2955 adults with mild-to-moderate hypertension receiving once-daily irbesartan, 1–900 mg, or placebo. This analysis showed that the antihypertensive effects of irbesartan increased with increasing dose and reached a plateau at 300 mg (Figure 1). Fifty-six per cent of patients showed a favourable response to irbesartan, 150 mg.[10]

**Figure 1.** Placebo-subtracted reductions in mean trough seated diastolic blood pressure (DBP; top) and seated systolic blood pressure (SBP; bottom) by 6–8 weeks' treatment with irbesartan, 1–900 mg.[10]

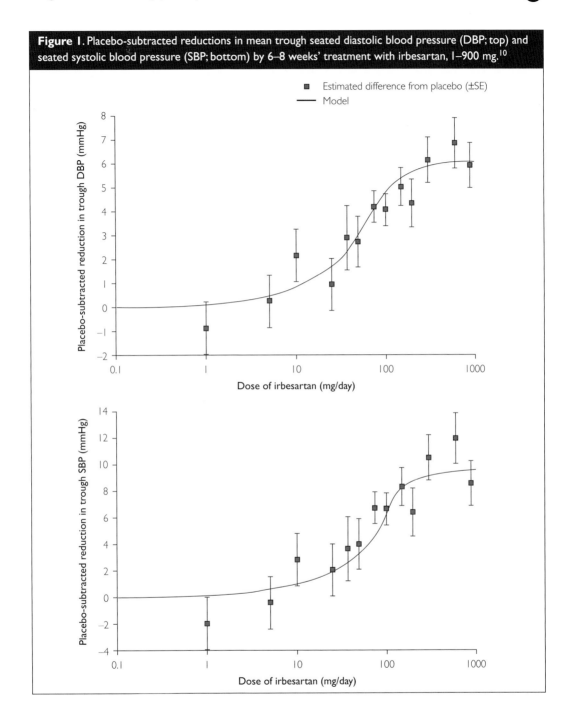

A study investigating the dose-dependent blood pressure-lowering effects of irbesartan found that the reduction was greater with a daily dose of 150 mg <u>titrated</u> to 300 mg than for 75 mg titrated to 150 mg.[11] A dose–response relationship was also observed in terms of therapeutic success, with 47% of the patients on the 75/150 mg regimen attaining a response, compared with 59% receiving the 150/300 mg regimen. This study shows that, if necessary, the irbesartan dose can be <u>titrated</u> up to a maximum of 300 mg/day in order to normalise blood pressure, with no apparent problematic drug accumulation.[11] Once-daily administration of irbesartan appears to be optimal in patients with hypertension, with an initial dose of 150 mg recommended for most patients.

## Irbesartan vs other angiotensin II receptor antagonists

The antihypertensive effects of irbesartan and other <u>angiotensin II receptor antagonists</u> have been compared in three large randomised trials, the findings of which are summarised in Table 1.[12–14] In these studies, irbesartan produced statistically superior reductions in blood pressure and response rates in patients with mild-to-moderate hypertension when compared with losartan (Figure 2) and valsartan.[12–14] It has been suggested that the improved <u>efficacy</u> of irbesartan compared with other agents in this class may be the result of greater $AT_1$-receptor antagonism.[14]

The antihypertensive effects of irbesartan, losartan, candesartan and valsartan have also been compared in a small, <u>double-blind, crossover study</u>.[15] In this study, 20 patients were randomised to receive irbesartan, 150 mg, losartan, 50 mg, candesartan, 8 mg, or valsartan, 80 mg, for 12 weeks, with four crossovers and a 4-week <u>placebo</u> <u>wash-out</u> period between drugs. A further 20 patients were randomised to receive the same initial doses of the four drugs, but if after 6 weeks their DBP was greater than 90 mmHg or the reduction in DBP was less than 10 mmHg, the dose was doubled. In the groups receiving the standard initial doses of the four drugs, blood pressure was consistently lower than during the placebo period. However, the decrease in blood pressure was greater in patients treated with irbesartan (14.1/9.9 mmHg) or valsartan (13.8/9.8 mmHg) than after treatment with losartan (9.9/6.9 mmHg). The decrease in blood pressure produced by candesartan (10.8/7.9 mmHg) was not significantly different from that produced by the other drugs. In the group of patients whose drug dose was doubled, all four agents were found to be equally effective in reducing blood pressure.[15]

## Irbesartan vs enalapril

It is interesting to compare the therapeutic efficacy of irbesartan with that of an ACE inhibitor, since such agents attenuate the effects of <u>angiotensin II</u> via distinct mechanisms. This has been investigated in two randomised, double-blind trials which compared the efficacy of irbesartan with the ACE inhibitor, enalapril, in patients with mild-to-moderate hypertension.[5,16]

In the first such study, patients (n=200) were randomised to 12 weeks' treatment with once-daily irbesartan, 75 mg, or enalapril, 10 mg, following a 4–5-week placebo lead-in period.[16] Doses were doubled at weeks 4 and 8 of the study period if seated DBP was greater than or equal to 90 mmHg. Irbesartan and enalapril were equally effective in lowering blood pressure over the 12-week study period, with blood pressure being normalised (<u>trough</u> DBP <90 mmHg) in 66 and

**Table 1.** Summary of large comparative studies of irbesartan and other angiotensin-II-receptor antagonists.[12–14]

| Drug regimen | Population | Main outcomes |
|---|---|---|
| Irbesartan, 150 or 300 mg/day, or losartan, 100 mg/day, or placebo 8 weeks' treatment[12] | Hypertension (seated DBP 95–110 mmHg) n=567 | • The antihypertensive effects of irbesartan, 150 mg, were comparable with those of losartan throughout the study.<br>• After 8 weeks' treatment, reductions in seated DBP and seated SBP from baseline were greater with irbesartan, 300 mg, than with losartan (differences of 5.1 and 3.0 mmHg, respectively; $p<0.01$ for both comparisons; Figure 1).<br>• There were no significant differences in rates of normalisation (trough seated DBP <90 mmHg) and response (normalisation or reduction in trough seated DBP ≥10 mmHg) between irbesartan, 300 mg, and losartan at week 8 (52 vs 42% and 63 vs 56%, respectively).<br>• Irbesartan, 300 mg, was associated with the lowest incidence of adverse events and discontinuations because of adverse events. |
| Irbesartan, 150–300 mg/day, or losartan, 50–100 mg/day 12 weeks' treatment[13] | Mild-to-moderate hypertension (stage 1, 2 or 3) n=370 | • At week 8, the mean decrease in trough seated DBP (the primary efficacy endpoint) was greater for irbesartan than losartan (10.2 vs 7.9 mmHg; $p<0.02$).<br>• Reductions in trough seated DBP and SBP were also greater with irbesartan than losartan at week 12 (13.8 vs 10.8 mmHg, $p<0.002$; 18.0 vs 13.9 mmHg, $p<0.02$).<br>• Response rates (normal trough seated DBP or reduction ≥10 mmHg) were greater with irbesartan (78%) than losartan (64%; $p<0.01$). |
| Irbesartan, 150 mg/day, or valsartan, 80 mg/day 8 weeks' treatment[14] | Mild-to-moderate hypertension (seated DBP 95–110 mmHg) n=426 | • Irbesartan produced greater reductions in trough diastolic ABP from baseline compared with valsartan (6.73 vs 4.84 mmHg; $p=0.035$).<br>• Significantly greater reductions in trough systolic ABP from baseline and mean 24-hour diastolic ABP were also associated with irbesartan (11.62 vs 7.5 mmHg, $p<0.01$; 6.36 vs 4.82 mmHg, $p=0.0023$).<br>• Irbesartan also produced greater reductions in office-measured seated DBP and seated SBP and self-measured morning diastolic blood pressure than valsartan ($p<0.01$ for all comparisons).<br>• Both drugs were well tolerated. Serious adverse events occurred in 1.4% of valsartan patients and 0.5% of irbesartan patients. None of these adverse events were considered to be related to the study drugs. |

ABP, ambulatory blood pressure; DBP, diastolic blood pressure; SBP, systolic blood pressure.

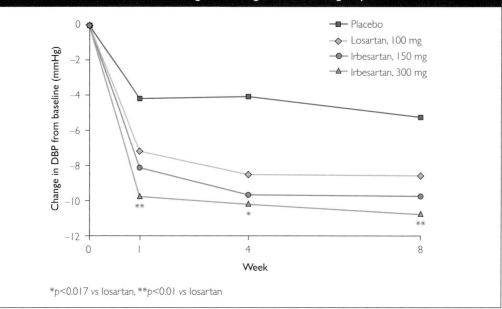

**Figure 2.** Adjusted mean changes from baseline in trough seated diastolic blood pressure (DBP) following 8 weeks' treatment with irbesartan, 150 mg and 300 mg, losartan, 100 mg, or placebo.[12]

*\*p<0.017 vs losartan, \*\*p<0.01 vs losartan*

63% of irbesartan- and enalapril-treated patients, respectively.[16] These results were supported by the second trial, which reported similar blood pressure reductions following 12 weeks' treatment with irbesartan, 150–300 mg, or enalapril, 10–20 mg. Thus, blood pressure control (daytime blood pressure <130/85 mmHg) was achieved by 40.5 and 33.9% of irbesartan- and enalapril-treated patients, respectively.[5] Moreover, in the second trial, irbesartan was significantly better tolerated than enalapril: the incidence of adverse events probably related to treatment was 9.2% with irbesartan compared with 24.6% with enalapril (*p*=0.026).[5]

The efficacy of irbesartan and enalapril has also been compared in patients with severe hypertension (seated DBP 115–130 mmHg), a population traditionally difficult to treat and often requiring combination therapy.[17] In this 12-week, double-blind trial, patients were randomised to irbesartan, 150 mg (n=121), or enalapril, 20 mg (n=61). The doses of irbesartan and enalapril were titrated to 300 mg and 40 mg, respectively, after 1 week if seated DBP remained above 106 mmHg, or after 2 weeks if seated DBP remained above 90 mmHg. If seated DBP was greater than 90 mmHg after this time, further antihypertensive drugs were added to the study regimens. Although reductions in seated trough blood pressure at week 12 were comparable between the two groups (approximately 30 mmHg), irbesartan therapy was associated with a reduced need for three or more adjunctive medications from week 6 compared with enalapril (67 *vs* 75%). Furthermore, irbesartan was significantly better tolerated than enalapril, the latter being associated with a significantly higher incidence of cough

> Irbesartan was significantly better tolerated than enalapril.

than irbesartan (13.1 *vs* 2.5%; *p*=0.007).[17] This is particularly pertinent when one considers that persistent cough is a common side-effect of ACE inhibitors and can be serious enough for patients to discontinue therapy.[18]

The efficacy of irbesartan and enalapril have also been compared in elderly patients (≥65 years of age) with mild-to-moderate hypertension (seated DBP 95–110 mmHg).[19] In this 8-week study, patients were randomised to receive either irbesartan, 150 mg (n=70), or enalapril, 10 mg (n=71), with a doubling of drug dose at week 4 for patients whose seated DBP remained above 90 mmHg. At the end of treatment, similar reductions in DBP and systolic blood pressure (SBP) were observed in the two treatment groups. Thus, mean reductions from baseline in seated DBP were 9.6 and 9.8 mmHg for the irbesartan and enalapril groups, respectively. Normalisation rates were also similar between groups (52.9 *vs* 54.9% for irbesartan and enalapril, respectively). There were no differences between groups in terms of serious adverse events, though irbesartan was associated with a significantly lower incidence of cough (4.3 *vs* 15.5%; *p*=0.046).[19]

Given that inflammation and thrombogenesis are important components of atherosclerosis, a 3-month study of patients with hypertension, documented coronary artery disease and recent coronary angioplasty (n=48) has specifically evaluated the relative anti-inflammatory effects of irbesartan (300 mg/day) and enalapril (20 mg/day).[20] This preliminary study has provided evidence that irbesartan (at this higher dosage) exerts stronger systemic anti-inflammatory and anti-aggregatory effects than does enalapril. However, further studies are required to investigate the anti-inflammatory properties of irbesartan in more detail.

## Irbesartan vs atenolol

Several studies have compared the clinical effects of irbesartan with those of the β-blocker, atenolol; the results of these studies are summarised in Table 2. These studies found that the blood pressure-lowering effect of irbesartan in hypertensive patients was similar to that of atenolol.[21–24] In addition, it appears that irbesartan has beneficial effects on a range of other cardiovascular parameters. For example, studies have shown that hypertension is often accompanied by abnormalities in haemostatic–fibrinolytic balance, which may predict future vascular events; irbesartan was associated with a more favourable modification of haemostatic–fibrinolytic status than atenolol.[22] Left ventricular hypertrophy (LVH) is a strong predictor of cardiovascular mortality, and regression of LVH by antihypertensive agents reduces the risk of cardiovascular complications. In patients with LVH, irbesartan treatment has been shown to produce a significantly greater reduction in left ventricular mass and improvement in cardiac electrical stability compared with atenolol.[23–25] For example, the Cardiovascular Irbesartan Project prospectively evaluated the relative effects of irbesartan and atenolol on LVH in patients with hypertension.[25] A total of 240 patients were allocated to 18 months' treatment with irbesartan (150–300 mg/day) or atenolol (50–100 mg/day). SBP and DBP were reduced by a similar extent in both

**Table 2.** Summary of comparative studies of irbesartan and atenolol.[21–24]

| Drug regimen | Population | Main outcomes |
|---|---|---|
| Irbesartan, 75–150 mg/day, or atenolol, 50–100 mg/day 24 weeks' treatment[21] | Mild-to-moderate hypertension (seated DBP 95–110 mmHg) n=231 | • Both treatments lowered BP from baseline ($p<0.05$), with no significant differences between treatments.<br>• Atenolol induced greater reductions in seated HR compared with irbesartan at week 12 ($p<0.05$).<br>• The incidence of serious adverse events and discontinuations because of adverse events was about twice as high with atenolol compared with irbesartan (3.3 *vs* 1.8% and 9.1 *vs* 4.5%, respectively). |
| Irbesartan, 75–300 mg/day, or atenolol, 25–150 mg/day 6 months' treatment[22] | Hypertension (≥140/90 mmHg) n=54 | • BP was significantly reduced with both irbesartan and atenolol at the end of the study ($p<0.05$), with no significant differences between treatments.<br>• Irbesartan was associated with a greater decrease in the plasma levels of the fibrinolytic/haemostatic markers fibrinogen, PAI-1 and thrombomodulin, compared with atenolol ($p<0.05$). |
| Irbesartan, 150–300 mg/day, or atenolol, 50–100 mg/day 48 weeks' treatment[23] | Mild-to-moderate hypertension (seated DBP 90–115 mmHg) and LVH n=115 | • Reductions in SBP and DBP at the end of treatment were similar in both treatment groups. Seated DBP was normalised (<90 mmHg) in 77 and 74% of patients in the irbesartan and atenolol groups, respectively, at 48 weeks.<br>• LVMI was significantly reduced ($p<0.001$) at 12, 24 and 48 weeks in the irbesartan group but only at 24 and 48 weeks in the atenolol group.<br>• The reduction in LVMI at week 48 was greater in the irbesartan group ($p=0.024$).<br>• The proportion of patients who attained normalised left ventricular mass (men ≤131 g/m$^2$; women ≤100 g/m$^2$) tended to be greater with irbesartan than for atenolol (47 *vs* 32%, respectively). |
| Irbesartan, 150–300 mg/day, or atenolol, 50–100 mg/day 48 weeks' treatment[24] | Mild-to-moderate hypertension (seated DBP 90–115 mmHg) and LVH n=115 | • Irbesartan significantly decreased QT and QTc dispersion at 48 weeks ($p<0.001$); whilst atenolol had only minor effects.<br>• The changes in QT and QTc dispersion with irbesartan were independent of changes in left ventricular mass, BP or HR, indicating structural and electrical cardiac remodelling. |

BP, blood pressure; DBP, diastolic BP; HR, heart rate; LVH, left ventricular hypertrophy; LVMI, left ventricular mass index; PAI-1, plasminogen activator inhibitor-1; SBP, systolic blood pressure.

treatment groups. At the end of the study, reductions in left ventricular mass (as determined by echocardiography) were reported only with irbesartan treatment, with differences between the two treatment groups apparent after 6 months of treatment. However, these reductions were shown to occur only in a subgroup of patients (n=59) within the highest quartile of baseline left ventricular mass. Voltage criteria for LVH (determined by electrocardiography [ECG]) were also consistently decreased exclusively with irbesartan treatment, and this occurred regardless of baseline values. Taken together these findings suggest that irbesartan may reduce the risk of cardiovascular events in hypertensive patients, particularly in those with LVH and irbesartan may be more effective than atenolol in these patients.[24,25]

> Irbesartan may reduce the risk of cardiovascular events in hypertensive patients, particularly in those with LVH.

The beneficial effects of irbesartan on vascular structure and function have been supported by a further study in which hypertensive patients (n=11) who had achieved good blood pressure control following 1 year's treatment with atenolol were switched to irbesartan treatment, also for 1 year.[26] Irbesartan treatment resulted in correction of patients' altered vascular structure (arterial resistance decreased from 8.44 to 6.46%; $p<0.01$) and endothelial function (normalisation of acetylcholine-induced endothelium-dependent relaxation), suggesting a vascular protective effect of the drug.[26] However, as comparatively few patients were involved in this trial, only tentative conclusions can be drawn.

## Irbesartan vs amlodipine

Very few clinical trials have been conducted that have specifically evaluated the relative blood pressure-lowering effects of irbesartan and the calcium-channel blocker, amlodipine. However, the large-scale Irbesartan Diabetic Nephropathy Trial (IDNT; see Clinical Efficacy in Patients with Diabetic Nephropathy), which enrolled hypertensive patients with nephropathy due to type 2 diabetes revealed that both irbesartan (300 mg/day) and amlodipine (10 mg/day) reduced blood pressure by a similar extent, although other antihypertensive agents were included in the different treatment arms in this study which may complicate this comparison.[27] A further 4-week study of 181 patients with mild-to-moderate hypertension also reported that irbesartan (150 mg/day) reduced blood pressure by a similar extent as amlodipine (5 mg/day).[28] Thus, DBP and SBP were reduced by 12/9 and 12/10 mmHg in the irbesartan and amlodipine groups, respectively.

Irbesartan has also been compared with amlodipine in an open-label assessment of their relative effects upon LV mass index in patients with untreated mild-to-moderate hypertension (DBP ≥100 mmHg) and LVH (n=60).[29] After 6 months' treatment with irbesartan (150–300 mg/day), the mean LV mass index (as determined by echocardiography) was reduced by a significantly greater extent than with amlodipine, 5–10 mg/day (–24.7 vs –11.6%; $p<0.0001$). The reduction in LV mass occurred despite there being no significant difference in blood pressure reduction in the two treatment groups (reductions in SBP/DBP of 18/22 and 15/19 mmHg for irbesartan and amlodipine, respectively).

### Irbesartan/hydrochlorothiazide combination therapy

A dose–response study of irbesartan has shown that about 56% of patients respond to irbesartan monotherapy at a dose of 150 mg/day and a further study has reported that 64% of patients had well-controlled blood pressure during long-term treatment with irbesartan (≤300 mg/day) alone.[10,30] Nevertheless, a substantial number of patients require additional antihypertensive agents to achieve their target blood pressure in clinical practice.[31] Thiazide diuretics are frequently used in combination regimens in patients who have not responded to monotherapy.[31] Consequently, several trials have investigated the effect of combining irbesartan with the diuretic hydrochlorothiazide (HCTZ).

The effect of adding HCTZ to irbesartan therapy has been assessed in two multicentre, double-blind, placebo-controlled studies.[32] After a placebo lead-in phase, patients with mild-to-moderate hypertension were randomised to irbesartan, 1–300 mg (n=731), or placebo (n=158), for 8 weeks. Patients whose blood pressure was not controlled at 8 weeks also received open-label HCTZ, 12.5 mg, for a further 2 weeks. The addition of HCTZ resulted in further dose-related decreases in blood pressure, with additional reductions in seated DBP ranging from 1.6 mmHg in the placebo group to 7.7 mmHg in the irbesartan, 300 mg, group (Figure 3).[32]

A similar beneficial effect on blood pressure with an irbesartan/HCTZ combination regimen has been observed in a study evaluating the effects of irbesartan in HCTZ-resistant hypertension.[33] In this study, patients initially received HCTZ, 25 mg, for 4 weeks. After this period, patients whose seated DBP remained elevated (93–110 mmHg; n=238)

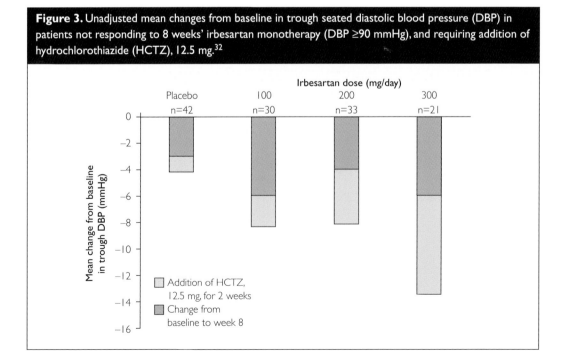

**Figure 3.** Unadjusted mean changes from baseline in trough seated diastolic blood pressure (DBP) in patients not responding to 8 weeks' irbesartan monotherapy (DBP ≥90 mmHg), and requiring addition of hydrochlorothiazide (HCTZ), 12.5 mg.[32]

were randomised to receive irbesartan, 75 mg, or placebo for a further 12 weeks. If seated DBP remained above 90 mmHg at 6 weeks, the dose of irbesartan was doubled. By week 12, the irbesartan/HCTZ combination had reduced seated DBP by an additional 7.1 mmHg compared with the placebo/HCTZ combination ($p<0.01$), with similar reductions in seated SBP. Furthermore, a greater percentage of patients receiving irbesartan/HCTZ achieved blood pressure normalisation compared with the placebo/HCTZ regimen (67 vs 29%; $p<0.01$).[33]

In patients whose hypertension was previously uncontrolled with monotherapy with a variety of antihypertensives or low-dose combination therapy (n=57), 12 weeks' fixed-dose combination treatment with irbesartan (300 mg/day) and hydrochlorothiazide (25 mg/day) led to significant reductions in 24-hour ambulatory blood pressure (–23/–13 mmHg; $p<0.0001$ vs baseline).[34] Moreover, the antihypertensive effect of this regimen was maintained over the entire dosing interval and was also homogeneous with respect to the circadian profile, as evidenced by the trough-to-peak ratios and the smoothness index.[34]

## Long-term treatment

The long-term efficacy of irbesartan has been evaluated in an analysis of five multicentre, open-label studies, which followed 1006 patients with hypertension (seated DBP 95–110 mmHg) for up to 2 years.[30] Patients received irbesartan monotherapy at an initial dose of 75 mg, titrated to 300 mg at 2–4-week intervals to achieve normalised blood pressure (seated DBP <90 mmHg). If normalised blood pressure was not achieved with irbesartan alone, adjunctive medications were added.

After 12 months' therapy, the mean reduction in seated SBP/DBP was 21.0/15.8 mmHg, a reduction that was sustained until the end of the follow-up period; however, the blood pressure reductions observed at 18 and 24 months were slightly lower (19/15 and 17/15 mmHg, respectively) than those achieved at 12 months. Normalisation and total-responder rates (normalised or ≥10 mmHg reduction in seated DBP) after 12 months' therapy were 83 and 90%, respectively, and remained at this level for the next 12 months (Figure 4). Similarly, the percentage of patients who achieved target blood pressure (<140/90 mmHg) remained stable from 6 months' therapy (66%) until the end of follow up. The findings of this study thus demonstrate that normalised blood pressure can be achieved and maintained by long-term therapy with irbesartan.[30]

## Patient compliance

Patient compliance with drug therapy is a critical issue in medicine, and is an essential factor in effective blood pressure control. Agents that are well tolerated and have favourable efficacy may provide more effective control of blood pressure by encouraging greater patient compliance. A retrospective study analysed the medical records of 2416 newly diagnosed hypertensive patients from Germany, France and the UK, in order to compare the rates of persistence (defined as the proportion of

A greater percentage of patients receiving irbesartan/HCTZ achieved blood pressure normalisation compared with the placebo/HCTZ regimen.

Normalised blood pressure can be achieved and maintained by long-term therapy with irbesartan.

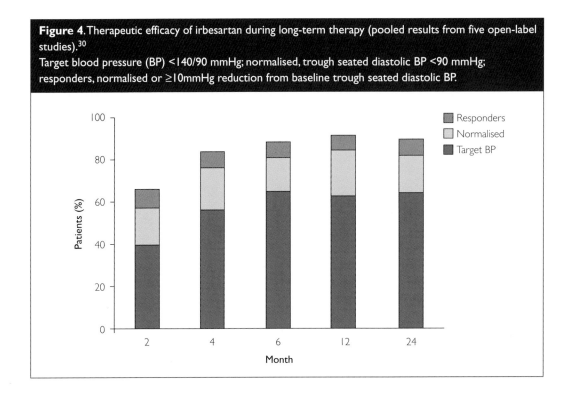

**Figure 4.** Therapeutic efficacy of irbesartan during long-term therapy (pooled results from five open-label studies).[30]
Target blood pressure (BP) <140/90 mmHg; normalised, trough seated diastolic BP <90 mmHg; responders, normalised or ≥10mmHg reduction from baseline trough seated diastolic BP.

Patients taking irbesartan showed significantly higher rates of persistence than those taking other <u>angiotensin II receptor antagonists</u>.

patients remaining on their initial therapy at 1 year) with irbesartan and other major classes of antihypertensives.[35] Wide variation in compliance was observed. Patients taking irbesartan showed significantly higher rates of persistence than those taking other <u>angiotensin II receptor antagonists</u> (60.8 *vs* 51.3%, *p*=0.009). Furthermore, patients taking irbesartan were more compliant with therapy than those taking one of the other drug classes. Comparable rates of persistence were observed for ACE inhibitors, <u>calcium-channel blockers</u> and β-<u>blockers</u> (42.0–49.7%; *p*<0.001 *vs* irbesartan). <u>Diuretic</u>-based treatment was associated with the lowest rate of persistence, with only 34.4% remaining on treatment at 1 year. This study also demonstrated that patients taking irbesartan were less likely to switch or require adjunctive therapy than those taking other classes of antihypertensive agents.

## Clinical efficacy in heart failure

Although ACE inhibitors are effective therapy for patients with heart failure, <u>morbidity</u> and <u>mortality</u> remain high, possibly because these agents do not produce a complete blockade of the actions of <u>angiotensin II</u>. Consequently, studies have investigated the potential role of angiotensin II receptor antagonists in this population.[a]

---

[a]Irbesartan is not licensed for this indication in the UK.

Preliminary data suggest that addition of irbesartan to conventional therapy may be beneficial in patients with heart failure.[36] In a 12-week pilot study involving 109 patients with heart failure (New York Heart Association [NYHA] functional class II and III), addition of irbesartan, 12.5–150 mg/day, to standard therapy (including ACE inhibitors) improved left ventricular ejection fraction (LVEF) and exercise tolerance time to a greater extent than placebo; the unadjusted change from baseline LVEF was 5.2 units in the irbesartan group and 2.4 units in the placebo group.[37]

In a second, larger 12-week study, the effects of irbesartan were evaluated in patients with heart failure in whom ACE inhibitors had been withdrawn.[38] Patients (n=218) with symptomatic heart failure (NYHA class II–IV) and LVEF of 40% or less who were receiving standard heart-failure medication (excluding ACE inhibitors) were randomised to receive irbesartan doses of 12.5–150 mg. The proportion of patients who died, were hospitalised for worsening heart failure or discontinued treatment because of worsening heart failure was significantly lower amongst patients treated with irbesartan, 75 or 150 mg/day, than those receiving irbesartan,12.5 or 37.5 mg/day (p=0.04).[38] Although further studies are clearly required to evaluate the effect of irbesartan in heart failure fully, these data suggest that the drug may be a promising new therapy for this condition.

> Although further studies are required to evaluate the effect of irbesartan in heart failure fully, these data suggest that the drug may be a promising new therapy for this condition.

## Clinical efficacy in patients with diabetic nephropathy

Results from several recent trials suggest that angiotensin II receptor antagonists are effective in protecting against the progression of nephropathy resulting from type 2 diabetes. The effects of irbesartan in this population have been investigated in one large and one smaller placebo-controlled trial.[39,40] In the larger study (the Irbesartan Microalbuminuria [IRMA II] trial), 590 patients with type 2 diabetes, hypertension (>135/85 mmHg) and persistent microalbuminuria (an early marker of diabetic nephropathy) were randomised to irbesartan, 150 or 300 mg/day, or placebo and were followed up for 2 years.[38] At the end of the follow-up period, the primary endpoint (time to onset of nephropathy) was reached in 5.2% of patients in the irbesartan, 300 mg, group and 9.7% of patients in the irbesartan, 150 mg, group, compared with 14.9% in the placebo group (p<0.001 and p=0.08 vs placebo, respectively). The reduction in blood pressure was also greater in the irbesartan, 150 and 300 mg, groups compared with placebo (143/83 mmHg and 141/83 mmHg vs 144/83 mmHg; p=0.004 for the comparison of SBP between the combined irbesartan groups and placebo).[39] However, a substudy of the IRMA II trial revealed no significant differences in blood pressure between the different treatment groups when patients (n=43) were evaluated using 24-hour ambulatory blood pressure monitoring.[41] Despite the similarity in blood-pressure responses, irbesartan (particularly at the higher dose) was associated with significantly lower albumin excretion rates. When a subgroup of patients in the IRMA II study had their antihypertensive treatments withdrawn after 2 years, the albumin excretion rate remained significantly reduced in patients previously exposed to irbesartan, 300 mg/day, suggesting that high-dose irbesartan treatment may confer long-term renoprotective effects.[42]

In the smaller placebo-controlled trial, patients with microalbuminuria – 64 with newly diagnosed hypertension (DBP 90–110 mmHg; SBP 140–180 mmHg) and 60 who were normotensive (<140/90 mmHg) – were randomised to twice-daily irbesartan, 150 mg, or placebo for 60 days. At the end of treatment, irbesartan had reduced microalbuminuria (assessed by the albumin excretion rate) in both hypertensive and normotensive diabetics compared with placebo ($p<0.01$). Irbesartan treatment also significantly reduced blood pressure in the hypertensive patients ($p<0.001$).[40]

The renoprotective effects of irbesartan have also been compared with those of the calcium-channel blocker, amlodipine, in the IDNT study.[27] In this study, 1715 patients with hypertension (>135/85 mmHg) and diabetic nephropathy (urine protein excretion >900 mg/24 hours) were randomised to irbesartan, 300 mg/day, amlodipine, 10 mg/day, or placebo. Treatment with irbesartan was associated with a 23% lower risk of the primary composite endpoint (doubling of the baseline serum creatinine concentration, development of end-stage renal disease, or death from any cause) than amlodipine ($p=0.006$), and a 20% lower risk than placebo ($p=0.02$).[27]

A separate analysis of data from the IDNT reported on the cardiovascular outcomes of patients enrolled into the study and revealed no differences in the composite cardiovascular endpoint between patients given irbesartan or amlodipine treatment.[43] However, irbesartan treatment was associated with a significantly lower incidence of heart failure compared with either placebo ($p=0.048$) or amlodipine treatment ($p=0.004$). In contrast, amlodipine (but not irbesartan) was associated with a significant reduction in the risk of myocardial infarction compared with placebo ($p=0.02$).[27]

The renoprotective effects of irbesartan in both the IRMA II and IDNT trials were independent of its blood pressure-lowering effects.[27,39]

> The renoprotective effects of irbesartan in both the IRMA II and IDNT trials were independent of its blood pressure-lowering effects.

## General practice studies

A large, open-label, observational study conducted in German clinical practice has prospectively evaluated the effects of irbesartan treatment (given as either monotherapy or in a fixed combination with hydrochlorothiazide) upon blood pressure, metabolic parameters and microalbuminuria in a total of 16,600 patients with hypertension and type 2 diabetes.[44] Mean reductions in SBP and DBP were 22.3 and 11.2 mmHg, respectively, and this blood pressure-lowering efficacy was maintained across various subgroups of the patient population (i.e. whether stratified by age, gender or the presence of micro/macrovascular complications). In addition, a relative risk reduction in the incidence of microalbuminuria of 32.9% was reported. Moreover, the mean 10-year estimated cardiovascular risk of the population decreased from 9.8% at baseline to 5.7% at the end of the study (a relative risk reduction of

58%). Irbesartan treatment also provided significant improvements in the majority of metabolic parameters (e.g. lipids, blood glucose and glycated haemoglobin). This analysis revealed that irbesartan was also very well tolerated, with only 0.3% of patients experiencing an adverse event.

## Safety

Irbesartan is generally well tolerated and has a safety and tolerability profile similar to placebo. The safety and tolerability of irbesartan in the treatment of mild-to-moderate hypertension has been evaluated in a pooled study of nine randomised, double-blind, placebo-controlled trials.[45] After a 4–5-week placebo lead-in phase, hypertensive patients (seated DBP 95–110 mmHg) were randomised to 4–12 weeks' treatment with either placebo (n=641) or irbesartan (n=1965), 1–900 mg/day.

Across the recommended clinical dose range, irbesartan was associated with a lower incidence of adverse events, serious adverse events and discontinuations because of adverse events than placebo, though these differences were not significant (Table 3). Overall, adverse events were reported by 56% of patients in both the irbesartan and placebo groups. The most commonly reported adverse events for irbesartan and placebo were headache (12.3 vs 16.6%), upper respiratory tract infection (8.5 vs 6.2%), musculoskeletal pain (6.6% in both groups) and dizziness (4.9 vs 5.0%). No relationship was noted between dose and adverse events or withdrawal rates. Furthermore, withdrawal of irbesartan was not associated with rebound hypertension or clinically important adverse events.[45] A further pooled study of seven randomised, double-blind, placebo-controlled trials of 2673 patients with mild-to-moderate hypertension (seated DBP 95–110 mmHg) has shown that irbesartan use was associated with a significant reduction in the incidence of headache compared with placebo ($p=0.003$).[46]

A postmarketing surveillance study of the safety of irbesartan has been conducted by primary-care physicians in Spain and has confirmed the good safety profile observed in controlled clinical trials.[47] A total of 4887 patients were enrolled into the study and were treated with irbesartan for 6 months (patients initially received 150 mg/day titrated

**Table 3.** Safety and tolerability of different doses of irbesartan in placebo-controlled trials.[45]

|  | Irbesartan[a] (n=1965) | Placebo (n=641) |
|---|---|---|
| Adverse events | 56.2 | 56.5 |
| Adverse drug experiences | 21.3 | 20.0 |
| Discontinuations because of adverse events | 3.3 | 4.5 |
| Serious adverse events | 1.0 | 1.9 |

[a]Includes irbesartan <75 mg to 900 mg treatment groups.

upward in 300 mg increments according to response). Adverse events were experienced by 2.2% of the study population over the course of the study, with only 0.1% of these patients experiencing more than one adverse event. Headache was the most commonly reported side-effect of treatment, which is consistent with the clinical trial programme of irbesartan.

A pooled analysis of five open-label studies found that irbesartan is well tolerated over long-term therapy of up to 2 years' duration.[30] Of the 1066 patients included in the study, only 0.6% discontinued because of treatment failure. The most common adverse events experienced by patients receiving long-term irbesartan therapy are shown in Table 4.[30]

The good tolerability profile of irbesartan in placebo-controlled trials has been confirmed in comparative trials. In comparative studies with atenolol, atenolol was associated with more adverse events and more withdrawals because of adverse events than irbesartan (3.3 *vs* 1.8% and 9.1 *vs* 4.5%, respectively).[21] Irbesartan treatment also resulted in significantly less cough than enalapril (2.5 *vs* 13.1%; *p*=0.007).[17] The low incidence of cough with irbesartan represents an important improvement in antihypertensive tolerability, since this side-effect is a major cause of discontinuation with ACE inhibitor therapy.[18] The tolerability of irbesartan appears to be comparable to that of other angiotensin II-receptor antagonists.[12–14]

## Drug interactions

Irbesartan has a low potential for interaction with co-prescribed drugs; no significant interactions have been identified between irbesartan and

**Table 4.** The most common adverse events experienced by patients receiving long-term (up to 2 years) irbesartan and irbesartan/hydrochlorothiazide (HCTZ) combination therapy.[30]

|  | Per cent of patients | | | |
|---|---|---|---|---|
|  | Irbesartan[a] (n=1006) | Irbesartan monotherapy (n=1006) | Irbesartan/ HCTZ (n=595) | Irbesartan/HCTZ± adjunctive therapy (n=288) |
| Musculoskeletal pain | 14.8 | 10.0 | 10.5 | 12.7 |
| Upper respiratory tract infection | 14.8 | 11.0 | 8.5 | 10.2 |
| Dizziness | 8.2 | 4.6 | 6.7 | 9.1 |
| Headache | 7.5 | 5.9 | 2.9 | 3.6 |
| Cough | 6.6 | 4.7 | 3.5 | 5.0 |
| Fatigue | 5.9 | 3.8 | 3.8 | 5.0 |
| Influenza | 5.5 | 4.1 | 3.2 | 3.6 |
| Pharyngitis | 5.5 | 4.3 | <2.0 | 2.2 |
| Sinus abnormality | 5.4 | 3.7 | 4.1 | 4.7 |
| Tracheobronchitis | 5.3 | 3.5 | 4.1 | 4.1 |
| Rash | 3.8 | <2.0 | 3.5 | 5.0 |

[a]Includes irbesartan 75–300 mg treatment groups.

HCTZ, nifedipine, simvastatin, tolbutamide, warfarin or digoxin.[48] However, irbesartan, 150 mg, has been reported to increase the steady-state peak plasma concentration of fluconazole by 19% and the AUC by 63%, though these increases are not thought to be clinically significant.[48]

## Pharmacoeconomics

A number of economic assessments of irbesartan treatment have been conducted from the perspective of a number of different countries and different healthcare systems. The vast majority of these data relate specifically to the economic consequences of irbesartan treatment for diabetic nephropathy rather than being actual assessments of its cost-effectiveness in the management of hypertension.

Given the substantial healthcare costs associated with the management of kidney disease and the nephroprotective role demonstrated for irbesartan in diabetic patients with hypertension, treatment with irbesartan has the potential to provide considerable cost savings in this patient population. Using data from the IDNT study, an economic analysis using a Markov model (previously used to determine the long-term clinical costs and cost outcomes in Belgium, Germany, France and the US),[28] determined the relative cost-effectiveness of irbesartan, amlodipine and control regimens from a UK perspective.[49] Mean costs and changes in life expectancy as a result of delay in end-stage renal disease over a 10-year period were determined, and revealed cost savings per patient of £5125 compared with amlodipine and £2919 compared with control. The associated reduction in progression to end stage renal disease led to improvements in projected discounted life expectancy of 0.07 and 0.21 years compared with amlodipine and control, respectively. Sensitivity analyses revealed that these results were robust when analysed under a wider range of assumptions concerning long-term treatment effectiveness and costs of complications and medications, and thus indicate that the conclusions of this study are applicable in a real-life scenario. These data are also consistent with pharmacoeconomic analyses performed in other countries.[28]

A further analysis (from a third-party payer perspective in the US) determined the relative benefits of early compared with late intervention with irbesartan in hypertensive patients with type 2 diabetes and microalbuminuria.[50] Again, data from the IDNT study were used to determine transition probabilities between the different health states within the Markov model. Early and late irbesartan treatment given to 1000 patients was projected to save US$11.9 million and US$3.3 million compared with the control arm. Early intervention with irbesartan in 1000 patients was projected to add 960 discounted life-years compared with 71 life years with late intervention. Again, the benefits of early intervention were maintained across a wide range of assumptions. Thus, this analysis supports earlier intervention with irbesartan to manage overt nephropathy in this patient population.

## Key points

● Irbesartan is a highly selective and potent <u>angiotensin II receptor antagonist</u>, which exerts its effects via its interaction with the type I angiotensin II ($AT_I$) receptor.

● Irbesartan produces greater functional antagonism of angiotensin II than the other agents in this class of drugs.

● The blood pressure-lowering <u>efficacy</u> of irbesartan appears to be superior to that of the angiotensin II receptor antagonists, losartan and valsartan.

● Irbesartan has similar antihypertensive efficacy to the ACE inhibitor, enalapril, the <u>β-blocker</u>, atenolol, and the <u>calcium-channel blocker</u>, amlodipine, but is better tolerated.

● Irbesartan reduces LV mass in hypertensive patients with LVH by a greater extent than atenolol and amlodipine.

● Irbesartan has beneficial cardioprotective effects, with preliminary studies indicating that it may be a promising new treatment for heart failure.

● Large-scale clinical trials have demonstrated that irbesartan has a renoprotective function in hypertensive patients with <u>diabetic nephropathy</u>. The use of irbesartan in this indication appears to be cost saving compared with amlodipine or standard antihypertensive treatment.

● Irbesartan has an excellent safety profile, and is well tolerated.

# References

A list of the published evidence which has been reviewed in compiling the preceding section of *BESTMEDICINE*.

1  Rodgers JE, Patterson JH. Angiotensin II-receptor blockers: clinical relevance and therapeutic role. *Am J Health Syst Pharm* 2001; **58**: 671–83.

2  Adams MA, Trudeau L. Irbesartan: review of pharmacology and comparative properties. *Can J Clin Pharmacol* 2000; **7**: 22–31.

3  Cleland JGF, Morgan K. Inhibition of the renin-angiotensin-aldosterone system in heart failure: new insights from basic clinical research. *Curr Opin Cardiol* 1996; **11**: 252–62.

4  Benz J, Oshrain C, Henry D *et al.* Valsartan, a new angiotensin II receptor antagonist: a double-blind study comparing the incidence of cough with lisinopril and hydrochlorothiazide. *J Clin Pharmacol* 1997; **37**: 101–7.

5  Coca A, Calvo C, Garcia-Puig J *et al.* A multicenter, randomized, double-blind comparison of the efficacy and safety of irbesartan and enalapril in adults with mild to moderate essential hypertension, as assessed by ambulatory blood pressure monitoring: the MAPAVEL Study (Monitorizacion Ambulatoria Presion Arterial APROVEL). *Clin Ther* 2002; **24**: 126–38.

6  Howerda NJ, Fogari R, Angeli P *et al.* Valsartan, a new angiotensin II antagonist for the treatment of essential hypertension: efficacy and safety compared with placebo and enalapril. *J Hypertens* 1996; **14**: 1147–51.

7  Belz GG, Butzer R, Kober S, Mang C, Mutschler E. Time course and extent of angiotensin II antagonism after irbesartan, losartan, and valsartan in humans assessed by angiotensin II dose response and radioligand receptor assay. *Clin Pharmacol Ther* 1999; **66**: 367–73.

8  Belz GG. Pharmacological differences among angiotensin II receptor antagonists. *Blood Press Suppl* 2001; **2**: 13–18.

9  Mazzolai L, Maillard M, Rossat J *et al.* Angiotensin II receptor blockade in normotensive subjects: A direct comparison of three $AT_1$ receptor antagonists. *Hypertension* 1999; **33**: 850–5.

10 Reeves RA, Lin CS, Kassler-Taub K, Pouleur H. Dose-related efficacy of irbesartan for hypertension: an integrated analysis. *Hypertension* 1998; **31**: 1311–16.

11 Guthrie R, Saini R, Herman T *et al.* Efficacy and tolerability of irbesartan, an angiotensin II receptor antagonist, in primary hypertension. *Clin Drug Invest* 1999; **15**: 217–27.

12 Kassler-Taub K, Littlejohn T, Elliott W, Ruddy T, Adler E. Comparative efficacy of two angiotensin II receptor antagonists, irbesartan and losartan in mild-to-moderate hypertension. Irbesartan/Losartan Study Investigators. *Am J Hypertens* 1998; **11(4 Pt 1)**: 445–53.

13 Oparil S, Guthrie R, Lewin AJ *et al.* An elective-titration study of the comparative effectiveness of two angiotensin II-receptor blockers, irbesartan and losartan. Irbesartan/Losartan Study Investigators. *Clin Ther* 1998; **20**: 398–409.

14 Mancia G, Korlipara K, van Rossum P, Villa G, Silvert B. An ambulatory blood pressure monitoring study of the comparative antihypertensive efficacy of two angiotensin II receptor antagonists, irbesartan and valsartan. *Blood Press Monit* 2002; **7**: 135–42.

15 Fogari R, Mugellini A, Zoppi A *et al.* A double-blind, crossover study of the antihypertensive efficacy of angiotensin II-receptor antagonists and their activation of the renin-angiotensin system. *Curr Ther Res Clin Exp* 2000; **61**: 669–79.

16 Mimran A, Ruilope L, Kerwin L *et al.* A randomised, double-blind comparison of the angiotensin II receptor antagonist, irbesartan, with the full dose range of enalapril for the treatment of mild-to-moderate hypertension. *J Hum Hypertens* 1998; **12**: 203–8.

17 Larochelle P, Flack JM, Marbury TC *et al.* Effects and tolerability of irbesartan versus enalapril in patients with severe hypertension. Irbesartan Multicenter Investigators. *Am J Cardiol* 1997; **80**: 1613–15.

18 *British National Formulary (BNF) 48.* London: The British Medical Association and the Royal Pharmaceutical Association of Great Britain. September, 2004.

19 Lacourciere Y. A multicenter, randomized, double-blind study of the antihypertensive efficacy and tolerability of irbesartan in patients aged ≥ 65 years with mild to moderate hypertension. *Clin Ther* 2000; **22**: 1213–24.

20 Schieffer B, Bunte C, Witte J *et al.* Comparative effects of AT1-antagonism and angiotensin-converting enzyme inhibition on markers of inflammation and platelet aggregation in patients with coronary artery disease. *J Am Coll Cardiol* 2004; **44**: 362–8.

21 Stumpe KO, Haworth D, Hoglund C *et al.* Comparison of the angiotensin II receptor antagonist irbesartan with atenolol for treatment of hypertension. *Blood Press* 1998; **7**: 31–7.

22 Makris TK, Stavroulakis GA, Krespi PG *et al.* Fibrinolytic/hemostatic variables in arterial hypertension: response to treatment with irbesartan or atenolol. *Am J Hypertens* 2000; **13**: 783–8.

23 Malmqvist K, Kahan T, Edner M *et al.* Regression of left ventricular hypertrophy in human hypertension with irbesartan. *J Hypertens* 2001; **19**: 1167–76.

24 Malmqvist K, Kahan T, Edner M, Bergfeldt L. Comparison of actions of irbesartan versus atenolol on cardiac repolarization in hypertensive left ventricular hypertrophy: results from the Swedish Irbesartan Left Ventricular Hypertrophy Investigation Versus Atenolol (SILVHIA). *Am J Cardiol* 2002; **90**: 1107–12.

25 Schneider MP, Klingbeil AU, Delles C *et al.* Effect of irbesartan versus atenolol on left ventricular mass and voltage: results of the CardioVascular Irbesartan Project. *Hypertension* 2004; **44**: 61–6.

26 Schiffrin EL, Park JB, Pu Q. Effect of crossing over hypertensive patients from a beta-blocker to an angiotensin receptor antagonist on resistance artery structure and on endothelial function. *J Hypertens* 2002; **20**: 71–8.

27 Lewis EJ, Hunsicker LG, Clarke WR *et al.* Renoprotective effect of the angiotensin-receptor antagonist irbesartan in patients with nephropathy due to type 2 diabetes. *N Engl J Med* 2001; **345**: 851–60.

28 Croom KF, Curran MP, Goa KL, Perry CM. Irbesartan: a review of its use in hypertension and in the management of diabetic nephropathy. *Drugs* 2004; **64**: 999–1028.

29 Gaudio C, Ferri FM, Giovannini M *et al.* Comparative effects of irbesartan versus amlodipine on left ventricular mass index in hypertensive patients with left ventricular hypertrophy. *J Cardiovasc Pharmacol* 2003; **42**: 622–8.

30 Littlejohn T, Saini R, Kassler-Taub K, Chrysant SG, Marbury T. Long-term safety and antihypertensive efficacy of irbesartan: pooled results of five open-label studies. *Clin Exp Hypertens* 1999; **21**: 1273–95.

31 Williams B, Poulter NR, Brown MJ *et al.* Guidelines for management of hypertension: report of the fourth working party of the British Hypertension Society, 2004-BHS IV. *J Hum Hypertens* 2004; **18**: 139–85.

32 Pool JL, Guthrie RM, Littlejohn TW *et al.* Dose-related antihypertensive effects of irbesartan in patients with mild-to-moderate hypertension. *Am J Hypertens* 1998; **11(4 Pt 1)**: 462–70.

33 Rosenstock J, Rossi L, Lin CS, MacNeil D, Osbakken M. The effects of irbesartan added to hydrochlorothiazide for the treatment of hypertension in patients non-responsive to hydrochlorothiazide alone. *J Clin Pharm Ther* 1998; **23**: 433–40.

34 Coca A, Calvo C, Sobrino J *et al.* Once-daily fixed-combination irbesartan 300 mg/hydrochlorothiazide 25 mg and circadian blood pressure profile in patients with essential hypertension. *Clin Ther* 2003; **25**: 2849–64.

35 Hasford J, Mimran A, Simons WR. A population-based European cohort study of persistence in newly diagnosed hypertensive patients. *J Hum Hypertens* 2002; **16**: 569–75.

36 Havranek EP. The effects of the angiotensin II receptor antagonist irbesartan in patients with congestive heart failure. *Cardiovasc Rev Rep* 1998; **19**: 29–33.

37 Tonkon M, Awan N, Niazi I *et al.* A study of the efficacy and safety of irbesartan in combination with conventional therapy, including ACE inhibitors, in heart failure. Irbesartan Heart Failure Group. *Int J Clin Pract* 2000; **54**: 11–14, 16–18.

38 Havranek EP, Thomas I, Smith WB *et al.* Dose-related beneficial long-term hemodynamic and clinical efficacy of irbesartan in heart failure. *J Am Coll Cardiol* 1999; **33**: 1174–81.

39 Parving HH, Lehnert H, Brochner-Mortensen J *et al.* Irbesartan in Patients with Type 2 Diabetes and Microalbuminuria Study Group. The effect of irbesartan on the development of diabetic nephropathy in patients with type 2 diabetes. *N Engl J Med* 2001; **345**: 870–8.

40 Sasso FC, Carbonara O, Persico M *et al.* Irbesartan reduces the albumin excretion rate in microalbuminuric type 2 diabetic patients independently of hypertension: a randomized double-blind placebo-controlled crossover study. *Diabetes Care* 2002; **25**: 1909–13.

41 Rossing K, Christensen PK, Andersen S *et al.* Comparative effects of Irbesartan on ambulatory and office blood pressure: a substudy of ambulatory blood pressure from the Irbesartan in Patients with Type 2 Diabetes and Microalbuminuria study. *Diabetes Care* 2003; **26**: 569–74.

42 Andersen S, Brochner-Mortensen J, Parving HH. Kidney function during and after withdrawal of long-term irbesartan treatment in patients with type 2 diabetes and microalbuminuria. *Diabetes Care* 2003; **26**: 3296–302.

43 Berl T, Hunsicker LG, Lewis JB *et al.* Cardiovascular outcomes in the Irbesartan Diabetic Nephropathy Trial of patients with type 2 diabetes and overt nephropathy. *Ann Intern Med* 2003; **138**: 542–9.

44 Bramlage P, Pittrow D, Kirch W. The effect of irbesartan in reducing cardiovascular risk in hypertensive type 2 diabetic patients: an observational study in 16,600 patients in primary care. *Curr Med Res Opin* 2004; **20**: 1625–31.

45 Simon TA, Gelarden RT, Freitag SA, Kassler-Taub KB, Davies R. Safety of irbesartan in the treatment of mild to moderate systemic hypertension. *Am J Cardiol* 1998; **82**: 179–82.

46 Hansson L, Smith DH, Reeves R, Lapuerta P. Headache in mild-to-moderate hypertension and its reduction by irbesartan therapy. *Arch Intern Med* 2000; **160**: 1654–8.

47 Morales-Olivas FJ, Aristegui I, Estan L *et al.* The KARTAN study: a postmarketing assessment of Irbesartan in patients with hypertension. *Clin Ther* 2004; **26**: 232–44.

48 Marino MR, Vachharajani NN. Drug interactions with irbesartan. *Clin Pharmacokinet* 2001; **40**: 605–14.

49 Palmer AJ, Annemans L, Roze S *et al.* An economic evaluation of the Irbesartan in Diabetic Nephropathy Trial (IDNT) in a UK setting. *J Hum Hypertens* 2004; **18**: 733–8.

50 Palmer AJ, Annemans L, Roze S *et al.* Cost-effectiveness of early irbesartan treatment versus control (standard antihypertensive medications excluding ACE inhibitors, other angiotensin-2 receptor antagonists, and dihydropyridine calcium channel blockers) or late irbesartan treatment in patients with type 2 diabetes, hypertension, and renal disease. *Diabetes Care* 2004; **27**: 1897–903.

# Acknowledgements

Figure 1 is adapted from Reeves *et al.*, 1998.[10]
Figure 4 is adapted from Littlejohn *et al.*, 1999.[30]

# 7. Drug review – Losartan (Cozaar®)

*Dr Richard Clark and Dr Sue Chambers*
*CSF Medical Communications Ltd*

## Summary

Losartan is an <u>angiotensin II receptor antagonist</u> that blocks the effects of angiotensin II at its type I (AT<sub>1</sub>) receptors. Clinical studies have shown that it is an effective antihypertensive agent, with comparable <u>efficacy</u> to <u>angiotensin-converting enzyme (ACE) inhibitors</u>, <u>calcium-channel blockers</u> and the <u>β-blocker</u> atenolol. A combination of losartan and the <u>thiazide</u> <u>diuretic</u> hydrochlorothiazide (HCTZ) reduces blood pressure to a greater extent than either drug alone. Thus, combination therapy can be considered for patients whose blood pressure is not adequately controlled with losartan <u>monotherapy</u>. In addition to its antihypertensive effects, losartan reduces <u>cardiovascular</u> <u>morbidity</u> and <u>mortality</u>, and the risk of stroke, in hypertensive patients with <u>left ventricular hypertrophy (LVH)</u>, and provides renoprotective effects in hypertensive patients with <u>nephropathy</u>. Losartan has proved to be well tolerated, and this has been attributed to its specificity and selectivity for AT<sub>1</sub> receptors. In particular, losartan produces a lower incidence of cough than ACE inhibitors.

## Introduction

Angiotensin II is a major component of the <u>renin–angiotensin system</u>. It plays an important role in <u>cardiovascular</u> <u>homeostasis</u> and, being a potent vasoconstrictor, is a major determinant of blood pressure. Drugs that block the renin–angiotensin system and the effects of angiotensin II have become well-accepted treatments for hypertension. Such drugs include ACE inhibitors and <u>angiotensin II receptor antagonists</u>. ACE inhibitors are effective antihypertensive agents, but the <u>enzyme</u> they inhibit is not very specific, and its inhibition leads to the accumulation of <u>bradykinin</u>. This inflammatory mediator may be responsible for some of the side-effects associated with the use of ACE inhibitors, such as cough.

Angiotensin II receptor antagonists are more specific than ACE inhibitors: they block the effects of angiotensin II generated by any pathway by competitively binding to $AT_1$ receptors. This specificity for $AT_1$ receptors translates into a more favourable side-effect profile.

In addition to its vasoconstrictor effects, angiotensin II mediates vascular hypertrophy and the development of atherosclerosis by stimulating the growth of vascular smooth muscle cells. It is also involved in the development of LVH, which is a major risk factor for cardiovascular morbidity and mortality, and plays a role in the progression of renal disease. Antihypertensive therapies that block the effects of angiotensin II have been shown to induce regression of LVH and to improve renal haemodynamics in patients with renal disease.[1–3]

> Losartan was the first oral angiotensin II receptor antagonist to be introduced into clinical practice.

Losartan was the first oral angiotensin II receptor antagonist to be introduced into clinical practice. It is a non-peptide drug that binds to $AT_1$ receptors, thus blocking the action of angiotensin II. Losartan is indicated in the UK for the treatment of hypertension, and also for reducing the risk of stroke in hypertensive patients with LVH and for providing renal protection in type 2 diabetic patients with nephropathy.

This section focuses on the clinical efficacy and safety of losartan and discusses the evidence that has accumulated for the drug in the context of data obtained from studies with other angiotensin II receptor antagonists and other antihypertensive agents, including ACE inhibitors, calcium-channel blockers and the β-blocker atenolol.

## Clinical efficacy in hypertension

### Dose-finding study

> ☞ Dose-ranging studies are particularly important to ensure that the optimum dose of a drug can be determined in order that benefit can be realised with the least risk of side-effects.

In a randomised, double-blind study of 576 patients with mild-to-moderate hypertension, patients received once-daily treatment with losartan at doses of 10, 25, 50, 100 or 150 mg, or enalapril, 20 mg, or placebo, for 8 weeks.[4] Losartan doses of 50–150 mg led to a reduction in blood pressure 24 hours after dosing compared with placebo ($p \leq 0.01$). The changes in blood pressure observed with the 50 mg dose were identical to those seen with 20 mg enalapril (maintenance dose), whilst losartan doses of 10 and 25 mg were not significantly different from placebo. The results of this study confirmed that once-daily dosing with losartan was effective, that the maximum reduction in blood pressure was achieved after 3–6 weeks of treatment and was maintained during the remainder of the 8-week treatment period. Based on the results of these trials the 50 mg dose was chosen as an appropriate starting dose.

### Open-label and placebo-controlled studies

Open-label and placebo-controlled studies have shown that losartan, 50 mg once daily, is an effective antihypertensive agent (Table 1).[5–14] The dose of losartan can be titrated to 100 mg/day for patients whose blood pressure is not adequately controlled with the lower dose.[5,6] In a study of patients with severe hypertension in which initial treatment with losartan alone was combined with HCTZ, a calcium antagonist and/or atenolol as necessary, losartan alone was found to be effective in 22% of patients and to be effective in a further 76% when concurrently

**Table 1.** Placebo-controlled or open-label trials investigating the antihypertensive efficacy of losartan.[5-14]

| Study | Study design | Study population | Dose regimen | Results | Conclusions |
|---|---|---|---|---|---|
| Weber et al., 1995[5] | Randomised, double-blind, placebo-controlled, dose comparison | Patients (n=122) with hypertension | Losartan, 50 or 100 mg o.d., or 50 mg b.d., for 4 weeks | All three doses of losartan were more effective than placebo in reducing blood pressure. The average 24-hour decreases were 9.2/6.9, 9.9/6.4 and 13.2/8.5 mmHg for 50 mg o.d., 100 mg o.d. and 50 mg b.d., respectively ($p < 0.01$ for all three doses vs placebo) | Losartan is an effective antihypertensive agent whether administered o.d. or b.d., and its effect is sustained over 24 hours |
| Dunlay et al., 1995[6] | Open-label, consecutive antihypertensive treatment | Patients (n=179) with severe hypertension | Initial therapy with losartan, 50 or 100 mg o.d., followed by the addition of HCTZ, a calcium-channel blocker, and/or atenolol as necessary, for 12 weeks | After 2 weeks, losartan significantly reduced diastolic blood pressure by a mean of 7.3 mmHg compared with baseline ($p < 0.001$), 24% of patients who achieved target blood pressure were on losartan monotherapy | Losartan is an effective initial therapy for patients with severe hypertension, and can be administered concurrently with HCTZ, calcium-channel blockers and atenolol |
| Byyny, 1996[7] | Randomised, double-blind, parallel-group, placebo-controlled | Patients (n=122) with mild-to-moderate hypertension | Losartan, 50 or 100 mg o.d., or 50 mg b.d., for 4 weeks. HCTZ, 12.5 mg, was added if necessary for a further 2 weeks | All doses of losartan reduced 24-hour diastolic and systolic blood pressure compared with placebo ($p < 0.01$). Response rates were 41, 54, 47 and 10% for losartan, 50 and 100 mg o.d., 50 mg b.d., and placebo, respectively | Losartan given once daily provides effective 24-hour control of blood pressure in hypertensive patients |
| Himmelmann et al., 1996[8] | Open-label treatment | Patients (n=19) with mild-to-moderate hypertension | Losartan, 50 mg o.d., for an average of 29 months. HCTZ, 6.5 or 12.5 mg o.d., was added to the treatment regimen after 4 weeks if necessary | Blood pressure decreased from 155.6/103.4 mmHg to 131.3/82.7 mmHg ($p < 0.001$) | Losartan is effective in reducing blood pressure during long-term treatment |

b.d., twice daily; HCTZ, hydrochlorothiazide; o.d., once daily.

**Table I.** Continued

| Study | Study design | Study population | Dose regimen | Results | Conclusions |
|---|---|---|---|---|---|
| Ikeda et al., 1997[9] | Randomised, double-blind, parallel-group, placebo-controlled | Patients (n=366) with mild-to-moderate hypertension | Losartan, 50 mg o.d., or losartan, 50 mg titrated to 100 mg o.d., after the first 6 weeks, or placebo, for 12 weeks | Active treatment significantly reduced trough and peak systolic and diastolic blood pressure at 6 weeks compared with placebo (p<0.01). At week 12, there was a slight additional fall in blood pressure with active treatment (p<0.01 vs placebo) but the difference between the two active treatment groups was not significant | Losartan, 50 or 100 mg o.d., was effective in reducing blood pressure in patients with mild-to-moderate hypertension. The 100 mg was no more effective than the 50 mg dose |
| Del Castillo et al., 1998[10] | Prospective, open-label | Hypertensive (n=76) renal transplant recipients | Losartan, 50 mg o.d., for 12 weeks. HCTZ, 25 mg, or furosemide, 40 mg, were added if necessary | After 12 weeks, losartan had significantly reduced mean arterial blood pressure from 113 to 102 mmHg (p<0.0001) | Losartan is effective in reducing blood pressure in hypertensive renal transplant recipients |
| Toto et al., 1998[11] | Open-label | Hypertensive patients (n=112) with chronic renal insufficiency | Losartan, 50 mg o.d. for 12 weeks. The dose was increased to 100 mg o.d. after 4 weeks if necessary, and a second antihypertensive drug was added after 8 weeks if required | At 12 weeks, the reduction in systolic/diastolic blood pressure averaged 14.7/12.1 mmHg in patients with mild renal insufficiency and 14.1/10.6 mmHg in those with moderate-to-severe renal insufficiency | Losartan was effective in reducing blood pressure in hypertensive patients with chronic renal disease |
| Hadjigavriel and Kyriakides, 1999[12] | Open-label | Hypertensive (n=20) renal transplant recipients | Losartan, 50 mg o.d., for 6 months. Some patients were already using other antihypertensive agents | Mean systolic blood pressure decreased by 17%, whilst mean diastolic blood pressure decreased by 27.5% (p<0.01 for both values) | Losartan is effective in reducing blood pressure in hypertensive renal transplant recipients |

b.d., twice daily; HCTZ, hydrochlorothiazide; o.d., once daily.

**Table 1.** Continued

| Study | Study design | Study population | Dose regimen | Results | Conclusions |
|---|---|---|---|---|---|
| Fernandez-Vega et al., 2001[13] | Prospective, open-label | Elderly (≥60 years) patients (n=504) with mild-to-moderate hypertension | Losartan, 50 mg o.d., for 6 weeks, increasing to losartan, 50 mg + HCTZ, 12.5 mg, o.d. if necessary for 6 weeks, and losartan, 100 mg + HCTZ, 25 mg, o.d. thereafter if necessary, for a total treatment period of 16 weeks | Blood pressure was controlled in 78% of patients after 16 weeks | A losartan-based regimen is effective in controlling blood pressure in elderly patients with hypertension |
| Cushman et al., 2002[14] | Randomised, double-blind, parallel-group, placebo-controlled | 308 patients with isolated systolic hypertension | Losartan, 50 mg o.d., increasing to losartan, 50 mg/HCTZ 12.5 mg, or losartan 100 mg/HCTZ 25 mg o.d, if necessary, or placebo, for 12 weeks | The decrease in mean trough systolic blood pressure was significantly greater with a losartan-based regimen than with placebo (p<0.001). The percentage of responders was also significantly greater with losartan (54% vs 28%; p<0.001) and the likelihood of responding to treatment was three-times greater than with placebo (p<0.001) | A losartan-based regimen showed superior antihypertensive efficacy to placebo in patients with isolated systolic hypertension |

b.d., twice daily; HCTZ, hydrochlorothiazide; o.d., once daily.

administered with other antihypertensive agents.[6] In another study, losartan was shown to be effective in reducing blood pressure during long-term (29 months) treatment.[8] Losartan has also been shown to provide effective blood pressure control in special patient groups, including the elderly, those with renal disease and renal transplant recipients.[10–13]

### Losartan vs other angiotensin II receptor antagonists

The results of studies comparing the antihypertensive efficacy of losartan and other angiotensin II receptor antagonists in patients with mild-to-moderate hypertension have been variable (Table 2).[15–30] Thus, in some studies, losartan has shown comparable antihypertensive efficacy to valsartan, candesartan and telmisartan,[16–18,23,29] but in other studies telmisartan and candesartan have proved to be superior.[20,22,24,25,28] In particular, candesartan appears to be better at controlling blood pressure after a missed dose.[22] In this study, the superiority of candesartan was attributed to its tighter binding to, and slower dissociation from, $AT_1$ receptors.

*Losartan has shown comparable antihypertensive efficacy to valsartan, candesartan and telmisartan.*

### Losartan vs ACE inhibitors

Clinical trials comparing the antihypertensive efficacy of losartan and ACE inhibitors suggest that losartan has a similar blood pressure-lowering effect to enalapril, captopril and fosinopril in patients with hypertension (Table 3).[31–41] Losartan also shows comparable antihypertensive efficacy to ACE inhibitors in hypertensive patients with diabetes or renal impairment.[34,36,38] In a study comparing losartan and quinapril in hypertensive patients with a previous history of stroke, the two drugs were equally effective in reducing daytime blood pressure, but losartan was significantly more effective in reducing nocturnal blood pressure ($p<0.05$).[39] In a study comparing losartan and perindopril, treatment with perindopril produced higher normalisation rates and response rates.[40] However, in this study, perindopril was combined with a diuretic whereas losartan was given alone, and studies have shown that a greater reduction in blood pressure can be achieved with losartan in combination with the diuretic HCTZ (see Clinical Efficacy in Combination with HCTZ).

*Losartan has a similar blood pressure-lowering effect to enalapril, captopril and fosinopril in patients with hypertension.*

### Losartan vs calcium-channel blockers

In clinical trials comparing losartan and calcium-channel blockers, losartan has proved comparable to nifedipine, felodipine, lercanidipine and amlodipine in reducing blood pressure in patients with mild-to-moderate hypertension (Table 4).[3,41–50] Losartan has also proved as effective as calcium-channel blockers in reducing blood pressure in elderly ($\geq$65 years of age) hypertensive patients.[49,50] In one study, losartan and amlodipine were found to be equally effective in reducing daytime blood pressure, but the antihypertensive effect of amlodipine appeared to last longer than that of losartan.[45]

*Losartan has proved comparable to nifedipine, felodipine, lercanidipine and amlodipine in reducing blood pressure in patients with mild-to-moderate hypertension.*

**Table 2.** Clinical studies comparing the antihypertensive efficacy of angiotensin II receptor antagonists in patients with mild-to-moderate hypertension.[15–30]

| Study | Study design | Number of patients | Treatment regimen | Results | Conclusions |
|---|---|---|---|---|---|
| **Valsartan** | | | | | |
| Hedner et al., 1999[16] | Randomised, double-blind, parallel-group, placebo-controlled | 1369 | Losartan, 50 mg o.d., or valsartan, 80 mg o.d., or placebo, for 8 weeks. Doses were doubled after 4 weeks if necessary | Both drugs produced similar decreases in mean blood pressure at 4 and 8 weeks compared with placebo. Significantly more patients responded to valsartan (62%) than losartan (55%; $p=0.02$) | Losartan and valsartan were equally effective in reducing blood pressure in patients with mild-to-moderate hypertension, but significantly more patients responded to valsartan than to losartan treatment |
| Monterroso et al., 2000[17] | Randomised, double-blind, parallel-group | 187 | Losartan, 50 mg o.d., or valsartan, 80 mg o.d., for 6 weeks | Both drugs significantly reduced systolic and diastolic blood pressure at 2, 4 and 6 weeks, but there was no significant difference between groups. A greater smoothness index suggested a smoother reduction in blood pressure with losartan. Response rates were 54% for losartan and 46% for valsartan | Losartan and valsartan had similar antihypertensive effects, but losartan produced a smoother reduction in blood pressure |
| Elliott et al., 2001[18] | Randomised, double-blind, parallel-group | 495 | Losartan, 50 mg o.d., or valsartan, 80 mg o.d., for 12 weeks | The two drugs were equally effective in reducing trough diastolic blood pressure after 12 weeks ($p<0.001$ for both drugs vs baseline). The percentage of patients reaching their target diastolic blood pressure was also similar for the two drugs (57 and 59%, respectively) | Losartan and valsartan are equally effective in reducing blood pressure in patients with mild-to-moderate hypertension |

HCTZ, hydrochlorothiazide; o.d., once daily.

**Table 2.** Continued

| Study | Study design | Number of patients | Treatment regimen | Results | Conclusions |
|---|---|---|---|---|---|
| **Candesartan** | | | | | |
| Andersson and Neldam, 1997 and 1998[19,20] | Randomised, double-blind, parallel-group, placebo-controlled | 337 | Losartan, 50 mg o.d., or candesartan, 8 or 16 mg o.d., or placebo, for 8 weeks | Losartan and candesartan, 8 mg, reduced trough diastolic blood pressure to a similar extent, but candesartan, 16 mg, was more effective than losartan in this respect (p=0.013) | Losartan, 50 mg o.d., and candesartan, 8 mg o.d., show similar antihypertensive efficacy, but candesartan, 16 mg o.d., is more effective than losartan, 50 mg o.d. |
| Gradman et al., 1999[21] | Randomised, double-blind, parallel-group | 332 | Losartan, 50 mg o.d., or candesartan, 16 mg o.d., for 8 weeks. Doses were doubled after 4 weeks if necessary | The reduction in trough diastolic blood pressure at 8 weeks was significantly greater with candesartan than losartan (p=0.016). Candesartan was also equally effective as losartan in reducing trough and peak systolic blood pressure. Response rates were 64% for candesartan and 54% for losartan, while the percentage of patients with controlled blood pressure were 54% and 43%, respectively | Candesartan was more effective than losartan in reducing diastolic blood pressure, but not systolic blood pressure |

HCTZ, hydrochlorothiazide; o.d., once daily.

**Table 2.** Continued

| Study | Study design | Number of patients | Treatment regimen | Results | Conclusions |
|---|---|---|---|---|---|
| Lacourcière et al., 1999[22] | Randomised, double-blind, parallel-group, placebo-controlled, forced-dose titration | 268 | Losartan, 50 mg o.d., or candesartan, 8 mg o.d., or placebo, for 4 weeks. Doses were doubled for a further 4 weeks | At 8 weeks, candesartan, 16 mg, reduced systolic blood pressure to a greater extent than losartan, 100 mg, during the daytime ($p<0.05$), night-time ($p<0.05$) and over 24 hours ($p<0.01$). It also reduced systolic and diastolic blood pressure to a greater degree between 0 and 36 hours ($p<0.01$ and $p<0.05$, respectively) and on the day of a missed dose ($p<0.001$ for both). Similar differences in systolic blood pressure reduction for candesartan, 8 mg, and losartan, 50 mg, were also reported | Candesartan is superior to losartan in reducing systolic blood pressure and in controlling systolic and diastolic blood pressure on the day of a missed dose |
| Manolis et al., 2000[23] | Randomised, double-blind, parallel-group | 1161 | Losartan, 50 mg o.d., titrated to 100 mg o.d. if necessary, or candesartan, 8 mg o.d. titrated to 16 mg o.d. if necessary, for 12 weeks | The reduction in blood pressure at 12 weeks was similar for the two drugs | Losartan and candesartan showed comparable antihypertensive efficacy |
| Bakris et al., 2001 (CLAIM study)[24] | Randomised, double-blind, parallel-group, forced titration | 654 | Losartan, 50 mg o.d., or candesartan, 16 mg o.d., for 2 weeks, followed by double doses for a further 6 weeks | Candesartan lowered trough systolic and diastolic blood pressure to a greater extent than losartan ($p<0.001$). Candesartan lowered peak blood pressure to a significantly greater extent ($p<0.05$). The percentage of responders was greater with candesartan (62.4 vs 54.0%; $p=0.033$) as was the percentage of patients who had their blood pressure adequately controlled (56.0 vs 46.9%; $p=0.023$) | Candesartan was more effective than losartan in controlling blood pressure |

HCTZ, hydrochlorothiazide; o.d., once daily.

**Table 2.** Continued

| Study | Study design | Number of patients | Treatment regimen | Results | Conclusions |
|---|---|---|---|---|---|
| Vidt et al., 2001[25] | Randomised, double-blind, parallel-group, forced titration | 611 | Losartan, 50 mg o.d., or candesartan, 16 mg o.d, for 2 weeks. Doses were then doubled for a further 6 weeks | After 8 weeks, candesartan had lowered trough blood pressure at 24 hours, peak pressure at 6 hours and pressure 48 hours post-dosing by a significantly greater extent losartan ($p<0.05$). Response rates were 52.1% for losartan and 58.8% for candesartan (difference not significant) | Candesartan is more effective than losartan in lowering blood pressure |
| **Irbesartan** | | | | | |
| Oparil et al., 1998[26] | Randomised, double-blind | 432 | Losartan, 50 mg o.d. titrated to 100 mg o.d. if necessary, or irbesartan, 150 mg o.d. titrated to 300 mg o.d. if necessary, for 12 weeks | The mean decrease in trough diastolic blood pressure was greater with irbesartan than losartan at 8 and 12 weeks ($p<0.02$ and 0.002, respectively). The mean decrease in systolic blood pressure was greater with irbesartan at 12 weeks ($p<0.02$) but not at 8 weeks. More patients responded to irbesartan (78%) than losartan (64%; $p<0$ | Irbesartan was significantly more effective than losartan in reducing trough diastolic blood pressure, and significantly more patients responded to irbesartan than to losartan |
| Kassler-Taub et al., 1998[27] | Randomised, double-blind, placebo-controlled | 567 | Losartan, 100 mg o.d., or irbesartan, 150 or 300 mg o.d., or placebo, for 8 weeks | The antihypertensive effects of losartan, 100 mg, and irbesartan, 150 mg, were similar, but irbesartan, 300 mg, produced a significantly greater decrease in trough diastolic and systolic blood pressure at 8 weeks than losartan ($p<0.01$ for diastolic and systolic values) | Losartan, 100 mg o.d., and irbesartan, 150 mg o.d., have similar antihypertensive effects, but irbesartan, 300 mg o.d., is significantly more effective |

HCTZ, hydrochlorothiazide; o.d., once daily.

**Table 2.** Continued

| Study | Study design | Number of patients | Treatment regimen | Results | Conclusions |
|---|---|---|---|---|---|
| **Telmisartan** | | | | | |
| Mallion et al, 1999[28] | Randomised, double-blind, parallel-group, placebo-controlled | 223 | Losartan, 50 mg o.d., telmisartan, 40 or 80 mg o.d., or placebo, for 6 weeks | All active treatments reduced blood pressure compared with placebo ($p<0.01$). The reductions in blood pressure 18–24 hours after dosing were greater with telmisartan than losartan ($p<0.05$ for both doses). Mean 24-hour blood pressure was better with telmisartan than with losartan ($p<0.05$ for both doses) | Telmisartan, 40 and 80 mg o.d., has a superior antihypertensive effect to losartan, 50 mg o.d. |
| Martina et al, 2003[29] | Prospective, randomised, double-blind | 30 | Losartan, 50 mg o.d., or telmisartan, 80 mg o.d., for 6 months. HCTZ, 12.5 mg, was added to the treatment regimens if necessary | Both drugs produced a similar reduction in blood pressure after 6 months | Losartan and telmisartan showed comparable antihypertensive efficacy |
| **Candesartan and valsartan** | | | | | |
| Fridman et al, 2002[15] | Randomised, double-blind, cross-over | 24 | Losartan, 50 mg o.d., or candesartan, 16 mg o.d., or valsartan, 80 mg o.d., for 4 weeks | Resting mean arterial pressure decreased to a greater extent with candesartan than with losartan or valsartan ($p<0.001$ for candesartan vs losartan and $p=0.004$ for candesartan vs valsartan for systolic blood pressure; $p=0.016$ for candesartan vs losartan and $p=0.062$ for candesartan vs valsartan for diastolic blood pressure) | Candesartan reduced resting systolic blood pressure to a significantly greater extent than losartan or valsartan, and reduced resting diastolic blood pressure to a significantly greater extent than losartan |

HCTZ, hydrochlorothiazide; o.d., once daily.

**Table 2.** Continued

| Study | Study design | Number of patients | Treatment regimen | Results | Conclusions |
|---|---|---|---|---|---|
| **Olmesartan, valsartan and irbesartan** | | | | | |
| Oparil et al., 2001[30] | Randomised, double-blind, parallel-group | 588 | Losartan, 50 mg o.d., olmesartan, 20 mg o.d., valsartan, 80 mg o.d., or irbesartan, 150 mg o.d, for 8 weeks | Olmesartan reduced cuff diastolic blood pressure to a greater degree than losartan ($p=0.0002$), valsartan ($p<0.0001$) and irbesartan ($p=0.04$). Differences between the other drugs were not significant. Reductions in cuff systolic blood pressure were similar for all four drugs. Olmesartan reduced mean 24-hour diastolic and systolic blood pressures to a greater degree than losartan and valsartan ($p<0.05$) but not irbesartan | Olmesartan was more effective than other angiotensin II receptor antagonists in reducing cuff diastolic but not systolic blood pressure. Olmesartan was more effective than losartan and valsartan, but not irbesartan, in reducing mean 24-hour diastolic and systolic blood pressures |

HCTZ, hydrochlorothiazide; o.d., once daily.

**Table 3.** Clinical studies comparing the antihypertensive efficacy of losartan and angiotensin-converting enzyme (ACE) inhibitors in hypertensive patients.[31-41]

| Study | Design | Patient population | Dose regimen | Results | Conclusions |
|---|---|---|---|---|---|
| **Enalapril** | | | | | |
| Tikkanen et al., 1995[31] | Randomised, double-blind, parallel-group | Patients (n=407) with mild-to-moderate hypertension | Losartan, 50 mg o.d., or enalapril, 20 mg o.d., for 12 weeks | Both drugs decreased systolic and diastolic blood pressure compared with baseline, and changes in trough blood pressure from baseline were similar for the two drugs. The response to treatment was also similar (excellent or good in 51 and 53% of losartan and enalapril patients, respectively) | Losartan and enalapril have a similar antihypertensive efficacy |
| Byyny et al., 1996[32] | Randomised, double-blind, placebo-controlled | Inpatients (n=100) with mild-to-moderate hypertension | Losartan, 50, 100 or 150 mg o.d., or enalapril, 10 mg o.d., or placebo, for 5 days | All three doses of losartan and enalapril reduced peak and trough systolic and diastolic blood pressure compared with placebo ($p<0.05$). The reductions in blood pressure were similar after 5 days of treatment | Losartan and enalapril have a similar antihypertensive efficacy |
| Ruff et al., 1996[33] | Randomised, double-blind, parallel-group | Patients (n=75) with severe hypertension | Losartan, 50 mg o.d. titrated to 100 mg o.d., if necessary, or enalapril, 10–40 mg o.d., for 12 weeks | After 12 weeks, the reduction in systolic blood pressure was greater with enalapril than with losartan ($p=0.037$) but the reduction in diastolic blood pressure was similar for the two drugs | The blood pressure-lowering effects of losartan and enalapril were generally similar in patients with severe hypertension |
| Kim et al., 2002[34] | Cross-over | Renal transplant recipients (n=50) with hypertension | Losartan or enalapril for 6 weeks (doses not specified) | Both drugs reduced mean arterial pressure by a similar extent ($p<0.05$ for both drugs vs baseline) | Losartan and enalapril show comparable antihypertensive efficacy in renal transplant patients |

b.d., twice daily; HCTZ, hydrochlorothiazide; o.d., once daily.

**Table 3.** Continued

| Study | Design | Patient population | Dose regimen | Results | Conclusions |
|---|---|---|---|---|---|
| **Captopril** | | | | | |
| Scholze et al., 1998[35] | Two-phase, randomised, double-blind | Patients (n=177) with mild-to-moderate hypertension | Captopril, 25 mg b.d., for 6 weeks, followed by losartan, 50 mg o.d., or continuing captopril for 6 weeks | Within 12 hours of the first dose of losartan, 31% of patients had two consecutive systolic blood pressure readings of 30 mmHg below their individual baseline value compared with 24% of patients who stayed on captopril | Losartan and captopril were equally effective in further reducing blood pressure after initial treatment with captopril |
| Schulz et al., 1999[36] | Randomised, double-blind, parallel-group | Patients (n=129) with mild-to-moderate hypertension and impaired renal function | Losartan, 50 mg o.d. possibly titrated to 100 mg o.d., or captopril, 25 mg b.d., possibly titrated to 50 mg b.d., for 12 weeks | Losartan and captopril reduced systolic and diastolic blood pressure by a similar degree | Losartan and captopril show similar antihypertensive efficacy in patients with renal impairment |
| **Verapamil and enalapril** | | | | | |
| Bakris et al., 2002[37] | Randomised, double-blind, placebo-controlled | Patients (n=406) with stage I–III hypertension | Losartan, 50 mg o.d. titrated to 100 mg o.d., extended-release verapamil, 240 mg titrated to 360 mg/day, or enalapril, 10 mg titrated to 20 mg/day, or placebo, for 8 weeks | Extended-release verapamil was more effective than losartan and enalapril in lowering morning systolic and diastolic blood pressure (p<0.001 for all comparisons). Verapamil and enalapril produced similar decreases in blood pressure over 24 hours. Losartan had a similar effect on systolic blood pressure, but was less effective in reducing diastolic blood pressure (p=0.004 vs verapamil). Verapamil was the only treatment to reduce heart rate (p<0.001). The decline in nocturnal blood pressure was similar for losartan and verapamil, and greater with enalapril (p=0.014) | Extended-release verapamil produces changes in blood pressure and heart rate that more closely match normal circadian rhythms of blood pressure than those seen with losartan and enalapril. Losartan was equally effective in reducing systolic blood pressure, but was less effective in reducing diastolic blood pressure than verapamil |

b.d., twice daily; HCTZ, hydrochlorothiazide; o.d., once daily.

**Table 3.** Continued

| Study | Design | Patient population | Dose regimen | Results | Conclusions |
|---|---|---|---|---|---|
| **Fosinopril** | | | | | |
| Kaygaci et al., 2002[38] | Randomised, open-label | Hypertensive patients (n=33) with type 2 diabetes | Losartan, 50 mg o.d., or fosinopril, 10 mg o.d., for 6 months | Both drugs reduced blood pressure by a similar extent after 1 and 6 months of treatment (losartan: $p<0.001$ vs baseline at 1 and 6 months; fosinopril: $p<0.05$ vs baseline at 1 and 6 months) | Losartan and fosinopril have similar antihypertensive effects in hypertensive patients with type 2 diabetes |
| **Quinapril** | | | | | |
| Okuguchi et al., 2002[39] | Prospective, randomised, cross-over | Patients (n=30) with hypertension and a previous history of stroke | Losartan, 50 mg o.d, or quinapril, 10 mg o.d., for 4 weeks | Reductions in daytime systolic and diastolic blood pressure were similar for the two drugs, but night-time blood pressures were lower with losartan than quinapril ($p<0.05$ for losartan vs quinapril for changes in systolic and diastolic blood pressure) | Losartan and quinapril were equally effective in reducing daytime blood pressure, but losartan was more effective in reducing nocturnal blood pressure in patients with a previous history of stroke |
| **Perindopril** | | | | | |
| Chanudet et al., 2001[40] | Prospective, randomised, double-blind, parallel-group | Patients (n=277) with essential hypertension | Losartan, 50 mg o.d., or perindopril, 2 mg, + indapamide (diuretic), 0.625 mg o.d., for 12 weeks | Normalisation rates were significantly higher in the perindopril group than in the losartan group (76.0% vs 60.0%; $p=0.009$), as were response rates (91.7 vs 81.8%, respectively; $p=0.025$). Average reductions in blood pressure were comparable. The decrease in average night-time systolic blood pressure was significantly greater in the perindopril group ($p=0.041$) | Perindopril in combination with a diuretic produced greater response rates and normalisation rates than losartan alone |

b.d., twice daily; HCTZ, hydrochlorothiazide; o.d., once daily.

**Table 3.** Continued

| Study | Design | Patient population | Dose regimen | Results | Conclusions |
|---|---|---|---|---|---|
| **Lisinopril** | | | | | |
| Campo et al., 2001[41] | Prospective, randomised, open-label | Patients (n=200) with mild hypertension | Losartan, 25–100 mg o.d., or lisinopril, 10–40 mg o.d., for 12 weeks; HCTZ, 12.5–25 mg, was added after 8 weeks if necessary. (This study also compared nisoldipine and atenolol.) | After 12 weeks, blood pressure reductions were comparable in all treatment groups. The percentage of patients who reached their target diastolic blood pressure was 60.8% for losartan and 68.8% for lisinopril | Losartan and lisinopril showed comparable antihypertensive efficacy |

b.d., twice daily; HCTZ, hydrochlorothiazide; o.d., once daily.

**Table 4.** Clinical studies comparing the antihypertensive efficacy of losartan and calcium-channel blockers in hypertensive patients.[3,41–50]

| Study | Design | Patient population | Treatment regimen | Results | Conclusions |
|---|---|---|---|---|---|
| **Amlodipine** | | | | | |
| Oparil et al., 1996[42] | Randomised, double-blind, parallel-group | Patients (n=190) with mild-to-moderate hypertension | Losartan, 50 mg o.d. with HCTZ added as necessary after 4 (12.5 mg) or 8 (25 mg) weeks, or amlodipine, 5 mg o.d. titrated to 10 mg o.d. after 4 weeks if necessary and HCTZ added (25 mg) after 8 weeks if necessary for 12 weeks | Reductions in trough diastolic blood pressure after 4, 8 and 12 weeks were comparable for the two drugs. Similar reductions in systolic blood pressure were observed. The percentage of patients reaching target diastolic blood pressure was also similar for the two drugs: 68% for losartan and 71% for amlodipine | Losartan with HCTZ added as necessary shows similar antihypertensive efficacy to amlodipine with HCTZ added as necessary in patients with mild-to-moderate hypertension |
| Fernandez-Andrade et al., 1998[3] | Randomised, double-blind, parallel-group, placebo-controlled | Patients (n=48) with hypertension and impaired renal function | Losartan, 50 mg o.d, or amlodipine, 5 mg o.d, for 12 weeks. Doses were doubled at 3 and 6 weeks if necessary, and HCTZ, 12.5 mg, was added to the losartan regimen if necessary | After 12 weeks, losartan produced a greater reduction in both systolic and diastolic blood pressure than amlodipine (p=0.009 and 0.008, respectively) | Losartan (with or without HCTZ) is more effective than amlodipine in reducing blood pressure in patients with renal impairment |
| Holdaas et al., 1998[43] | Randomised, prospective, double-blind, placebo-controlled, cross-over | Patients (n=15) with hypertension and non-diabetic renal disease | Losartan, 50 mg o.d, or amlodipine, 5 mg o.d. for 4 weeks. The doses were doubled after 1 week if necessary | Mean arterial blood pressure decreased from baseline with both drugs (p<0.01 for both drugs vs baseline) | Losartan and amlodipine were equally effective in reducing blood pressure in hypertensive patients with renal disease |
| Ishimitsu et al., 2002[44] | Randomised, cross-over | Patients (n=15) with essential hypertension | Losartan, 50–100 mg o.d, or amlodipine, 2.5–10 mg o.d, for 12–16 weeks | Reductions in average 24-hour blood pressure and daytime blood pressure were comparable for the two drugs. The reduction in average 24-hour systolic blood pressure was lower with amlodipine (p<0.05) | Losartan and amlodipine were equally effective in reducing daytime blood pressure, but the antihypertensive effect of amlodipine lasted for longer than that of losartan |

GITS, gastrointestinal therapeutic system; HCTZ, hydrochlorothiazide; o.d., once daily.

**Table 4.** Continued

| Study | Design | Patient population | Treatment regimen | Results | Conclusions |
|---|---|---|---|---|---|
| Volpe et al., 2003[45] | Prospective, randomised, double-blind, parallel-group | Patients (n=857) with isolated systolic hypertension | Losartan, 50 mg o.d. titrated to 100 mg o.d. at 12 weeks if necessary and HCTZ added if necessary at weeks 6 (12.5 mg) and 12 (25 mg), or amlodipine, 5 mg o.d. increasing to 10 mg if necessary at 6 weeks and HCTZ (25 mg) being added if necessary at 12 weeks, for a total treatment period of 18 weeks | At week 18, the mean change in systolic blood pressure from baseline was 27.4 mmHg for losartan and 28.1 mmHg for amlodipine. The response rates were 73.9% and 75.4%, respectively | Losartan and amlodipine showed comparable antihypertensive efficacy in patients with isolated systolic hypertension |
| Phillips et al. 2003[46] | Randomised, double-blind, parallel-group | Patients (n=440) with mild-to-moderate hypertension | Losartan, 50 mg o.d., or amlodipine, 5 mg o.d, for 18 weeks. If necessary, HCTZ, 12.5 mg, was added to the losartan regimen, and the dose of amlodipine was doubled | 42.3% of losartan and 43.6% of amlodipine subjects achieved target diastolic blood pressure at the lower dose. Of those receiving the higher doses, 42% of losartan/HCTZ subjects and 59% of amlodipine subjects (p=0.009) achieved target blood pressure. Overall, 63.8% of amlodipine subjects and 55.1% of losartan subjects achieved target blood pressure (difference not significant). Changes in 24-hour ambulatory blood pressure were similar for the two groups | Both losartan and amlodipine were equally effective in reducing blood pressure |

GITS, gastrointestinal therapeutic system; HCTZ, hydrochlorothiazide; o.d., once daily.

**Table 4.** Continued

| Study | Design | Patient population | Treatment regimen | Results | Conclusions |
|---|---|---|---|---|---|
| **Nifedipine** | | | | | |
| Weir et al., 1996[47] | Randomised, double-blind, parallel-group | Patients (n=223) with hypertension | Losartan, 50 mg o.d. with HCTZ added if necessary at weeks 4 (12.5 mg) and 8 (25 mg), or nifedipine GITS, 30 mg o.d. titrated to 60 mg at 4 weeks and 90 mg at 8 weeks if necessary, for 12 weeks | Reductions in trough diastolic blood pressure and systolic blood pressure at weeks 4, 8 and 12 were comparable for the two drugs. The percentage of patients reaching target diastolic pressure was also similar: 74% for losartan, 68% for nifedipine | Losartan and nifedipine GITS, with HCTZ added as necessary, show comparable antihypertensive efficacy |
| Conlin et al., 1998[48] | Randomised, double-blind, parallel-group | Elderly (≥65 years) patients (n=140) with diastolic hypertension | Losartan, 50 mg o.d. with HCTZ, 12.5 or 25 mg, added if necessary, or nifedipine GITS, 30 mg o.d. increasing to 60 or 90 mg o.d. if necessary, for 12 weeks | The reduction in trough diastolic blood pressure at 4 weeks was greater with nifedipine ($p<0.05$), but those at 8 and 12 weeks were similar for the two drugs. A similar percentage of patients in each group achieved their target pressure (81% for losartan, 90% for nifedipine) | Losartan and nifedipine GITS showed comparable antihypertensive efficacy in elderly patients with diastolic hypertension |
| **Felodipine** | | | | | |
| Chan et al., 1995[49] | Randomised, double-blind | Elderly (≥65 years of age) patients (n=132) with mild-to-moderate hypertension | Losartan 50 mg o.d. titrated to 100 mg o.d., or extended-release felodipine, 5 mg o.d. titrated to 10 mg o.d., for 12 weeks | After 6 weeks, extended-release felodipine had reduced diastolic blood pressure to a greater extent than losartan ($p<0.01$), but the mean reduction in diastolic blood pressure after 12 weeks was similar for the two drugs. Reductions in systolic blood pressure after 6 and 12 weeks were also similar for the two drugs | Losartan and extended-release felodipine were equally effective in reducing blood pressure in elderly hypertensive patients after 12 weeks |

GITS, gastrointestinal therapeutic system; HCTZ, hydrochlorothiazide; o.d., once daily.

**Table 4.** Continued

| Study | Design | Patient population | Treatment regimen | Results | Conclusions |
|---|---|---|---|---|---|
| **Lercanidipine** | | | | | |
| James et al., 2002[50] | Randomised, double-blind | Patients (n=265) with mild-to-moderate hypertension | Losartan 50 mg o.d. titrated to 100 mg o.d. if necessary, or lercanidipine, 10 mg o.d. titrated to 20 mg o.d. if necessary, for 16 weeks | After 16 weeks, 65% of losartan-treated patients had achieved normalised diastolic blood pressure and 78% had responded to treatment. Corresponding figures for lercanidipine were 71 and 81%, respectively. In patients who required dose titration, the response to lercanidipine was greater than that to losartan (57 vs 40%) | Losartan and lercanidipine showed comparable antihypertensive efficacy |
| **Nisoldipine** | | | | | |
| Campo et al., 2001[41] | Prospective, randomised, open-label | Patients (n=200) with mild hypertension | Losartan, 25–100 mg o.d., or nisoldipine, 5–20 mg o.d. for 12 weeks. HCTZ, 12.5–25 mg, was added after 8 weeks if necessary. (This study also compared lisinopril and atenolol.) | After 12 weeks, blood pressure reductions were comparable in all treatment groups. The percentage of patients who reached their target diastolic blood pressure was 60.8% for losartan and 62.2% for nisoldipine | Losartan and nisoldipine showed comparable antihypertensive efficacy |

GITS, gastrointestinal therapeutic system; HCTZ, hydrochlorothiazide; o.d., once daily.

## Losartan vs β-blockers

The antihypertensive efficacy of losartan has been compared with that of the β-blocker atenolol in a number of studies, principally the Losartan Intervention for Endpoint Reduction in Hypertension (LIFE) study and its substudies (Table 5).[41,51–57] The LIFE study enrolled over 9000 patients with hypertension and signs of LVH on electrocardiogram (ECG) to treatment with losartan or atenolol for at least 4 years. The principal objective of the study was to determine cardiovascular morbidity and mortality in this patient population, but blood pressure readings were also performed in both treatment groups. The results of LIFE and its substudies, together with other studies that have compared the antihypertensive efficacy of losartan and atenolol indicate that the two drugs reduce blood pressure by a similar magnitude in patients with hypertension, in patients with hypertension plus signs of LVH, and in those with hypertension plus signs of LVH and diabetes. The data relating to cardiovascular outcomes are presented in more detail in subsequent sections of this review.

# Clinical efficacy in patients with LVH

In addition to raised blood pressure, hypertension is associated with structural changes in the cardiovascular system, including LVH. This condition is well established as a major risk factor for cardiovascular disease, and hence cardiovascular morbidity and mortality. Angiotensin II has an important influence on cardiac structure and function, stimulating cell proliferation and growth. Thus, antagonism of this compound may help to improve LVH, and reduce cardiovascular morbidity and mortality. Indeed, the effects of losartan on these parameters have been investigated in a number of clinical studies.

## Effects on left ventricular mass

The majority of studies have shown that losartan has a beneficial effect on LVH, leading to a reduction in left ventricular mass (LVM) and other associated parameters (Table 6).[1,8,29,53,55,58–62] Furthermore, comparative studies suggest that losartan is more effective in this respect than the ACE inhibitor enalapril, the calcium-channel blocker amlodipine, the β-blocker atenolol and the thiazide diuretic HCTZ.[1,53,55,58,60,61] In a study comparing losartan and telmisartan, the two drugs were equally effective in reducing LVM.[29]

> Losartan has a more beneficial effect on LVH than ACE inhibitors, calcium-channel blockers, β-blockers and HCTZ.

## Effects on left ventricular performance

Two substudies of LIFE investigated the effects of antihypertensive therapy with losartan or atenolol on left ventricular performance. In one study of 728 hypertensive patients with LVH, left ventricular diastolic filling was improved after 1 year of antihypertensive therapy with losartan or atenolol.[63] In another study of hypertensive patients with LVH (n=679), 3 years of antihypertensive therapy with losartan or

**Table 5. Clinical studies comparing the antihypertensive efficacy of losartan and the β-blocker atenolol in hypertensive patients.**[41,51–57]

| Study | Design | Patient population | Treatment regimen | Results | Conclusions |
|---|---|---|---|---|---|
| Dahlof et al., 1995[51] | Prospective, randomised, double-blind, parallel-group | Patients (n=202) with mild-to-moderate hypertension | Losartan or atenolol, 50 mg o.d. titrated to 100 mg o.d. if necessary, for 12 weeks | The reduction in trough diastolic blood pressure at weeks 6 and 12 was similar for the two drugs. A similar percentage of patients responded to treatment with each drug | Losartan and atenolol were equally effective in reducing diastolic blood pressure in patients with mild-to-moderate hypertension |
| Farsang et al., 2000[52] | Randomised, double-blind | Patients (n=273) with isolated systolic hypertension | Losartan or atenolol, 50 mg o.d., for 16 weeks. HCTZ, 12.5 mg, added as necessary after 8 and 12 weeks | After 16 weeks, losartan and atenolol had reduced systolic blood pressure by a similar degree and 67% of losartan patients and 64% of atenolol patients remained on monotherapy throughout the study | Losartan and atenolol showed a similar effect on systolic blood pressure in patients with isolated systolic hypertension |
| Campo et al., 2001[41] | Prospective, randomised, open-label | Patients (n=200) with mild hypertension | Losartan, 25–100 mg o.d., or atenolol, 25–100 mg o.d., for 12 weeks. HCTZ, 12.5–25 mg, was added after 8 weeks if necessary. (This study also compared lisinopril and nisoldipine.) | After 12 weeks, blood pressure reductions were comparable in all treatment groups. The percentage of patients who reached their target diastolic blood pressure was 60.8% for losartan and 64.6% for atenolol | Losartan and atenolol showed comparable antihypertensive efficacy |
| Dahlof et al., 2002 (REGAAL substudy)[53] | Randomised, double-blind | Patients (n=225) with hypertension and LVH | Losartan, 50 mg o.d., or atenolol, 50 mg o.d., both titrated to 100 mg if necessary and HCTZ, 12.5 or 25 mg o.d., added if necessary, for 36 weeks | The changes from baseline for diastolic blood pressure were greater in the atenolol group at weeks 6 and 36 (p=0.016), but the two drugs achieved similar blood pressure readings at week 36 | Losartan and atenolol showed similar blood pressure-lowering effects in hypertensive patients with LVH |

HCTZ, hydrochlorothiazide; LIFE, Losartan Intervention for Endpoint Reduction in Hypertension Study; LVH, left ventricular hypertrophy; o.d., once daily; REGAAL, Losartan LVH Regression Study.

**Table 5.** Continued

| Study | Design | Patient population | Treatment regimen | Results | Conclusions |
|---|---|---|---|---|---|
| Dahlof et al., 2002 (LIFE study)[54] | Randomised, double-blind, parallel-group | Patients (n=9193) with hypertension and signs of LVH | Losartan or atenolol, 50 mg o.d. titrated to 100 mg o.d. if necessary and HCTZ, 12.5 or 25 mg, added as necessary, for at least 4 years | Blood pressure (systolic and diastolic) was reduced by a similar amount for the two drugs. Target systolic blood pressure was achieved in 49% of losartan patients and 46% of atenolol patients. Target diastolic blood pressure was achieved in 89% of patients in both groups | Losartan and atenolol showed similar blood pressure-lowering effects in patients with signs of LVH |
| Kjeldsen et al., 2002 (LIFE substudy)[55] | Randomised, double-blind, parallel-group | Patients (n=1326) with isolated systolic hypertension and LVH | Losartan or atenolol, 50 mg o.d. titrated to 100 mg o.d. if necessary and HCTZ, 12.5 or 25 mg, added as necessary, for at least 4 years | Blood pressure was reduced by 28/9 mmHg in both groups | Losartan and atenolol were equally effective in reducing blood pressure in patients with isolated systolic hypertension and LVH |
| Lindholm et al., 2002 (LIFE substudy)[56] | Randomised, double-blind, parallel-group | Patients (n=1195) with diabetes, hypertension and signs of LVH | Losartan or atenolol, 50 mg o.d. titrated to 100 mg o.d. if necessary and HCTZ, 12.5 or 25 mg, added as necessary, for at least 4 years | Mean blood pressure fell by 17/11 and 19/11 mmHg for losartan and atenolol, respectively. 85% of losartan patients and 82% of atenolol patients reached their target diastolic blood pressure by the end of the study. Corresponding figures for systolic blood pressure were 38% and 34%, respectively | Losartan and atenolol were equally effective in reducing blood pressure in patients with diabetes and signs of LVH |
| Devereux et al., 2003 (LIFE substudy)[57] | Randomised, double-blind, parallel-group | Patients (n=6886) with hypertension and signs of LVH but no clinical evidence of vascular disease | Losartan or atenolol, 50 mg o.d. titrated to 100 mg o.d. if necessary and HCTZ, 12.5 or 25 mg, added as necessary, for at least 4 years | By the end of the study, systolic and diastolic blood pressure had fallen by comparable amounts for the two drugs. Target blood pressure was achieved in 50% of losartan patients and 47% of atenolol patients | Losartan and atenolol were equally effective in reducing blood pressure in patients with LVH but no clinical evidence of vascular disease |

HCTZ, hydrochlorothiazide; LIFE, Losartan Intervention for Endpoint Reduction in Hypertension Study; LVH, left ventricular hypertrophy; o.d., once daily; REGAAL, Losartan LVH Regression Study.

**Table 6.** Clinical studies investigating the effects of losartan on left ventricular mass (LVM) in hypertensive patients with left ventricular hypertrophy (LVH).[1,8,29,53,55,58–62]

| Study | Design | Patient population | Treatment regimens | Results | Conclusions |
|---|---|---|---|---|---|
| **Losartan-based regimen** | | | | | |
| Himmelmann et al., 1996[8] | Open-label, prospective | Patients (n=19) with mild-to-moderate hypertension | Losartan, 50 mg o.d., for a mean of 29.3 months. HCTZ, 6.25 or 12.5 mg, added if necessary after 4 and 6 weeks, respectively. A calcium-channel blocker added if necessary after 8 weeks | LV internal diameter decreased significantly (p=0.006), interventricular septal thickness increased significantly (p=0.001), and posterior wall thickness increased significantly (p=0.023). LVM showed no significant change | LV wall thickness increased but LVM showed no significant change with losartan treatment |
| **Losartan vs telmisartan** | | | | | |
| Martina et al., 2003[29] | Prospective, randomised, double-blind | Patients (n=30) with mild-to-moderate hypertension | Losartan, 50 mg o.d., or telmisartan, 80 mg o.d., for 6 months. HCTZ, 12.5 mg, was added to the treatment regimen if necessary | After 6 months, the mean LVM index had decreased significantly from 115 to 101 g/m² with telmisartan (p=0.04) and from 117 to 101 g/m² with losartan (p=0.009) | Losartan and telmisartan reduced LVM and were equally effective in doing so |
| **Losartan vs enalapril** | | | | | |
| De Rosa et al., 2002[59] | Randomised, double-blind, parallel-group | Patients (n=50) with World Health Organization stage II hypertension | Losartan, 12.5 mg o.d. titrated to 25 and then 50 mg o.d., or enalapril, 5 mg titrated to 10 and then 20 mg o.d., for 3 years | Both drugs significantly reduced LVM, and septal and posterior wall thickness (p<0.001 for all parameters). The observed reductions were similar for the two drugs | Losartan and enalapril reduced LVM, and were equally effective in doing so |

HCTZ, hydrochlorothiazide; LIFE, Losartan Intervention for Endpoint Reduction in Hypertension Study; LVH, left ventricular hypertrophy; LVM, left ventricular mass; o.d., once daily; REGAAL, Losartan LVH Regression Study.

## Table 6. Continued

| Study | Design | Patient population | Treatment regimens | Results | Conclusions |
|---|---|---|---|---|---|
| **Losartan vs amlodipine** | | | | | |
| Martina et al, 1999[1] | Randomised, double-blind | Patients (n=25) with mild-to-moderate hypertension | Losartan, 50 mg o.d. titrated to 50 mg + HCTZ, 12.5 mg, or amlodipine, 5 mg titrated to 10 mg, for 16 weeks | Losartan significantly decreased LVM (p=0.003) and LVM index (p=0.01). Amlodipine had no significant effect | Losartan but not amlodipine reduced LVM as early as 16 weeks after the initiation of therapy |
| **Losartan vs enalapril and amlodipine** | | | | | |
| Shibasaki et al, 2002[60] | Randomised, double-blind | Hypertensive patients (n=30) with end-stage renal disease | Losartan, 50 mg o.d., or enalapril, 5 mg o.d, or amlodipine, 5 mg o.d, for 6 months | LVM index decreased in the losartan and enalapril groups, but not in the amlodipine group. The decrease achieved with losartan was greater than that achieved with the other two drugs (p=0.034 for losartan vs enalapril; p=0.026 for losartan vs amlodipine) | Losartan has a greater LVH-reducing effect than enalapril and amlodipine in hypertensive patients with end-stage renal disease |
| **Losartan vs HCTZ** | | | | | |
| Tedesco et al, 1998[61] | Randomised, double-blind | Patients (n=77) with mild-to-moderate hypertension | Losartan, 50 mg o.d., or HCTZ, 25 mg o.d, for 22 months | Losartan, but not HCTZ, produced a reduction in LVM index at 10 and 22 months (reduction 9 $g/m^2$ at 10 months, p<0.04; reduction 11 $g/m^2$ at 22 months, p<0.02) | Losartan but not HCTZ reduced LVM in hypertensive patients |
| **Losartan vs atenolol** | | | | | |
| Dahlof et al, 2002 (REGAAL substudy)[53] | Randomised, double-blind | Hypertensive patients (n=225) with LVH | Losartan, 50 mg o.d, or atenolol, 50 mg o.d, both titrated to 100 mg if necessary and HCTZ, 12.5 or 25 mg o.d, added if necessary, for 36 weeks | Losartan significantly reduced the LVM index after 36 weeks (p<0.001) whereas atenolol did not. The decrease in LVM index was greater with losartan than atenolol (p<0.001) | Losartan but not atenolol reduced LVM in hypertensive patients with LVH |

HCTZ, hydrochlorothiazide; LIFE, Losartan Intervention for Endpoint Reduction in Hypertension Study; LVH, left ventricular hypertrophy; LVM, left ventricular mass; o.d., once daily; REGAAL, Losartan LVH Regression Study;

**Table 6.** Continued

| Study | Design | Patient population | Treatment regimens | Results | Conclusions |
|---|---|---|---|---|---|
| **Losartan vs atenolol** | | | | | |
| Kjeldsen et al., 2002 (LIFE substudy)[55] | Randomised, double-blind, parallel group | Patients (n=1326) with isolated systolic hypertension and LVH | Losartan or atenolol, 50 mg o.d. titrated to 100 mg o.d. if necessary, and HCTZ, 12.5 or 25 mg, added as necessary, for at least 4 years | Losartan reduced LVH by a greater extent than atenolol (p<0.001) | Losartan was superior to atenolol in reducing LVH |
| Devereux et al. 2004. (LIFE substudy)[58] | Randomised, double-blind, parallel-group | Hypertensive patients (n=960) with LVH | Losartan or atenolol, 50 mg o.d. titrated to 100 mg o.d. if necessary, and HCTZ, 12.5 or 25 mg, added as necessary for at least 4 years | Losartan reduced the LVM index by a greater extent than atenolol (−21.7 vs −17.7 g/m²; p=0.021). This superiority of losartan was maintained when patients were stratified according to gender, age and severity of LVH at baseline | Antihypertensive treatment regimens containing losartan resulted in greater regression of LVH than conventional atenolol treatment |
| **Losartan or atenolol** | | | | | |
| Devereux et al., 2002 (LIFE substudy)[62] | Randomised, double-blind, parallel group | Hypertensive patients (n=754) with LVH | Losartan or atenolol, 50 mg o.d. if necessary and HCTZ, 12.5 or 25 mg, added as necessary, for at least 4 years | After 1 year of antihypertensive therapy (either drug), LVM had decreased by 27 g (p<0.001). After 2 years, LVM had decreased by a further 11 g (p<0.001 vs year 1). LVM index and relative wall thickness also decreased significantly after 1 and 2 years (p<0.001 for all comparisons) | Sustained blood pressure reduction in hypertensive patients with LVH leads to a reduction in LVM |

HCTZ, hydrochlorothiazide; LIFE, Losartan Intervention for Endpoint Reduction in Hypertension Study; LVH, left ventricular hypertrophy; LVM, left ventricular mass; o.d., once daily; REGAAL, Losartan LVH Regression Study.

atenolol led to a decrease in LVM, an increase in left ventricular midwall shortening and contractility and an increase in left ventricular stroke volume ($p<0.001$ for all parameters).[64]

## Effects on cardiovascular morbidity and mortality

The LIFE study is one of only a few major outcomes studies to demonstrate a significant difference in the effects of two different antihypertensive agents upon major cardiovascular outcomes. Thus, in the main LIFE study and in its substudies, losartan has proved to be superior to the β-blocker atenolol in reducing cardiovascular morbidity and mortality in hypertensive patients with LVH (Table 7).[54–57] In these studies, the primary composite endpoint of cardiovascular death, stroke or myocardial infarction occurred in significantly fewer losartan-treated patients than atenolol-treated patients (11 *vs* 13%; relative risk reduction 13%; $p=0.021$). The difference between the two treatment groups was principally attributable to a more substantial reduction in the incidence of fatal and non-fatal stroke with losartan than with atenolol (5 *vs* 7%; relative risk reduction 25%; $p=0.001$). The incidence of cardiovascular death and myocardial infarction was not different between the two treatment groups. Thus, in conclusion, the LIFE study has demonstrated larger benefits for losartan over atenolol with regard to stroke prevention, despite broadly similar blood pressure reductions being achieved with both agents. As a direct consequence of the findings of the LIFE study, losartan is now licensed in the UK for stroke prevention in patients with hypertension and LVH.

> The LIFE study has demonstrated larger benefits for losartan over atenolol with regard to stroke prevention, despite broadly similar blood pressure reductions being achieved with both agents.

Given the substantial burden that stroke imposes in terms of death and disability, the findings of the LIFE study may have significant implications for clinical practice. Recent guidelines from the British Hypertension Society (*www.bhsoc.org*), have acknowledged the findings of the LIFE study, and have highlighted the potential benefits of angiotensin II receptor antagonist treatment in stroke prevention in such patients.

The impact of widespread implementation of a losartan-based treatment regimen on stroke prevention has been estimated in individuals across the European Union (EU) who meet the inclusion and exclusion criteria of the LIFE study.[65] About 7.8 million individuals aged 55–80 years across the EU are estimated to have hypertension and ECG-diagnosed LVH. According to data from LIFE, approximately 125,000 first strokes would be prevented over a 5.5-year treatment period if these patients were treated with losartan. Therefore, it would appear that a losartan-based treatment strategy has the potential to provide a substantial public health benefit in terms of reducing the burden of morbidity and mortality associated with stroke.

In patients with diabetes, the effects of losartan treatment on cardiovascular mortality and morbidity were more pronounced than in the non-diabetic population. Thus, there was a 24% reduction in the risk of reaching the primary composite endpoint of cardiovascular death, stroke or myocardial infarction with losartan (18 *vs* 23%; $p=0.017$).[56] Cardiovascular mortality and all-cause mortality were also reduced with

**Table 7.** Results of studies comparing the effects of losartan and atenolol on cardiovascular morbidity and mortality in hypertensive patients with left ventricular hypertrophy (LVH).[54–57]

| Study | Patient population | Results | Conclusions |
| --- | --- | --- | --- |
| Dahlof et al, 2002[54] | Hypertensive patients (n=9193) with LVH | Cardiovascular death, stroke or myocardial infarction occurred in 11% of losartan-treated patients and 13% of atenolol-treated patients (p=0.021). Death from cardiovascular disease occurred in 4% of losartan-treated patients and 5% of atenolol-treated patients (NS). Fatal or non-fatal stroke occurred in 5 and 7% of patients, respectively (p=0.001). Furthermore, 4% of patients in both groups had a fatal or non-fatal myocardial infarction (NS) | Losartan was more effective than atenolol in reducing cardiovascular morbidity and mortality, and in reducing the risk of stroke, in hypertensive patients with LVH |
| Kjeldsen et al, 2002[55] | Patients (n=1326) with isolated systolic hypertension and LVH | Cardiovascular death, stroke or myocardial infarction was reduced by 25% with losartan compared with atenolol (p=0.02). Compared with atenolol, patients receiving losartan showed a reduction in cardiovascular mortality (p=0.01), a reduction in fatal and non-fatal stroke (p=0.02) and a reduction in total mortality (p=0.046) | Losartan was more effective than atenolol in reducing cardiovascular morbidity and mortality in patients with isolated systolic hypertension and LVH |
| Lindholm et al, 2002[56] | Hypertensive patients (n=1195) with diabetes and LVH | Cardiovascular death, stroke or myocardial infarction occurred in 17.6% of losartan-treated patients and 22.8% of atenolol-treated patients (p=0.031). Death from cardiovascular disease occurred in 6.5 and 10.0% of patients, respectively (p=0.028). All-cause mortality rates were 10.7 and 17.1%, respectively (p=0.002) | Losartan was more effective than atenolol in reducing cardiovascular morbidity and mortality in hypertensive patients with diabetes |
| Devereux et al, 2003[57] | Hypertensive patients (n=688) with LVH but no clinical evidence of vascular disease | The primary composite endpoint occurred in 8.3% of losartan-treated patients and 10.2% of atenolol-treated patients (p=0.008). Cardiovascular death occurred in 3.0 and 3.8% of patients, respectively (NS). Fatal or non-fatal stroke occurred in 3.7 and 5.5% of patients, respectively (p<0.001) and fatal or non-fatal myocardial infarction occurred in 3.2 and 2.9% of patients, respectively (NS) | Losartan was more effective than atenolol in reducing cardiovascular morbidity and mortality, and the risk of stroke, in hypertensive patients with LVH but no clinical evidence of vascular disease |

NS, not significant.

losartan, by 37% (*p*=0.028) and 39% (*p*=0.002) respectively.[56] Thus, these data indicate that hypertensive diabetics with LVH appear to derive more benefit from treatment with losartan than with atenolol.

### Effects on the risk of diabetes

The risk of new-onset diabetes in patients with hypertension who receive antihypertensive therapy was investigated in a substudy of LIFE.[66] Of the 9222 patients who were randomised to receive antihypertensive therapy with losartan or atenolol in LIFE, 7998 did not have diabetes at baseline and were therefore at risk of developing the condition during the study. Using a prediction scoring method, the authors of the substudy showed that new-onset diabetes occurred in significantly fewer losartan-treated patients than atenolol-treated patients (6 *vs* 8%; *p*<0.001). Thus, antihypertensive therapy with losartan was associated with a lower risk of developing diabetes than treatment with atenolol.

> Antihypertensive therapy with losartan was associated with a lower risk of developing diabetes than treatment with atenolol.

## Clinical efficacy in renal protection

Hypertension plays a major role in the progression of chronic renal disease and contributes towards morbidity and mortality in haemodialysis patients. Furthermore, angiotensin II appears to be involved in the progression of renal damage.[11] Thus, by reducing blood pressure and by inhibiting the actions of angiotensin II in the kidney, losartan has the potential to offer protection against the progression of renal disease. Indeed, numerous studies have shown that losartan has renoprotective effects that are mediated through regulation of glomerular haemodynamics and a reduction in proteinuria. Open and placebo-controlled studies have shown that losartan significantly reduces albuminuria and the risk of end-stage renal disease in hypertensive patients with nephropathy and/or diabetes, renal transplant recipients and children with chronic renal disease.[12,24,67–71] Comparative studies have shown that losartan is superior to captopril and amlodipine in improving renal function in hypertensive patients with or without renal impairment.[3,36,43,72] Furthermore, losartan has similar renoprotective effects to enalapril and fosinopril in such patients.[34,38,73,74] In one comparative study, losartan was shown to be superior to enalapril in improving renal function.[59]

> Losartan is superior to captopril and amlodipine in improving renal function in hypertensive patients.

In addition, a substudy of the LIFE trial has demonstrated that losartan elicits a greater reduction in albuminuria over time than does atenolol.[75]

## Clinical efficacy in combination with HCTZ

Although losartan is effective in reducing blood pressure when given as monotherapy, some patients with more resistant hypertension require two different antihypertensive drugs to control their blood pressure. Losartan administered concomitantly with the thiazide diuretic HCTZ has been established as a suitable combination because of the complementary and different pharmacological mechanisms of action of the two drugs. A number of clinical studies have shown that a

A combination of losartan and HCTZ can be considered for patients whose blood pressure is not adequately controlled with losartan monotherapy, including those with diabetes and renal dysfunction.

combination of losartan and HCTZ reduces blood pressure to a greater extent than either drug alone (Table 8).[5,6,70,76–81] Furthermore, combination therapy has been shown to reduce albuminuria in hypertensive, diabetic patients with nephropathy to a greater extent than monotherapy with either drug.[70] Thus, a combination of losartan and HCTZ can be considered for patients whose blood pressure is not adequately controlled with losartan monotherapy, including those with diabetes and renal dysfunction. Losartan is available in combination with HCTZ for this purpose.

In comparative trials, a combination of losartan and HCTZ has shown comparable antihypertensive efficacy to the angiotensin II receptor antagonist telmisartan, the ACE inhibitor enalapril and the calcium-channel blockers amlodipine and nifedipine gastrointestinal therapeutic system (GITS) (Table 9).[42,47,48,82–84] In one study, however, a combination of telmisartan and HCTZ appeared to have greater antihypertensive efficacy than a combination of losartan and HCTZ.[85]

## Clinical efficacy in combination with nifedipine

The combination of nifedipine and losartan appear to improve the control of blood pressure compared with either monotherapy.

A recent 8-week, randomised, double-blind study has evaluated the relative efficacy of a combination of low-dose nifedipine (20 mg/day) and losartan (50 mg/day) compared with either agent given as monotherapy.[86] A total of 300 patients with mild-to-moderate hypertension were randomised to treatment with either the combination or the individual monotherapy. All three treatment regimens significantly lowered mean 24-hour diastolic blood pressure, though losartan monotherapy appeared to lower blood pressure by a lesser extent than in patients receiving the combination (–10.6, –8.4 and –5.4 mmHg for the combination, nifedipine monotherapy and losartan monotherapy, respectively; $p<0.05$ for the combination vs losartan). Similar observations were reported with regard to 24-hour mean systolic blood pressure, daytime blood pressure, and night-time blood pressure. In addition, the smoothness index (as a measure of the homogeneity of the blood-pressure lowering response) was greatest in the combination arm than with either monotherapy, and this difference was significant when compared with losartan (for diastolic blood pressure) and for both monotherapies with regard to systolic blood pressure. All treatment regimens were well tolerated in this study. Thus, the combination of nifedipine and losartan appear to improve the control of blood pressure compared with either monotherapy.

## Safety

The safety and tolerability of losartan have been investigated in numerous clinical trials. The results of these trials have shown that losartan has an excellent safety profile. This has been attributed to the drug's specificity and selectivity for $AT_1$ receptors.[87]

**Table 8.** Studies investigating the antihypertensive efficacy of losartan in combination with the diuretic hydrochlorothiazide (HCTZ).[5,6,70,76–81]

| Study | Design | Patient population | Treatment regimens | Results | Conclusions |
|---|---|---|---|---|---|
| Dunlay et al., 1995[6] | Open-label | Patients (n=179) with severe hypertension | Initial therapy with losartan, 50 or 100 mg o.d, followed by the addition of HCTZ, 12.5 or 25 mg o.d, a calcium-channel blocker; and/or atenolol as necessary, for 12 weeks | Of the patients who achieved target diastolic blood pressure, 24% were on losartan monotherapy, 41% were on losartan + HCTZ, and 4% required losartan + HCTZ + a calcium-channel blocker | The addition of HCTZ to losartan provided further blood pressure control in patients whose blood pressure could not be controlled on losartan alone |
| Weber et al., 1995[5] | Randomised, double-blind, placebo-controlled | Hypertensive patients (n=122) | Losartan, 50 or 100 mg o.d, or 50 mg b.d, or placebo, for 4 weeks. Patients whose blood pressure was not controlled after this time also received HCTZ, 12.5 mg, for a further 2 weeks | The addition of HCTZ produced a further reduction in blood pressure in all four treatment groups | The addition of HCTZ to losartan provided further reductions in blood pressure beyond those achieved with losartan monotherapy |
| MacKay et al., 1996[76] | Randomised, double-blind, parallel-group, placebo-controlled | Patients (n=703) with essential hypertension | Losartan, 50 mg o.d; HCTZ, 12.5 mg o.d; losartan, 50 mg, + HCTZ, 6.25 or 12.5 mg o.d; or placebo; for 12 weeks | Combination therapy (with 12.5 mg HCTZ) produced a greater reduction in blood pressure than with either drug alone (p<0.001). The blood pressure reduction with losartan, 50 mg, + HCTZ, 6.25 mg, was no different from that achieved with either drug alone | A combination of losartan, 50 mg, and HCTZ, 12.5 mg, produced a greater reduction in blood pressure than either drug alone |
| Ruilope et al., 1996[77] | Randomised, double-blind | Patients (n=312) with moderate-to-severe hypertension whose blood pressure was not controlled with losartan monotherapy | Losartan, 50 mg, + HCTZ, 6.25, 12.5 or 25 mg o.d, or losartan, 50 mg, + placebo, for 12 weeks | The reduction in blood pressure observed with losartan + HCTZ, 6.25 mg, was no different from that observed with losartan + placebo. However, the reductions in blood pressure with losartan + 12.5 or 25 mg HCTZ were greater than those with losartan/placebo (p<0.05) | The addition of HCTZ, 12.5 or 25 mg, to losartan produced effective control of blood pressure in a substantial majority of patients who showed only a partial response to losartan monotherapy |

o.d, once daily.

**Table 8.** Continued

| Study | Design | Patient population | Treatment regimens | Results | Conclusions |
|---|---|---|---|---|---|
| Flack et al., 2001[78] | Randomised, double-blind, parallel-group, placebo-controlled | African-American patients (n=440) with mild-to-moderate hypertension | Losartan, 50–150 mg o.d.; or losartan, 50 mg, + HCTZ 12.5 mg o.d.; or losartan, 100 mg, + HCTZ, 25 mg o.d.; or placebo; for 12 weeks | Response rates were 45.8% with losartan alone; 62.7% with losartan + HCTZ; and 27.2% with placebo. The reduction in diastolic and systolic blood pressure with losartan/HCTZ was greater than with losartan alone (p<0.01) | A combination of losartan and HCTZ gives a greater reduction in blood pressure than losartan alone |
| Oparil et al., 2001[79] | Open-label | Patients (n=131) with severe hypertension | Losartan, 50 mg, + HCTZ, 12.5 mg o.d, increased to 100/25 mg if necessary, for 12 weeks. Felodipine and/or atenolol were then added if blood pressure was still not controlled | Combination therapy reduced blood pressure compared with baseline (p<0.01). By 12 weeks, 35% were still taking losartan/ HCTZ, and 48% were taking 100/25 mg + felodipine | Losartan/HCTZ alone or in combination with other antihypertensive agents is effective and generally well tolerated in patients with severe hypertension |
| de Pablos-Velasco et al., 2002[70] | Randomised, open-label | Patients (n=90) with type 2 diabetes, hypertension and microalbuminuria | Losartan, 50 mg o.d, for 4 weeks. If further blood pressure control required, patients titrated to 100 mg o.d, or losartan, 50 mg, + HCTZ, 12.5 mg for a further 4 weeks | After the additional 4 weeks, patients receiving losartan, 100 mg, showed a further reduction in blood pressure (p<0.001 vs 50 mg). Combination therapy reduced blood pressure even further (p<0.001 vs 50 mg). Albuminuria decreased with losartan, 100 mg (p=0.002 vs 50 mg), and decreased even further with losartan/HCTZ (p<0.001 vs 50 mg) | When blood pressure is not controlled with losartan, 50 mg, increasing the dose to 100 mg or adding HCTZ achieves a further reduction in blood pressure and albuminuria in hypertensive, diabetic patients with nephropathy |

o.d., once daily.

**Table 8.** Continued

| Study | Design | Patient population | Treatment regimens | Results | Conclusions |
|---|---|---|---|---|---|
| Gradman et al., 2002[80] | Randomised, double-blind, placebo-controlled, parallel-group | Patients (n=446) with moderate-to-severe hypertension | Losartan, 50/HCTZ 12.5 mg o.d., or losartan, 100/HCTZ 25 mg o.d., or placebo, for 8 weeks | Trough diastolic blood pressure showed a greater reduction with active treatments than with placebo (p<0.001 for both treatments). The reduction with losartan 100/HCTZ 25 was greater than with losartan 50/HCTZ 12.5 (p<0.001). Response rates were 86.7, 78.9 and 50.0% for 100/25, 50/12.5 and placebo groups, respectively | A combination of losartan and HCTZ was effective and well tolerated in patients with moderate-to-severe hypertension. Higher doses of the two drugs provided greater antihypertensive efficacy than the lower doses |
| Dickson et al., 2003[81] | Open-label | Hypertensive patients (n=32) with mild-to-moderate renal impairment | Losartan, 50 mg + HCTZ 12.5 mg o.d., for 4 weeks. This was increased to 100/25 mg if necessary for a further 8 weeks | Combination therapy reduced systolic and diastolic blood pressure (p<0.01 vs baseline). Of the 28 patients with measurements at 12 weeks 46% remained on losartan 50/HCTZ 12.5, 21% were on the higher doses, and 33% required additional antihypertensive medication | Losartan + HCTZ was effective in controlling blood pressure and well tolerated in hypertensive patients with mild-to-moderate renal impairment |

o.d., once daily.

**Table 9.** Studies comparing the antihypertensive efficacy of a combination of losartan and hydrochlorothiazide (HCTZ) with that of other antihypertensive agents. [42,47,48,82–85]

| Study | Design | Patient population | Treatment regimens | Results | Conclusions |
|---|---|---|---|---|---|
| **Telmisartan** | | | | | |
| Lacourciere et al., 2003[85] | Prospective, randomised, open-label, blinded-endpoint | Patients (n=397) with mild-to-moderate hypertension | Losartan, 50 mg, + HCTZ, 12.5 mg o.d., or telmisartan, 40 mg + HCTZ, 12.5 mg o.d., or telmisartan, 80 mg + HCTZ, 12.5 mg o.d., for 6 weeks | Both telmisartan regimens reduced systolic and diastolic blood pressure by a greater degree than losartan during the last 6 hours of the dosing interval ($p<0.05$), and reduced mean 24-hour systolic blood pressure by a greater degree ($p<0.001$). Only the higher dose of telmisartan lowered mean 24-hour diastolic blood pressure by a greater degree than losartan ($p<0.001$) | Telmisartan/HCTZ shows greater antihypertensive efficacy than losartan/HCTZ |
| Neutel et al., 2003[82] | Randomised, prospective, open, parallel-group, blinded-endpoint | Patients (n=714) with mild-to-moderate hypertension | Losartan, 50 mg, + HCTZ, 12.5 mg o.d., or telmisartan, 80 mg o.d., for 6 weeks | Reductions in diastolic and systolic blood pressure were similar for the two groups | Losartan/HCTZ and telmisartan show comparable antihypertensive efficacy in patients with mild-to-moderate hypertension |
| **Enalapril** | | | | | |
| Townsend et al., 1995[83] | Randomised, double-blind, parallel-group | Patients (n=268) with mild-to-moderate hypertension | Losartan, 50 mg o.d., for 8 weeks. HCTZ, 12.5 mg, added if necessary for a further 4 weeks, or enalapril, 5 mg o.d. for 4 weeks, 10 mg o.d., for a further 4 weeks if necessary, and HCTZ, 25 mg o.d. added if necessary after another 4 weeks | Both treatments significantly reduced systolic and diastolic blood pressure after 4, 8 and 12 weeks. The percentage of patients reaching target diastolic blood pressure was similar for the two groups. The mean decrease in diastolic blood pressure was greater with losartan than enalapril in black patients ($p=0.02$) and elderly patients ($p=0.03$) | Losartan with or without HCTZ showed comparable antihypertensive efficacy to enalapril with or without HCTZ. Losartan appeared to be more effective in special patient groups |

GITS, gastrointestinal therapeutic system; o.d., once daily.

**Table 9.** Continued

| Study | Design | Patient population | Treatment regimens | Results | Conclusions |
|---|---|---|---|---|---|
| **Enalapril** | | | | | |
| Naidoo et al., 1999[84] | Randomised, double-blind, parallel-group | Patients (n=349) with uncontrolled moderate-to-severe hypertension | Losartan 100 mg/HCTZ 25 mg o.d., or enalapril 10 mg/HCTZ 25 mg o.d., for 12 weeks | The reduction in diastolic blood pressure compared with baseline was similar for the two drug combinations. Trough diastolic blood pressure was normalised in 63% of patients receiving losartan/HCTZ and in 58% of those receiving enalapril/HCTZ | Losartan in combination with HCTZ shows comparable antihypertensive efficacy to enalapril in combination with HCTZ |
| **Amlodipine** | | | | | |
| Oparil et al., 1996[42] | Randomised, double-blind, parallel-group | Patients (n=190) with essential hypertension | Losartan, 50 mg o.d. with HCTZ, 12.5 mg added if necessary after 4 weeks, and HCTZ, 25 mg, added if necessary after 8 weeks, or amlodipine, 5 mg o.d., increased to 10 mg o.d. if necessary after 4 weeks and HCTZ, 25 mg, added if necessary after 8 weeks, for a total treatment period of 12 weeks | Reductions in systolic blood pressure and trough diastolic blood pressure were comparable between the two groups at 4, 8 and 12 weeks. The percentage of patients reaching target diastolic blood pressure was also comparable: 68% for losartan and 71% for amlodipine | Losartan with or without HCTZ showed comparable antihypertensive efficacy to amlodipine with or without HCTZ in patients with essential hypertension |
| **Nifedipine GITS** | | | | | |
| Weir et al., 1996[47] | Randomised, double-blind, parallel-group | Patients (n=223) with essential hypertension | Losartan, 50 mg o.d., titrated to 50 mg + HCTZ, 12.5 mg, after 4 weeks and 50 mg + HCTZ, 25 mg after 8 weeks, or nifedipine GITS, 30 mg o.d., titrated to 60 mg after 4 weeks and 90 mg after 8 weeks, for a total treatment period of 12 weeks | The reductions in systolic blood pressure and trough diastolic blood pressure were comparable after 4, 8 and 12 weeks. The percentage of patients reaching target diastolic blood pressure was also comparable: 74% for losartan and 68% for nifedipine GITS | Losartan with or without HCTZ shows comparable antihypertensive efficacy to nifedipine GITS in patients with essential hypertension |

GITS, gastrointestinal therapeutic system; o.d., once daily.

**Table 9.** Continued

| Study | Design | Patient population | Treatment regimens | Results | Conclusions |
|---|---|---|---|---|---|
| Conlin et al., 1998[48] | Randomised, double-blind, parallel-group | Elderly (≥65 years) patients (n=140) with diastolic hypertension | Losartan, 50 mg o.d., titrated to 50 mg + HCTZ, 12.5 mg, after 4 weeks and 50 mg + HCTZ, 25 mg, after 8 weeks, or nifedipine GITS, 30 mg o.d., titrated to 60 mg after 4 weeks and 90 mg after 8 weeks, for a total treatment period of 12 weeks | The reduction in diastolic blood pressure at 4 weeks was greater with nifedipine than losartan ($p<0.05$), but the reductions at 8 and 12 weeks were comparable. Reductions in systolic blood pressure were comparable at all time points. The percentage of patients reaching target diastolic blood pressure was also comparable: 81% for losartan and 90% for nifedipine GITS | Losartan with or without HCTZ shows antihypertensive efficacy comparable with nifedipine GITS in elderly patients with diastolic hypertension |

GITS, gastrointestinal therapeutic system; o.d., once daily.

## Adverse events

In a review of safety data from 16 <u>double-blind</u> trials, in which approximately 2900 hypertensive patients received treatment with losartan, headache (14.1%), upper respiratory tract infection (6.5%), dizziness (4.1%), asthenia/fatigue (3.8%) and cough (3.1%) were the most frequently reported <u>adverse events</u>.[87] The incidence of these adverse events was comparable with those observed in patients who received <u>placebo</u> (Figure 1). The most frequent adverse events considered to be related to treatment were headache (4.2%), dizziness (2.4%) and asthenia/fatigue (2.0%). Of these, only dizziness occurred more frequently in losartan-treated patients than among those who received placebo (1.3%).[87]

In the same review, the profile of adverse events observed with other antihypertensive agents was generally similar to that observed with losartan. However, notable differences were: a higher incidence of asthenia/fatigue with other agents (6.7% for ACE inhibitors, 5.9% for atenolol, 5.5% with HCTZ vs 3.8% for losartan), apart from a lower incidence (zero) with the <u>calcium-channel blocker</u> felodipine; a higher incidence of cough with ACE inhibitors (8.8 vs 3.1% for losartan); a higher incidence of dizziness (7.4 vs 2.4%) and insomnia (4.4 vs 1.1%) with atenolol than for losartan, respectively; and a higher incidence of oedema (14.0 vs 1.7%) and diarrhoea (4.7 vs 1.9%) with felodipine than losartan, respectively.

The percentage of patients who withdrew from treatment due to adverse events was 2.3% for losartan, this figure being comparable with that observed with ACE inhibitors (2.5%) and HCTZ (3.0%), and much lower than that observed with atenolol (8.8%) and felodipine (9.3%).

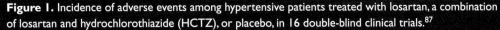

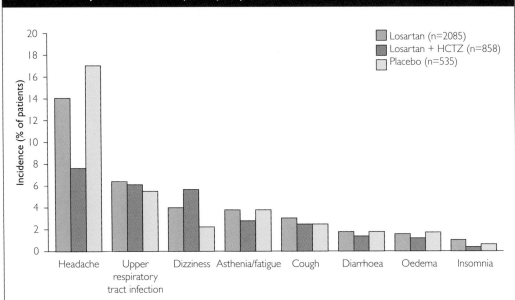

**Figure 1.** Incidence of adverse events among hypertensive patients treated with losartan, a combination of losartan and hydrochlorothiazide (HCTZ), or placebo, in 16 double-blind clinical trials.[87]

The lower incidence of cough with losartan compared with ACE inhibitors is not unexpected. A chronic dry cough is the most common adverse event associated with ACE inhibitors due to the fact that they increase levels of bradykinin in the lungs. This, in turn, increases bronchial sensitivity and induces a cough.[88] Angiotensin II receptor antagonists have no direct effect on bradykinin levels and thus do not produce the dry cough experienced with ACE inhibitors. Indeed, several comparative trials have confirmed that the incidence of dry cough is significantly lower with losartan than with ACE inhibitors (Table 10).[4,31,74,88–91]

## Laboratory parameters

No clinically relevant or unexpected changes in laboratory variables have occurred during treatment with losartan in clinical trials. The most common abnormal laboratory parameter has been increased levels of alanine aminotransferase (1.9% of patients).[87] This increase has tended to be small and transient in nature. Hyperkalaemia has been reported in 1.5% of losartan-treated patients, which is comparable with the incidence among patients treated with ACE inhibitors (1.3%).

## Safety in combination with HCTZ

In a review of 16 clinical trials the incidence of adverse events with a combination of losartan and HCTZ tended to be lower than that observed with losartan alone (Figure 1).[87] The only exception to this was a higher incidence of dizziness with combined treatment (5.7 vs 4.1%). As with losartan alone, the incidence of asthenia/fatigue (2.9%) and cough (2.6%) was lower with combined losartan/HCTZ treatment than with other antihypertensive agents. A total of 2.8% of patients who

**Table 10.** Incidence of dry cough in clinical trials comparing losartan and angiotensin-converting enzyme (ACE) inhibitors.[4,31,74,88–91]

| Study[a] | ACE inhibitor | Incidence of cough with ACE inhibitor (%) | Incidence of cough with losartan (%) | p-value |
|---|---|---|---|---|
| Lacourciere et al., 1994[89] | Lisinopril | 71.7 | 29.2 | <0.01 |
| Ramsay and Yeo, 1995[90] | Lisinopril | 72 | 29 | <0.01 |
| Chan et al., 1997[91] | Lisinopril | 97 | 18 | <0.001 |
| Paster et al., 1998[88] | Lisinopril | 87.5 | 36.7 | <0.0001 |
| Gradman et al., 1995[4] | Enalapril | 8 | 3 | Not given |
| Tikkanen et al., 1995[31] | Enalapril | 12.2 | 1.0 | <0.01 |
| Lacourciere et al., 2000[74] | Enalapril | 14 | 0 | 0.006 |

[a]The incidence of cough was determined by a self- or nurse-administered symptom questionnaire with the exception of studies by Lacourciere et al., and Gradman et al., which both reported the incidence of cough through the reporting of cough as an adverse event.

received combination therapy withdrew from treatment due to adverse events, which was comparable to the figures with losartan (2.3%) and HCTZ (3.0%) alone. As expected, combination therapy was associated with an increase in serum uric acid concentrations (3.5%) and a decrease in serum potassium concentrations (3.2%). The incidence of these events was comparable to those observed with HCTZ alone (3.9 and 4.3%, respectively).

In a study comparing losartan/HCTZ and nifedipine GITS in elderly hypertensive patients, patients receiving nifedipine experienced significantly more adverse events than patients receiving losartan/HCTZ (54 *vs* 36%; *p*<0.05), and significantly more patients receiving nifedipine experienced swollen ankles (24 *vs* 5%; *p*=0.001).[64] Thus, a combination of losartan and HCTZ was better tolerated than nifedipine GITS in elderly hypertensive patients.

The incidence of adverse events with a combination of losartan and HCTZ tended to be lower than that observed with losartan alone.

### Special patient groups

In studies published since the 1995 review of clinical trials, losartan has proved to be well tolerated in patients with renal impairment, in renal transplant recipients, in patients with diabetes and associated nephropathy, in elderly patients and in children.[10,11,36,49,71,74,87] In one study, 13 out of 52 children (25%) with chronic proteinuric renal disease experienced an adverse event.[71] Most of the events improved or resolved with dose adjustment, although nine out of the 52 children (17%) discontinued with treatment because of adverse events.[71]

# Pharmacoeconomics

A US economic study has evaluated the cost-effectiveness of losartan given with conventional antihypertensive therapy (excluding ACE inhibitors and other angiotensin II receptor antagonists) in providing renal protection in diabetic patients with end-stage renal disease.[92] The results showed that such treatment reduced the number of days with end-stage renal disease by 33.6 days per patient over 3.5 years (*p*=0.004 *vs* placebo plus conventional therapy) and consequently reduced the cost associated with end-stage renal disease by $5144 per patient (*p*=0.003). After taking into account the cost of losartan, the net saving was $3522 per patient over 3.5 years (*p*=0.041). This equates to £2515 per patient over 3.5 years.[93] Thus, treatment with losartan reduced the incidence of end-stage renal disease and also produced substantial cost savings in diabetic patients with end-stage renal disease.

Treatment with losartan reduced the incidence of end-stage renal disease and also produced substantial cost savings in diabetic patients with end-stage renal disease.

## Key points

- Losartan is a non-peptide angiotensin II receptor antagonist that acts by directly blocking the effects of angiotensin II at its $AT_1$ receptors.

- Losartan is indicated for the treatment of hypertension, for reducing the risk of stroke in hypertensive patients with LVH, and for providing renal protection in patients with type 2 diabetes and nephropathy.

- After oral administration, losartan is metabolised in the liver into an active metabolite. This metabolite is responsible for most of the antihypertensive effect of the drug.

- Losartan inhibits the vasoconstrictor actions of angiotensin II in a dose-dependent manner. The effect lasts for more than 24 hours, suggesting that once-daily dosing is appropriate.

- Open and placebo-controlled studies have shown that losartan, 50 mg once daily, is an effective antihypertensive agent. The dose can be titrated to 100 mg once daily for patients whose blood pressure is not controlled at the lower dose.

- Studies comparing the antihypertensive efficacies of losartan and other angiotensin II receptor antagonists have conflicting results: some studies suggest that losartan is as effective as other angiotensin II receptor antagonists, whilst other studies suggest that irbesartan, candesartan and telmisartan are superior.

- Studies comparing the blood pressure-lowering effects of losartan and other antihypertensive agents suggest that losartan has comparable efficacy to ACE inhibitors, calcium-channel blockers and the β-blocker atenolol.

- Losartan has a beneficial effect on LVH, leading to a reduction in LVM and an improvement in left ventricular performance. Comparative studies suggest that losartan is more effective in this respect than ACE inhibitors, calcium-channel blockers and atenolol.

- Losartan is superior to atenolol in reducing cardiovascular morbidity and mortality, particularly the risk of stroke, in hypertensive patients with LVH.

- Losartan has renoprotective effects that are mediated through the regulation of glomerular haemodynamics and a decrease in proteinuria. Losartan appears to be superior in this respect to other antihypertensive agents.

- A combination of losartan and the thiazide diuretic HCTZ reduces blood pressure by a greater extent than either drug alone. Such therapy can be considered in patients whose blood pressure is not controlled by losartan alone. Losartan is available in combination with HCTZ for this purpose.

- Losartan was well tolerated in clinical trials, with a safety profile comparable with that of placebo. The only adverse event to occur more frequently with losartan was dizziness.

- The safety profile of losartan was generally comparable with that of other antihypertensive agents, though it was associated with a much lower incidence of cough and asthenia/fatigue than ACE inhibitors.

- The safety profile of losartan and HCTZ in combination is comparable with that of losartan alone.

# References

A list of the published evidence which has been reviewed in compiling the preceding section of *BESTMEDICINE*.

1 Martina B, Dieterle T, Weinbacher M, Battegay E. Effects of losartan titrated to losartan/hydrochlorothiazide and amlodipine on left ventricular mass in patients with mild-to-moderate hypertension. A double-blind randomized controlled study. *Cardiology* 1999; **92**: 110–14.

2 Fauvel JP, Velon S, Berra N *et al.* Effects of losartan on renal function in patients with essential hypertension. *J Cardiovasc Pharmacol* 1996; **28**: 259–63.

3 Fernandez-Andrade C, Russo D, Iversen B *et al.* Comparison of losartan and amlodipine in renally impaired hypertensive patients. *Kidney Int Suppl* 1998; **68**: S120–4.

4 Gradman AH, Arcuri KE, Goldberg AI *et al.* A randomized, placebo-controlled, double-blind, parallel study of various doses of losartan potassium compared with enalapril maleate in patients with essential hypertension. *Hypertension* 1995; **25**: 1345–50.

5 Weber MA, Byyny RL, Pratt JH *et al.* Blood pressure effects of the angiotensin II receptor blocker, losartan. *Arch Intern Med* 1995; **155**: 405–11.

6 Dunlay MC, Fitzpatrick V, Chrysant S *et al.* Losartan potassium as initial therapy in patients with severe hypertension. *J Hum Hypertens* 1995; **9**: 861–7.

7 Byyny RL. Antihypertensive efficacy of the angiotensin II AT1-receptor antagonist losartan: results of a randomized, double-blind, placebo-controlled, parallel-group trial using 24-hour blood pressure monitoring. Ambulatory blood pressure monitoring study group. *Blood Press Suppl* 1996; **2**: 71–7.

8 Himmelmann A, Svensson A, Bergbrant A, Hansson L. Long-term effects of losartan on blood pressure and left ventricular structure in essential hypertension. *J Hum Hypertens* 1996; **10**: 729–34.

9 Ikeda LS, Harm SC, Arcuri KE, Goldberg AI, Sweet CS. Comparative antihypertensive effects of losartan 50 mg and losartan 50 mg titrated to 100 mg in patients with essential hypertension. *Blood Press* 1997; **6**: 35–43.

10 del Castillo D, Campistol JM, Guirado L *et al.* Efficacy and safety of losartan in the treatment of hypertension in renal transplant recipients. *Kidney Int Suppl* 1998; **68**: S135–9.

11 Toto R, Shultz P, Raij L *et al.* Efficacy and tolerability of losartan in hypertensive patients with renal impairment. *Hypertension* 1998; **31**: 684–91.

12 Hadjigavriel M, Kyriakides G. Efficacy and safety of losartan in renal transplant recipients. *Transplant Proc* 1999; **31**: 3300–1.

13 Fernandez-Vega F, Abellan J, Sanz de Castro S *et al.* A study on the efficacy and safety of losartan in elderly patients with mild to moderate essential hypertension. *Int Urol Nephrol* 2001; **32**: 519–23.

14 Cushman WC, Brady WE, Gazdick LP, Zeldin RK. The effect of a losartan-based treatment regimen on isolated systolic hypertension. *J Clin Hypertens (Greenwich)* 2002; **4**: 101–7.

15 Fridman KU, Elmfeldt D, Wysocki M, Friberg PR, Andersson OK. Influence of AT1 receptor blockade on blood pressure, renal haemodynamics and hormonal responses to intravenous angiotensin II infusion in hypertensive patients. *Blood Press* 2002; **11**: 244–52.

16 Hedner T, Oparil S, Rasmussen K *et al.* A comparison of the angiotensin II antagonists valsartan and losartan in the treatment of essential hypertension. *Am J Hypertens* 1999; **12**: 414–7.

17 Monterroso VH, Rodriguez Chavez V, Carbajal ET *et al.* Use of ambulatory blood pressure monitoring to compare antihypertensive efficacy and safety of two angiotensin II receptor antagonists, losartan and valsartan. Losartan trial investigators. *Adv Ther* 2000; **17**: 117–31.

18 Elliott WJ, Calhoun DA, DeLucca PT *et al.* Losartan versus valsartan in the treatment of patients with mild to moderate essential hypertension: data from a multicenter, randomized, double-blind, 12-week trial. *Clin Ther* 2001; **23**: 1166–79.

19 Andersson OK, Neldam S. A comparison of the antihypertensive effects of candesartan cilexetil and losartan in patients with mild to moderate hypertension. *J Hum Hypertens* 1997; **11(Suppl 2)**: S63–4.

20 Andersson OK, Neldam S. The antihypertensive effect and tolerability of candesartan cilexetil, a new generation angiotensin II antagonist, in comparison with losartan. *Blood Press* 1998; **7**: 53–9.

21 Gradman AH, Lewin A, Bowling BT *et al.* Comparative effects of candesartan cilexetil and losartan in patients with systemic hypertension. Candesartan versus losartan efficacy comparison (CANDLE) study group. *Heart Dis* 1999; **1**: 52–7.

22 Lacourciere Y, Asmar R. A comparison of the efficacy and duration of action of candesartan cilexetil and losartan as assessed by clinic and ambulatory blood pressure after a missed dose, in truly hypertensive patients: a placebo-controlled, forced titration study. Candesartan/losartan study investigators. *Am J Hypertens* 1999; **12**: 1181–7.

23 Manolis AJ, Grossman E, Jelakovic B *et al.* Effects of losartan and candesartan monotherapy and losartan/hydrochlorothiazide combination therapy in patients with mild to moderate hypertension. Losartan trial investigators. *Clin Ther* 2000; **22**: 1186–203.

24 Bakris G, Gradman A, Reif M *et al.* Antihypertensive efficacy of candesartan in comparison to losartan: the CLAIM study. *J Clin Hypertens (Greenwich)* 2001; **3**: 16–21.

25 Vidt DG, White WB, Ridley E *et al*. A forced titration study of antihypertensive efficacy of candesartan cilexetil in comparison to losartan: CLAIM study II. *J Hum Hypertens* 2001; **15**: 475–80.

26 Oparil S, Guthrie R, Lewin AJ *et al*. An elective-titration study of the comparative effectiveness of two angiotensin II-receptor blockers, irbesartan and losartan. Irbesartan/losartan study investigators. *Clin Ther* 1998; **20**: 398–409.

27 Kassler-Taub K, Littlejohn T, Elliott W, Ruddy T, Adler E. Comparative efficacy of two angiotensin II receptor antagonists, irbesartan and losartan in mild-to-moderate hypertension. Irbesartan/losartan study investigators. *Am J Hypertens* 1998; **11**: 445–53.

28 Mallion J, Siche J, Lacourciere Y. ABPM comparison of the antihypertensive profiles of the selective angiotensin II receptor antagonists telmisartan and losartan in patients with mild-to-moderate hypertension. *J Hum Hypertens* 1999; **13**: 657–64.

29 Martina B, Dieterle T, Sigle JP, Surber C, Battegay E. Effects of telmisartan and losartan on left ventricular mass in mild-to-moderate hypertension. A randomized, double-blind trial. *Cardiology* 2003; **99**: 169–70.

30 Oparil S, Williams D, Chrysant SG, Marbury TC, Neutel J. Comparative efficacy of olmesartan, losartan, valsartan, and irbesartan in the control of essential hypertension. *J Clin Hypertens (Greenwich)* 2001; **3**: 283–91.

31 Tikkanen I, Omvik P, Jensen HA. Comparison of the angiotensin II antagonist losartan with the angiotensin converting enzyme inhibitor enalapril in patients with essential hypertension. *J Hypertens* 1995; **13**: 1343–51.

32 Byyny RL, Merrill DD, Bradstreet TE, Sweet CS. An inpatient trial of the safety and efficacy of losartan compared with placebo and enalapril in patients with essential hypertension. *Cardiovasc Drugs Ther* 1996; **10**: 313–19.

33 Ruff D, Gazdick LP, Berman R, Goldberg AI, Sweet CS. Comparative effects of combination drug therapy regimens commencing with either losartan potassium, an angiotensin II receptor antagonist, or enalapril maleate for the treatment of severe hypertension. *J Hypertens* 1996; **14**: 263–70.

34 Kim W, Lee S, Kang SK *et al*. Effects of angiotensin converting enzyme inhibitor and angiotensin II receptor antagonist therapy in hypertensive renal transplant recipients. *Transplant Proc* 2002; **34**: 3223–4.

35 Scholze J, Stapff M. Start of therapy with the angiotensin II antagonist losartan after immediate switch from pretreatment with an ACE inhibitor. *Br J Clin Pharmacol* 1998; **46**: 169–72.

36 Schulz E, Bech JN, Pedersen EB, Muller GA. A randomized, double-blind, parallel study on the safety and antihypertensive efficacy of losartan compared to captopril in patients with mild to moderate hypertension and impaired renal function. *Nephrol Dial Transplant* 1999; **14(Suppl 4)**: 27–8.

37 Bakris G, Sica D, Ram V *et al*. A comparative trial of controlled-onset, extended-release verapamil, enalapril, and losartan on blood pressure and heart rate changes. *Am J Hypertens* 2002; **15**: 53–7.

38 Kavgaci H, Sahin A, Onder Ersoz H, Erem C, Ozdemir F. The effects of losartan and fosinopril in hypertensive type 2 diabetic patients. *Diabetes Res Clin Pract* 2002; **58**: 19–25.

39 Okuguchi T, Osanai T, Fujiwara N *et al*. Effect of losartan on nocturnal blood pressure in patients with stroke: comparison with angiotensin converting enzyme inhibitor. *Am J Hypertens* 2002; **15**: 998–1002.

40 Chanudet X, De Champvallins M. Antihypertensive efficacy and tolerability of low-dose perindopril/indapamide combination compared with losartan in the treatment of essential hypertension. *Int J Clin Pract* 2001; **55**: 233–9.

41 Campo C, Segura J, Fernandez ML *et al*. A prospective comparison of four antihypertensive agents in daily clinical practice. *J Clin Hypertens (Greenwich)* 2001; **3**: 139–44.

42 Oparil S, Barr E, Elkins M *et al*. Efficacy, tolerability, and effects on quality of life of losartan, alone or with hydrochlorothiazide, versus amlodipine, alone or with hydrochlorothiazide, in patients with essential hypertension. *Clin Ther* 1996; **18**: 608–25.

43 Holdaas H, Hartmann A, Berg KJ, Lund K, Fauchald P. Renal effects of losartan and amlodipine in hypertensive patients with non-diabetic nephropathy. *Nephrol Dial Transplant* 1998; **13**: 3096–102.

44 Ishimitsu T, Minami J, Yoshii M *et al*. Comparison of the effects of amlodipine and losartan on 24-hour ambulatory blood pressure in hypertensive patients. *Clin Exp Hypertens* 2002; **24**: 41–50.

45 Volpe M, Junren Z, Maxwell T *et al*. Comparison of the blood pressure-lowering effects and tolerability of losartan- and amlodipine-based regimens in patients with isolated systolic hypertension. *Clin Ther* 2003; **25**: 1469–89.

46 Phillips RA, Kloner RA, Grimm RH, Weinberger M. The effects of amlodipine compared to losartan in patients with mild to moderately severe hypertension. *J Clin Hypertens (Greenwich)* 2003; **5**: 17–23.

47 Weir MR, Elkins M, Liss C *et al*. Efficacy, tolerability, and quality of life of losartan, alone or with hydrochlorothiazide, versus nifedipine GITS in patients with essential hypertension. *Clin Ther* 1996; **18**: 411–28.

48 Conlin PR, Elkins M, Liss C *et al*. A study of losartan, alone or with hydrochlorothiazide *vs* nifedipine GITS in elderly patients with diastolic hypertension. *J Hum Hypertens* 1998; **12**: 693–9.

49 Chan JC, Critchley JA, Lappe JT *et al*. Randomised, double-blind, parallel study of the anti-hypertensive efficacy and safety of losartan potassium compared with felodipine ER in elderly patients with mild to moderate hypertension. *J Hum Hypertens* 1995; **9**: 765–71.

50 James IG, Jones A, Davies P. A randomised, double-blind, double-dummy comparison of the efficacy and tolerability of lercanidipine tablets and losartan tablets in patients with mild to moderate essential hypertension. *J Hum Hypertens* 2002; **16**: 605–10.

51 Dahlof B, Keller SE, Makris L *et al*. Efficacy and tolerability of losartan potassium and atenolol in patients with mild to moderate essential hypertension. *Am J Hypertens* 1995; **8**: 578–83.

52 Farsang C, Garcia-Puig J, Niegowska J *et al*. The efficacy and tolerability of losartan versus atenolol in patients with isolated systolic hypertension. Losartan ISH Investigators Group. *J Hypertens* 2000; **18**: 795–801.

53 Dahlof B, Zanchetti A, Diez J *et al*. Effects of losartan and atenolol on left ventricular mass and neurohormonal profile in patients with essential hypertension and left ventricular hypertrophy. *J Hypertens* 2002; **20**: 1855–64.

54 Dahlof B, Devereux RB, Kjeldsen SE *et al*. Cardiovascular morbidity and mortality in the Losartan Intervention For Endpoint reduction in hypertension study (LIFE): a randomised trial against atenolol. *Lancet* 2002; **359**: 995–1003.

55 Kjeldsen SE, Dahlof B, Devereux RB *et al*. Effects of losartan on cardiovascular morbidity and mortality in patients with isolated systolic hypertension and left ventricular hypertrophy: a Losartan Intervention for Endpoint Reduction (LIFE) substudy. *JAMA* 2002; **288**: 1491–8.

56 Lindholm LH, Ibsen H, Dahlof B *et al*. Cardiovascular morbidity and mortality in patients with diabetes in the Losartan Intervention For Endpoint reduction in hypertension study (LIFE): a randomised trial against atenolol. *Lancet* 2002; **359**: 1004–10.

57 Devereux RB, Dahlof B, Kjeldsen SE *et al*. Effects of losartan or atenolol in hypertensive patients without clinically evident vascular disease: a substudy of the LIFE randomized trial. *Ann Intern Med* 2003; **139**: 169–77.

58 Devereux RB, Dahlof B, Gerdts E *et al*. Regression of hypertensive left ventricular hypertrophy by losartan compared with atenolol: the Losartan Intervention for Endpoint Reduction in Hypertension (LIFE) trial. *Circulation* 2004; **110**: 1456-62.

59 De Rosa ML, Cardace P, Rossi M, Baiano A, de Cristofaro A. Comparative effects of chronic ACE inhibition and AT1 receptor blocked losartan on cardiac hypertrophy and renal function in hypertensive patients. *J Hum Hypertens* 2002; **16**: 133–40.

60 Shibasaki Y, Masaki H, Nishiue T *et al*. Angiotensin II type 1 receptor antagonist, losartan, causes regression of left ventricular hypertrophy in end-stage renal disease. *Nephron* 2002; **90**: 256–61.

61 Tedesco MA, Ratti G, Aquino D *et al*. Effects of losartan on hypertension and left ventricular mass: a long-term study. *J Hum Hypertens* 1998; **12**: 505–10.

62 Devereux RB, Palmieri V, Liu JE *et al*. Progressive hypertrophy regression with sustained pressure reduction in hypertension: the Losartan Intervention For Endpoint Reduction study. *J Hypertens* 2002; **20**: 1445–50.

63 Wachtell K, Bella JN, Rokkedal J *et al*. Change in diastolic left ventricular filling after one year of antihypertensive treatment: the Losartan Intervention For Endpoint Reduction in Hypertension (LIFE) Study. *Circulation* 2002; **105**: 1071–6.

64 Wachtell K, Palmieri V, Olsen MH *et al*. Change in systolic left ventricular performance after 3 years of antihypertensive treatment: the Losartan Intervention for Endpoint (LIFE) Study. *Circulation* 2002; **106**: 227–32.

65 Dahlof B, Burke TA, Krobot K *et al*. Population impact of losartan use on stroke in the European Union (EU): projections from the Losartan Intervention For Endpoint reduction in hypertension (LIFE) study. *J Hum Hypertens* 2004; **18**: 367–73.

66 Lindholm LH, Ibsen H, Borch-Johnsen K *et al*. Risk of new-onset diabetes in the Losartan Intervention For Endpoint reduction in hypertension study. *J Hypertens* 2002; **20**: 1879–86.

67 Brenner BM, Cooper ME, de Zeeuw D *et al*. Effects of losartan on renal and cardiovascular outcomes in patients with type 2 diabetes and nephropathy. *N Engl J Med* 2001; **345**: 861–9.

68 Gansevoort RT, de Zeeuw D, Shahinfar S, Redfield A, de Jong PE. Effects of the angiotensin II antagonist losartan in hypertensive patients with renal disease. *J Hypertens Suppl* 1994; **12**: S37–42.

69 Lozano JV, Llisterri JL, Aznar J, Redon J. Losartan reduces microalbuminuria in hypertensive microalbuminuric type 2 diabetics. *Nephrol Dial Transplant* 2001; **16(Suppl 1)**: 85–9.

70 de Pablos-Velasco PL, Pazos Toral F, Esmatjes JE *et al*. Losartan titration versus diuretic combination in type 2 diabetic patients. *J Hypertens* 2002; **20**: 715–19.

71 Ellis D, Vats A, Moritz ML *et al*. Long-term antiproteinuric and renoprotective efficacy and safety of losartan in children with proteinuria. *J Pediatr* 2003; **143**: 89–97.

72 Iino Y, Hayashi M, Kawamura T *et al*. Interim evidence of the renoprotective effect of the angiotensin II receptor antagonist losartan versus the calcium channel blocker amlodipine in patients with chronic kidney disease and hypertension: a report of the Japanese Losartan Therapy Intended for Global Renal Protection in Hypertensive Patients (JLIGHT) Study. *Clin Exp Nephrol* 2003; **7**: 221–30.

73 Andersen S, Tarnow L, Rossing P, Hansen BV, Parving HH. Renoprotective effects of angiotensin II receptor blockade in type 1 diabetic patients with diabetic nephropathy. *Kidney Int* 2000; **57**: 601–6.

74 Lacourciere Y, Belanger A, Godin C *et al.* Long-term comparison of losartan and enalapril on kidney function in hypertensive type 2 diabetics with early nephropathy. *Kidney Int* 2000; **58**: 762–9.

75 Ibsen H, Wachtell K, Olsen MH *et al.* Does albuminuria predict cardiovascular outcome on treatment with losartan versus atenolol in hypertension with left ventricular hypertrophy? A LIFE substudy. *J Hypertens* 2004; **22**: 1805–11.

76 MacKay JH, Arcuri KE, Goldberg AI, Snapinn SM, Sweet CS. Losartan and low-dose hydrochlorothiazide in patients with essential hypertension. A double-blind, placebo-controlled trial of concomitant administration compared with individual components. *Arch Intern Med* 1996; **156**: 278–85.

77 Ruilope LM, Simpson RL, Toh J *et al.* Controlled trial of losartan given concomitantly with different doses of hydrochlorothiazide in hypertensive patients. *Blood Press* 1996; **5**: 32–40.

78 Flack JM, Saunders E, Gradman A *et al.* Antihypertensive efficacy and safety of losartan alone and in combination with hydrochlorothiazide in adult African Americans with mild to moderate hypertension. *Clin Ther* 2001; **23**: 1193–208.

79 Oparil S, Aurup P, Snavely D, Goldberg A. Efficacy and safety of losartan/hydrochlorothiazide in patients with severe hypertension. *Am J Cardiol* 2001; **87**: 721–6.

80 Gradman AH, Brady WE, Gazdick LP, Lyle P, Zeldin RK. A multicenter, randomized, double-blind, placebo-controlled, 8-week trial of the efficacy and tolerability of once-daily losartan 100 mg/hydrochlorothiazide 25 mg and losartan 50 mg/hydrochlorothiazide 12.5 mg in the treatment of moderate-to-severe essential hypertension. *Clin Ther* 2002; **24**: 1049–61.

81 Dickson TZ, Zagrobelny J, Lin CC *et al.* Pharmacokinetics, safety, and antihypertensive efficacy of losartan in combination with hydrochlorothiazide in hypertensive patients with renal impairment. *J Clin Pharmacol* 2003; **43**: 591–603.

82 Neutel JM, Kolloch RE, Plouin PF, Meinicke TW, Schumacher H. Telmisartan *vs* losartan plus hydrochlorothiazide in the treatment of mild-to-moderate essential hypertension – a randomised ABPM study. *J Hum Hypertens* 2003; **17**: 569–75.

83 Townsend R, Haggert B, Liss C, Edelman JM. Efficacy and tolerability of losartan versus enalapril alone or in combination with hydrochlorothiazide in patients with essential hypertension. *Clin Ther* 1995; **17**: 911–23.

84 Naidoo DP, Sareli P, Marin F *et al.* Increased efficacy and tolerability with losartan plus hydrochlorothiazide in patients with uncontrolled hypertension and therapy-related symptoms receiving two monotherapies. *Adv Ther* 1999; **16**: 187–99.

85 Lacourciere Y, Gil-Extremera B, Mueller O, Byrne M, Williams L. Efficacy and tolerability of fixed-dose combinations of telmisartan plus HCTZ compared with losartan plus HCTZ in patients with essential hypertension. *Int J Clin Pract* 2003; **57**: 273–9.

86 Kuschnir E, Bendersky M, Resk J *et al.* Effects of the combination of low-dose nifedipine GITS 20 mg and losartan 50 mg in patients with mild to moderate hypertension. *J Cardiovasc Pharmacol* 2004; **43**: 300–5.

87 Goldberg AI, Dunlay MC, Sweet CS. Safety and tolerability of losartan potassium, an angiotensin II receptor antagonist, compared with hydrochlorothiazide, atenolol, felodipine ER, and angiotensin-converting enzyme inhibitors for the treatment of systemic hypertension. *Am J Cardiol* 1995; **75**: 793–5.

88 Paster RZ, Snavely DB, Sweet AR *et al.* Use of losartan in the treatment of hypertensive patients with a history of cough induced by angiotensin-converting enzyme inhibitors. *Clin Ther* 1998; **20**: 978–89.

89 Lacourciere Y, Brunner H, Irwin R *et al.* Effects of modulators of the renin-angiotensin-aldosterone system on cough. Losartan cough study group. *J Hypertens* 1994; **12**: 1387–93.

90 Ramsay LE, Yeo WW. ACE inhibitors, angiotensin II antagonists and cough. The losartan cough study group. *J Hum Hypertens* 1995; **9(Suppl 5)**: S51–4.

91 Chan P, Tomlinson B, Huang TY *et al.* Double-blind comparison of losartan, lisinopril, and metolazone in elderly hypertensive patients with previous angiotensin-converting enzyme inhibitor-induced cough. *J Clin Pharmacol* 1997; **37**: 253–7.

92 Herman WH, Shahinfar S, Carides GW *et al.* Losartan reduces the costs associated with diabetic end-stage renal disease: the RENAAL study economic evaluation. *Diabetes Care* 2003; **26**: 683–7.

93 Weaver J, Vora J, O'Hare P, Robinson P, Gerth W. Losartan reduces the costs associated with dialysis and transplantation: implications of RENAAL study in the United Kingdom. *J Hum Hypertens* 2002; **16**: 13.

# 8. Drug review – Olmesartan (Olmetec®)

*Dr Richard Clark*
*CSF Medical Communications Ltd*

## Summary

A wide range of <u>angiotensin II receptor antagonists</u> are available for the treatment of hypertension. Olmesartan medoxomil (hereafter referred to as olmesartan) is the seventh member of this class to be licensed in the UK. It has been tested extensively in clinical trials, some of which have compared it with other antihypertensives, including other <u>angiotensin II receptor antagonists</u>. These studies have shown olmesartan to be more effective in reducing <u>systolic blood pressure (SBP)</u> or <u>diastolic blood pressure (DBP)</u> compared with losartan, valsartan or irbesartan. Other direct clinical comparisons have also reported that olmesartan is associated with superior control of hypertension when compared with the <u>calcium-channel blocker</u>, amlodipine, and the <u>angiotensin-converting enzyme (ACE) inhibitor</u>, captopril. Olmesartan was also reported to be at least as effective as the β-blocker, atenolol. Importantly, olmesartan provides consistent 24-hour control of blood pressure with a convenient once-daily dosing schedule. Olmesartan is generally well tolerated with a similar <u>safety and tolerability</u> profile to the other angiotensin II receptor antagonists.

## Introduction

Angiotensin II plays an important role in <u>cardiovascular</u> <u>homeostasis</u>, and, being a potent <u>vasoconstrictor</u>, appears to be a major determinant of blood pressure in both <u>normotensive</u> and hypertensive individuals. As such, angiotensin II is thought to be an important mediator in the <u>pathogenesis</u> of essential hypertension. Drugs that modify the <u>renin–angiotensin system</u>, such as the ACE inhibitors and the angiotensin II receptor antagonists, have become well-accepted treatments for hypertension in recent years. However, treatment with ACE inhibitors is associated with an accumulation of <u>bradykinin</u>, due to the non-specific nature of the ACE <u>enzyme</u>. Bradykinin is an inflammatory mediator and vasodilator that, aside from its physiological effects, can result in adverse events such as cough, and more rarely, angioedema, which are both associated with ACE inhibitor treatment.

Angiotensin II receptor antagonists are more specific than ACE inhibitors in terms of their inhibitory action on angiotensin II. This is because they block the effects of angiotensin II generated by non-ACE pathways (e.g. those catalysed by the enzyme chymase) by binding to the type 1 angiotensin II ($AT_1$) receptor. This specificity for the $AT_1$ receptor translates into a more favourable side-effect profile.

In addition to its vasoconstrictor effects, angiotensin II mediates vascular hypertrophy and the development of atherosclerosis by stimulating the proliferation of vascular smooth muscle cells. Angiotensin II is also implicated in the development of left ventricular hypertrophy (LVH), which is a major independent risk factor for cardiovascular morbidity and mortality, and also plays a role in the progression of renal disease.[1] Antihypertensive modalities that block the effects of angiotensin II have been shown to induce regression of LVH and have hepato- and renoprotective effects.[2,3]

Olmesartan is a non-peptide prodrug. The active form of olmesartan binds selectively to the $AT_1$ receptor, thus blocking the action of angiotensin II. Olmesartan is licensed in the UK for the treatment of essential hypertension.

This review focuses on the efficacy and safety of olmesartan and discusses the significant evidence for the drug in the context of data obtained from studies with other antihypertensive agents including other angiotensin II receptor antagonists, ACE inhibitors, calcium-channel blockers, β-blockers and the thiazide diuretic, hydrochlorothiazide (HCTZ).

## Clinical efficacy and tolerability

### Placebo-controlled and dose-ranging studies

A meta-analysis of seven randomised, double-blind, placebo-controlled, dose-ranging trials assessed the efficacy and safety of olmesartan in patients with mild-to-moderate hypertension.[4] A total of 3055 patients comprised the efficacy population with 3095 included in the safety assessment. Patients received daily doses of olmesartan ranging from 2.5 to 80 mg/day for 6–52 weeks. The proportion of patients classified as responders (those achieving a DBP of 90 mmHg or lower, or whose DBP fell by at least 10 mmHg) increased with the dose of olmesartan in the range of 2.5–40 mg/day. All doses of olmesartan were more effective in lowering DBP than placebo ($p \leq 0.009$). Olmesartan doses of 20 or 40 mg/day were more effective at lowering DBP than the 5 mg ($p=0.001$ and $p<0.001$, respectively) and the 10 mg daily doses ($p=0.012$ and $p=0.011$, respectively). After adjustment for the placebo effect, the greatest mean decrease in DBP was associated with the 80 mg dose (7.7 mmHg; Figure 1). The SBP-lowering effect of olmesartan increased with increasing dose across the 2.5–80 mg/day range after adjustment for placebo (Figure 1). All doses of olmesartan were more effective than

**Figure 1.** The effect of olmesartan, administered once daily, on diastolic blood pressure (DBP; left) and systolic blood pressure (SBP; right), showing mean changes from baseline (plus standard error) following adjustment for the placebo effect.[4]

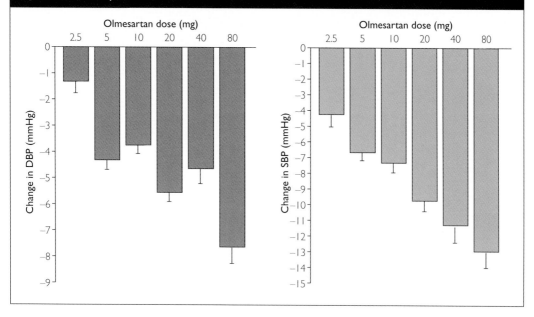

placebo in terms of SBP normalisation (SBP ≤140 mmHg; $p \leq 0.001$). All doses of olmesartan were reportedly well tolerated, with more withdrawals occurring amongst those receiving placebo than olmesartan (14 *vs* 9%, respectively). A similar incidence of treatment-emergent adverse events occurred in the placebo and olmesartan groups (47 and 52%, respectively). Although at first glance this appears rather high in comparison with most other trials of angiotensin II receptor antagonists, which generally report rates of approximately 15–20%, this is likely to reflect data collection methods used in the olmesartan trials, as adverse event rates were equally high in the placebo group.[4] Furthermore, the incidence of treatment-emergent adverse events seemed unrelated to the dose of olmesartan.

These trials have demonstrated that once-daily treatment with olmesartan is more effective in reducing blood pressure than placebo at doses as low as 2.5 mg/day. However, the licensed dose range in the UK (10–40 mg/day) provides greater reductions in blood pressure than lower doses without a concomitant increase in adverse events.

A further meta-analysis of data derived from seven randomised, double-blind, placebo controlled studies, has evaluated olmesartan's antihypertensive efficacy across a large cohort of patients with essential hypertension (n=1777).[5] In addition, the effects of olmesartan upon pulse pressure (i.e. the difference between SBP and DBP) in all patients with wide pulse pressures at baseline (>55 mmHg; n=917) and in an elderly subpopulation of patients with wide baseline pulse pressures (≥65 years; n=296) were also examined in this meta-analysis. This assessment is of particular interest because baseline pulse pressure is a significant independent predictor of cardiovascular morbidity and mortality in older individuals regardless of their baseline SBP. Olmesartan, at doses of 20 and 40 mg/day, elicited significant reductions in SBP relative to placebo in the total patient cohort (mean reductions: –15.1 and –17.6 mmHg, respectively; *p*<0.0001 *vs* placebo). In patients with wide baseline pulse pressure, the reductions in SBP were even more pronounced (mean reductions in SBP: –17.7 and –22.0 mmHg; mean reductions in pulse pressure: –7.4 and –8.8 mmHg; olmesartan 20 and 40 mg, respectively; both parameters *p*<0.0001 *vs* placebo). In addition, in the elderly patient population with wide pulse pressures at baseline, olmesartan reduced SBP and pulse pressures by a similar extent as observed in the younger patient population (SBP: –21.8 and –22.5 mmHg; pulse pressures: –6.7 and –7.6 mmHg; all *p*<0.05 *vs* placebo). Olmesartan at both doses and in all populations was equally well tolerated, though there were slightly more reports of headache in the wide pulse pressure group. Thus, in conclusion, olmesartan reduces SBP and pulse pressure in a broad patient population with essential hypertension, including elderly patients with wide pulse pressures at baseline.

> Olmesartan reduces SBP and pulse pressure in a broad patient population with essential hypertension, including elderly patients with wide pulse pressures at baseline.

## 24-hour blood pressure control

Ideal characteristics for an antihypertensive treatment include the provision of 24-hour blood pressure control, attenuation of the early morning surge in blood pressure and maintenance of normal circadian patterns of blood pressure. It has been established that blood pressure varies according to circadian patterns such that blood pressure is at its lowest at 3 am, and then starts to rise again during the early hours of the morning before waking, with the sharpest increase between 6 am and 9 am.[6] Cerebral haemorrhage and myocardial infarction (MI) may be precipitated by rapid increases in blood pressure, such as those that occur in the morning in both normotensive and hypertensive patients. Significantly, it has been reported that most strokes occur between 8 am and noon, whilst most MIs occur between 6 am and noon.[7,8] Furthermore, cardiovascular risk is related to patients' overall blood pressure load (the magnitude of blood pressure elevation and the duration of raised blood pressure).[9] Although the current emphasis in hypertension management is to 'treat to target blood pressure', the need for effective 24-hour blood pressure control should also be emphasised. The sixth annual report of the Joint National Committee (JNC-VI) stated that optimal drug formulations should provide 24-hour efficacy with a once-daily dose, with at least 50% of the peak effect remaining at the end of 24 hours.[10] Thus, a good antihypertensive should provide consistent and smooth reductions in blood pressure over 24 hours, reducing the risk of blood pressure variability. The variation in blood pressure over 24 hours can be evaluated by the use of ambulatory blood pressure monitoring (ABPM).

ABPM has been used in an 8-week, randomised, placebo-controlled, double-blind trial to examine the effect of olmesartan given to patients

> A good antihypertensive should provide consistent and smooth reductions in blood pressure over 24 hours, reducing the risk of blood pressure variability.

(n=334) with moderate-to-severe hypertension.[11] Patients received olmesartan, 5, 20, or 80 mg, once daily, or olmesartan, 2.5, 10 or 40 mg, twice daily, or placebo. Treatment with all doses of olmesartan, given either once or twice daily, resulted in reductions in mean 24-hour DBP, and daytime (8 am–8 pm) or night-time (8 pm–8 am) DBP compared with those who were given placebo (all comparisons $p<0.0001$; Figure 2). The consistency and duration of blood pressure reductions was assessed by measuring the trough-to-peak (T/P) ratio of the 24-hour diastolic and systolic records after 8 weeks of treatment. These ratios were all greater than 50% for once- or twice-daily doses. Thus, the T/P diastolic ratio ranges were 57–73% and T/P systolic ratios were 58–63%. In conclusion, olmesartan provides a consistent and smooth reduction in blood pressure over 24 hours, satisfying the requirements of the JNC-VI guidelines. Moreover, this study has shown that a once-daily dosing schedule appeared to be as effective as a twice-daily regimen.

> Olmesartan provides a consistent and smooth reduction in blood pressure over 24 hours and a once-daily dosing schedule appeared to be as effective as a twice-daily regimen.

## Olmesartan vs other angiotensin II receptor antagonists

A randomised, double-blind, parallel-group study compared the effects of olmesartan, 10 mg/day, or losartan, 50 mg/day, for up to 6 months in patients with mild-to-moderate hypertension (n=316).[12] Doses of olmesartan or losartan were doubled at week 4 as necessary, whilst HCTZ (dose: 12.5–25 mg/day) could be added to either treatment group, if

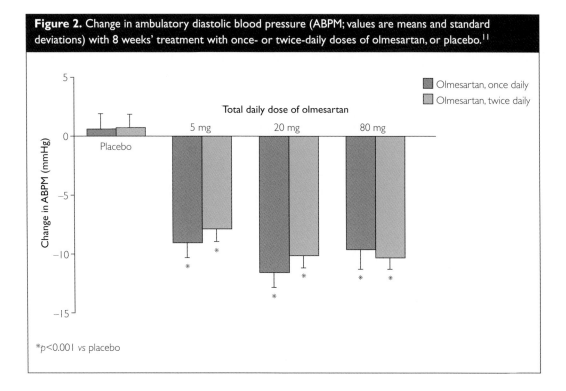

**Figure 2.** Change in ambulatory diastolic blood pressure (ABPM; values are means and standard deviations) with 8 weeks' treatment with once- or twice-daily doses of olmesartan, or placebo.[11]

*p<0.001 vs placebo

**Table 1.** Comparison of the effects of olmesartan, 10–20 mg/day, and losartan, 50–100 mg/day, after 12 weeks' treatment.[12]

| Outcome | Olmesartan | Losartan | Two-sided 95% confidence interval |
|---|---|---|---|
| Mean change from baseline in DBP (mmHg) | −10.6 | −8.5 | −3.6, −0.5 |
| Mean change from baseline in SBP (mmHg) | −14.9 | −11.6 | −6.0, −0.6 |
| Patients receiving lower dose[a] (%) | 58.2 | 36.8 | – |
| Patients receiving higher dose[b] (%) | 41.8 | 63.2 | – |

[a]Olmesartan, 10 mg/day; losartan, 50 mg/day
[b]Olmesartan, 20 mg/day; losartan, 100 mg/day
DBP, diastolic blood pressure; SBP, systolic blood pressure.

required, after 12 weeks. The main findings of this trial after 12 weeks' treatment are summarised in Table 1. Greater reductions in DBP and SBP were obtained after 12 weeks with olmesartan than with losartan (Table 1; no *p*-values reported). In addition, a greater proportion of patients required titration to the higher dose of losartan than the higher dose of olmesartan (no *p*-value reported). Furthermore, fewer patients receiving olmesartan required the addition of HCTZ to their treatment regimen (35 *vs* 48%; no *p*-value reported). By week 24, 20% of patients in the olmesartan group were receiving the 20 mg dose without HCTZ and 35% were receiving the 20 mg dose with the addition of 12.5 or 25 mg HCTZ. By week 24 in the losartan group, 29% of patients were receiving the 100 mg dose without HCTZ and 48% were receiving the 100 mg dose with 12.5 or 25 mg HCTZ. Thus, even after 24 weeks, more patients required dose titration and concomitant HCTZ treatment in the losartan than the olmesartan group.

A US-based, randomised, double-blind, parallel-group trial compared 8 weeks' treatment with the recommended starting doses of various angiotensin II receptor antagonists (olmesartan, 20 mg/day,[a] losartan, 50 mg/day, valsartan, 80 mg/day, and irbesartan, 150 mg/day).[13] These doses reflect the standard maintenance doses of angiotensin II receptor antagonists used in the UK. Patients participating in this trial (n=588) had DBPs between 100 and 115 mmHg and a mean daytime DBP of between 90 and 119 mmHg. Treatment with all four angiotensin II receptor antagonists resulted in significant decreases in both DBP and SBP from baseline after 8 weeks (*p*<0.001 for all groups). However, the mean reduction in cuff DBP achieved with olmesartan (11.5 mmHg) was significantly greater than that with losartan (8.2 mmHg; *p*=0.0002), valsartan (7.9 mmHg; *p*<0.0001) or with irbesartan (9.9 mmHg; *p*=0.0412). Mean reductions in SBP after 8 weeks were: olmesartan, 11.3 mmHg; losartan, 9.5 mmHg; valsartan, 8.4 mmHg; irbesartan, 11.0 mmHg. The

---

[a]Recommended starting dose in the US; in the UK the recommended starting dose is 10 mg/day.

differences in reductions in SBP provided by the different agents, however, were not significant. After 2 weeks' treatment, olmesartan proved to be more effective than losartan, valsartan or irbesartan in lowering DBP (10.7, 7.6, 9.0 and 9.0 mmHg, respectively) or SBP (13.0, 8.9, 9.2 and 10.8 mmHg, respectively). The differences in these blood pressure reductions were significant in favour of olmesartan ($p\leq0.05$) for all comparisons after 2 weeks.

This study also investigated ABPM and generated results similar to the clinic blood pressure data (Figure 3). The reduction in mean 24-hour DBP provided by olmesartan was greater than the reductions achieved with losartan and valsartan (8.5, 6.2 and 5.6 mmHg, respectively; $p<0.05$ for both comparisons). A similar pattern was observed for reductions in systolic ABPM: olmesartan reduced mean 24-hour SBP by 12.5 mmHg compared with 9.0 and 8.1 mmHg for losartan and valsartan, respectively ($p<0.05$ for both comparisons). No significant difference was observed between olmesartan and irbesartan for 24-hour DBP (8.5 vs 7.4 mmHg; $p=0.087$) or SBP (12.5 vs 11.3 mmHg; p-value not reported), although numerically superior values were obtained in those receiving olmesartan. The consistency of 24-hour blood pressure control was assessed by calculating a T/P ratio for each agent. For DBP this ratio was highest (superior) for olmesartan (0.69), followed by losartan, irbesartan and valsartan (0.64, 0.62 and 0.55, respectively). For DBP, T/P ratios were similar for olmesartan and losartan (0.68 and 0.69, respectively), and higher for olmesartan than those for valsartan (0.48) and irbesartan (0.60). However, no statistical analyses were performed on the T/P ratios for either SBP or DBP.

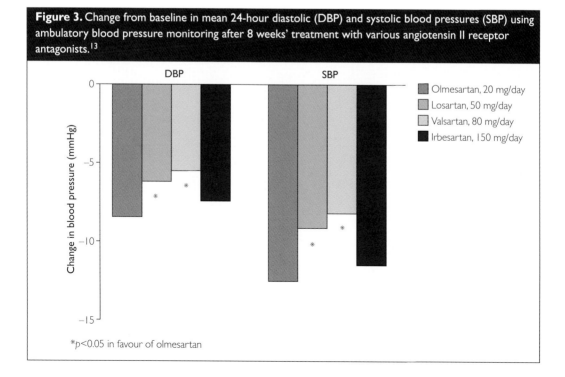

**Figure 3.** Change from baseline in mean 24-hour diastolic (DBP) and systolic blood pressures (SBP) using ambulatory blood pressure monitoring after 8 weeks' treatment with various angiotensin II receptor antagonists.[13]

*$p<0.05$ in favour of olmesartan

All treatments in this study were generally well tolerated. The overall incidence of <u>adverse events</u> was similar in all treatment groups (30.6, 32.0, 44.8 and 35.6% for olmesartan, losartan, valsartan and irbesartan groups, respectively), though numerically the fewest events occurred in the olmesartan group. Upper respiratory tract infection, headache, fatigue, back pain and dizziness were the most common complaints across the treatment groups.

The antihypertensive <u>efficacy</u> of olmesartan has been compared with that of candesartan in a randomised, <u>double-blind</u>, parallel-group study of 643 patients with predominantly mild-to-moderate hypertension.[14] Patients were randomised to once-daily treatment with olmesartan, 20 mg, or candesartan, 8 mg, for a total of 8 weeks. Again, these doses reflect the standard maintenance doses of both agents used in the UK. Both treatments reduced daytime DBP from <u>baseline</u> (the primary efficacy <u>endpoint</u>) as determined by ABPM. However, olmesartan proved to be significantly more effective than candesartan at all time intervals assessed ($p \leq 0.0126$). Thus, respective mean reductions in daytime DBP at weeks 1, 2 and 8 were 6.7, 8.4 and 9.3 mmHg with olmesartan compared with 5.3, 6.0 and 7.8 mmHg with candesartan. Likewise, olmesartan provided greater reductions in mean 24-hour DBP, and mean daytime and 24-hour SBP than candesartan. Thus, for each of these parameters and at each time interval the decrease from baseline with olmesartan was 1.5–2.5 mmHg greater than that achieved with candesartan. There were no significant differences between treatment groups with regard to <u>trough</u>-sitting DBP and SBP. Both treatments were well tolerated, with 9.4% of patients experiencing adverse events in the olmesartan group compared with 12.3% in the candesartan group.

Thus, in conclusion, in general these studies have demonstrated that olmesartan appears to be more effective than losartan, valsartan, irbesartan and candesartan at reducing SBP and DBP, and is as equally well tolerated.

> Olmesartan appears to be more effective than losartan, valsartan, irbesartan and candesartan, at reducing SBP and DBP and is as equally well tolerated.

## Olmesartan vs calcium-channel blockers

A randomised, double-blind, parallel-group trial compared 8 weeks' treatment with olmesartan, 20 mg/day, amlodipine, 5 mg/day, or <u>placebo</u>, in patients with mild-to-moderate hypertension (n=440).[15] Patients were evaluated using ABPM at baseline and after 8 weeks' treatment, as well as standard clinic blood pressure measurements. Both olmesartan and amlodipine produced greater reductions in <u>ambulatory</u> and standard clinic DBP and SBP than placebo treatment ($p<0.001$). Mean reductions from baseline in diastolic ABPM were similar for patients treated with olmesartan or amlodipine (7.7 and 7.0 mmHg, respectively), as were reductions in systolic ABPM (12.2 and 12.3 mmHg, respectively). Similar reductions with olmesartan or amlodipine treatment were also observed in standard clinic DBPs (10.8 and 10.1 mmHg, respectively) and SBPs (10.3 and 10.3 mmHg, respectively). However, more patients treated with olmesartan than amlodipine achieved the SBP and DBP targets (<130 and <85 mmHg, respectively; Table 2).

**Table 2.** Control of blood pressure after 8 weeks' treatment with olmesartan, 20 mg/day, or amlodipine, 5 mg/day.[15]

| Outcome | Responders (%) | | |
| --- | --- | --- | --- |
| | Olmesartan | Amlodipine | p-value[a] |
| ABPM responders[b] | 71.3 | 69.8 | NS |
| Ambulatory DBP <85 mmHg | 48.0 | 38.4 | 0.01 |
| Ambulatory SBP <130 mmHg | 33.9 | 17.4 | 0.02 |
| Standard clinic BP responders[b] | 49.7 | 50.8 | NS |
| Standard clinic DBP <85 mmHg | 20.0 | 13.4 | 0.03 |
| Standard clinic SBP <130 mmHg | 24.6 | 15.6 | 0.04 |

[a]All p-values are for olmesartan vs amlodipine.

[b]Responders had a DBP <90 mmHg or a decrease in DBP of ≥10 mmHg from baseline.

ABPM, ambulatory blood pressure monitoring; BP, blood pressure; DBP, diastolic blood pressure; NS, not significant; SBP, systolic blood pressure.

Both agents were well tolerated, with a similar incidence of treatment-emergent adverse events between groups (olmesartan, 35%; amlodipine, 36%; placebo, 26%; p>0.05 for all pairwise comparisons). However, a significantly higher incidence of nausea was associated with amlodipine than olmesartan treatment (2.7 vs 0%; p=0.039). Consistent with its side-effect profile, amlodipine was associated with a numerically higher incidence of oedema compared with olmesartan, although this difference did not reach statistical significance (9.1 vs 4.3%).

These studies compared the minimum starting doses of olmesartan and amlodipine in the US. However, in the UK the starting dose for olmesartan is 10 mg/day, and as such it is perhaps of more relevance in the UK to conduct a comparison between this dose of olmesartan and a 5 mg daily dose of amlodipine. Therefore, these results should be interpreted with caution.

In summary, olmesartan, 20 mg/day, is more effective than amlodipine, 5 mg/day, in controlling SBP or DBP to stringent targets (<130 and <85 mmHg, respectively) in patients with mild-to-moderate hypertension, and may be better tolerated.

> Olmesartan, 20 mg/day, is more effective than amlodipine, 5 mg/day, in controlling SBP or DBP to stringent targets.

## Olmesartan vs β-blockers

The recommended UK starting doses for olmesartan (10 mg/day) and atenolol (50 mg/day), both in combination with HCTZ (25 mg/day), were compared over a 12-week period in a randomised, double-blind trial in patients (n=328) with moderate-to-severe hypertension.[12] Doses of olmesartan and atenolol were doubled after 4 weeks, as necessary. Reductions from baseline in DBP were similar for patients receiving the olmesartan–HCTZ combination or the atenolol–HCTZ combination (17.3 and 17.2 mmHg, respectively). Furthermore, decreases in SBP and DBP of approximately 14–15 and 12 mmHg, respectively, were obtained for both agents after only 2 weeks' treatment. Similar proportions of patients required their dose of olmesartan and atenolol to be doubled (26.2 and 28.1%, respectively), whilst a similar proportion of patients receiving olmesartan or atenolol experienced adverse events (35.4 and 36.6%, respectively).

In conclusion, olmesartan and atenolol demonstrated equivalent efficacy, tolerability and safety in a population of patients with moderate-to-severe hypertension.

### Olmesartan vs ACE inhibitors

Olmesartan, 5–20 mg once daily, has been compared with the ACE inhibitor, captopril, 12.5–50 mg twice daily, over a 12-week period in a randomised, double-blind, parallel-group trial in patients (n=291) with mild-to-moderate hypertension.[12] Initial doses (olmesartan, 5 mg once daily or captopril, 12.5 mg twice daily) were doubled at weeks 4 and 8, if required. The confidence intervals in Table 3 indicate that olmesartan is superior to captopril in terms of SBP and DBP reductions.

Furthermore, fewer patients in the olmesartan than the captopril group were titrated to the highest dose (25.0 vs 54.9%, respectively). By week 12, only 14% of patients receiving captopril remained on the starting dose compared with 42% of patients in the olmesartan group on the starting dose. Both agents were well tolerated, with a similar proportion of patients in the olmesartan or captopril groups experiencing adverse events (61 and 62%, respectively). Thus, olmesartan, 5–20 mg once daily, is more effective than the ACE inhibitor captopril, 12.5–50 mg twice daily. Furthermore, olmesartan has a more convenient once-daily dosing schedule. However, the practical relevance of the comparison in this study is questionable given the availability of longer-acting ACE inhibitors that can be administered on a once-daily basis.

**Table 3.** Comparison of the antihypertensive effects of olmesartan, 5–20 mg once daily, and captopril, 12.5–50 mg twice daily, after 12 weeks' treatment.[12]

| Outcome | Olmesartan | Captopril | Two-sided 95% confidence interval |
|---|---|---|---|
| Mean change from baseline in DBP (mmHg) | –9.9 | –6.8 | –3.6, –0.5 |
| Mean change from baseline in SBP (mmHg) | –14.9 | –7.1 | –10.4, –4.7 |
| Patients (%) receiving: | | | |
| • low dose[a] | 41.7 | 14.1 | – |
| • middle dose[b] | 33.3 | 31.0 | – |
| • high dose[c] | 25.0 | 54.9 | – |

[a]Olmesartan, 5 mg once daily; captopril, 12.5 mg twice daily.
[b]Olmesartan, 10 mg once daily; captopril, 25 mg twice daily.
[c]Olmesartan, 20 mg once daily; captopril, 50 mg twice daily.
DBP, diastolic blood pressure; SBP, systolic blood pressure.

## Olmesartan in combination with HCTZ

An 8-week, randomised, <u>double-blind</u>, <u>factorial-design study</u> investigated olmesartan <u>monotherapy</u> and various combinations of olmesartan and HCTZ in patients with hypertension (DBP of 100–115 mmHg).[16] Patients (n=502) were randomised to 12 groups: <u>placebo</u>, olmesartan monotherapy (10, 20 or 40 mg/day), HCTZ monotherapy (12.5 or 25 mg/day), or one of six groups of olmesartan–HCTZ combination therapy. The reductions in SBP and DBP for all 12 treatment groups are shown in Figure 4, and generally appear to be dose related. The proportion of patients classed as responders (<u>trough</u> DBP <90 mmHg, or a reduction from <u>baseline</u> of ≥10 mmHg) was also dose related and was the highest in the olmesartan, 40 mg, plus HCTZ, 25 mg, group (92.3%). All doses of olmesartan and HCTZ were generally well tolerated, with no significant or clinically relevant differences in the rate of treatment-emergent <u>adverse events</u> between groups.

A 24-week, <u>open-label</u> trial investigated the effectiveness of a 'stepped-care' approach for the treatment of hypertension in patients (n=201) with a DBP of 90–109 mmHg.[17] All patients received olmesartan, 20 mg/day for 4 weeks. At subsequent 4-week intervals the drug regimen was modified in patients whose blood pressure remained above 130/85 mmHg in the following manner: up-<u>titration</u> of olmesartan dose to 40 mg/day; addition of HCTZ 12.5 mmHg; up-titration of HCTZ dose to 25 mg/day; addition of amlodipine, 5 mg/day; up-titration of amlodipine dose to 10 mg/day. After 8 weeks of treatment, 58.7% of patients reached blood pressure targets of less

> The proportion of patients classed as responders was dose related and was the highest in the olmesartan, 40 mg, plus HCTZ, 25 mg, group (92.3%).

**Figure 4.** Reductions in diastolic blood pressure (DBP; left) and systolic blood pressure (SBP; right) after 8 weeks' treatment with either placebo, olmesartan or hydrochlorothiazide (HCTZ) monotherapies, or various combinations of olmesartan and HCTZ.[16]

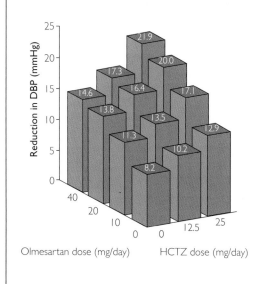
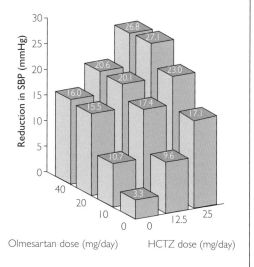

than or equal to 140/90 mmHg. Furthermore, the percentage of responders (DBP <90 mmHg or decreased by ≥10 mmHg) was 83.8%. After 24 weeks' treatment the mean reduction in blood pressure was 33.7/18.2 mmHg with 87.7% of patients achieving the target blood pressure (≤130/85 mmHg) whilst 93.3% achieved a less stringent target (≤140/90 mmHg).

This trial provides evidence that although olmesartan is effective in treating many patients to blood pressure targets, a stepped-care approach incorporating initial olmesartan treatment is remarkably effective. Furthermore, a stepped-care approach is now recommended by the latest published guidelines as the most effective way to treat patients to their target blood pressure.[18–20]

## Long-term treatment

The effect of treating patients with stepped doses (5–40 mg/day) of olmesartan, where required, for up to 1 year, has been evaluated in 26 hypertensive patients who had blood pressures of at least 160/95 mmHg.[21] SBPs and DBPs decreased by 28.8 and 15.8 mmHg, respectively, after 12 months' treatment. Long-term olmesartan treatment was generally well tolerated in this study with only one patient discontinuing treatment due to adverse events.

## Anti-atherosclerotic and organ-protective effects

Olmesartan has demonstrated the potential to confer anti-atherosclerotic effects in addition to its effect on blood pressure in a primate model.[22,23] Likewise, olmesartan has also demonstrated renal-protective effects in animal models, and hepatic-protective effects in vitro.[2,3,24,25] However, these areas are beyond the scope of this review, which focuses primarily on olmesartan's antihypertensive effects and clinical, rather than preclinical data.

## Anti-inflammatory effects

The anti-inflammatory effects of olmesartan monotherapy and olmesartan in combination with pravastatin have been examined in a double-bind, randomised clinical trial of patients with hypertension and micro-inflammation (n=199).[26] Six weeks of olmesartan monotherapy (20 mg/day) was associated with significant reductions in levels of high-sensitivity C-reactive protein (–15.1%; $p<0.005$), high-sensitivity tumour necrosis factor-$\alpha$ (–8.9%; $p<0.02$), interleukin-6 (–14.0%; $p<0.05$) and monocyte chemotactic protein-1 (–6.5%), whilst placebo did not exert any effects on these markers of inflammation. These anti-inflammatory properties were maintained when pravastatin (20 mg/day) was added to the treatment regimen after 6 weeks of olmesartan monotherapy. However, pravastatin alone did not exert any anti-inflammatory effects in this study. Thus, olmesartan monotherapy significantly reduces biochemical markers of vascular inflammation in hypertensive patients as early as 6 weeks after initiation of treatment.

Olmesartan monotherapy significantly reduces biochemical markers of vascular inflammation in hypertensive patients.

This anti-inflammatory property may contribute to an overall beneficial effect of olmesartan upon cardiovascular outcomes.

## Safety and tolerability

Olmesartan treatment is generally well tolerated with an incidence of adverse events that is similar to patients receiving placebo. Thus, in a meta-analysis of seven randomised, placebo-controlled clinical trials the overall incidence of adverse events was 51.5 and 47.2% in patients (safety population: n=3095) receiving olmesartan or placebo, respectively.[4] Furthermore, there was no dose-related increase in adverse events. The most common adverse event reported in these studies was headache, which occurred in 7.8 and 9.4% of the olmesartan and placebo groups, respectively. Other commonly occurring adverse events were upper respiratory tract infection, influenza-like symptoms, bronchitis and dizziness, all experienced by a similar percentage of patients in the olmesartan and placebo groups. The majority (89%) of these adverse events were considered to be either mild or moderate in severity.

## Pharmacoeconomics

The cost-effectiveness of olmesartan treatment has been compared with that for other angiotensin II receptor antagonists (irbesartan, losartan and valsartan) in a US managed-care setting.[27] A randomised, double-blind trial directly comparing angiotensin II receptor antagonists was used as a source of comparative data, and the reduction in the risk of cardiovascular events was estimated from the Framingham Heart Study.[13] The probability of particular cardiovascular events occurring given certain clinical parameters, such as DBP, was predicted using an accelerated failure time Weibull model. Olmesartan was predicted to reduce the costs due to cardiovascular disease by US$906,000, US$3,397,000 and US$2,969,000 compared with irbesartan, valsartan and losartan, respectively. Limitations of this study include the extrapolation of results from an 8-week comparative trial to a longer-term outcome and that only starting doses of angiotensin II receptor antagonists were compared. However, olmesartan has the potential to reduce the overall cost of medical care for hypertensive patients compared with other angiotensin II receptor antagonists, and these data may also be applicable to patients in countries other than the US, although further pharmacoeconomic analyses from a UK-based healthcare perspective would be desirable to confirm these observations.

You are strongly urged to consult your doctor before taking, stopping or changing any of the products reviewed or referred to in *BESTMEDICINE* or any other medication that has been prescribed or recommended by your doctor.

Olmesartan has the potential to reduce the overall cost of medical care for hypertensive patients compared with other angiotensin II receptor antagonists.

## Key points

- Olmesartan is a non-peptide prodrug, whose active form binds selectively and non-competitively to $AT_1$ receptors.

- Doses of olmesartan between 2.5 and 80 mg/day were associated with greater blood pressure reductions than treatment with <u>placebo</u>.

- Olmesartan exhibits a dose-related effect on SBP and DBP, although the incidence of <u>adverse events</u> does not appear to increase with increasing dose.

- Olmesartan also reduces pulse pressure in a broad hypertensive patient population including elderly patients with a wide pulse pressure at <u>baseline</u>.

- Olmesartan provides consistent and smooth control of blood pressure over a 24-hour period as measured by ABPM.

- A once-daily dose of olmesartan was as effective as a twice-daily regimen in terms of reducing <u>ambulatory</u> blood pressure.

- Greater reductions in DBP and SBP were obtained with olmesartan than with losartan, valsartan, irbesartan and candesartan.

- Olmesartan provides superior control of blood pressure compared with the <u>calcium-channel blocker</u>, amlodipine, or the ACE inhibitor, captopril. Olmesartan, in combination with HCTZ, also appears to be at least as effective as the <u>β-blocker</u>, atenolol, also in combination with HCTZ.

- Combining initial olmesartan treatment with sequential additional treatment with HCTZ and amlodipine (as required) provides a very effective stepped-care approach to treating hypertension to stringent targets in the vast majority of patients.

- Olmesartan treatment is generally well tolerated, with an incidence of adverse events in clinical trials that was similar to patients receiving placebo.

- The overall incidence of adverse events was similar in patients receiving olmesartan, losartan, valsartan or irbesartan.

- Pharmacoeconomic data have indicated that olmesartan may reduce healthcare costs by a greater extent than losartan, irbesartan or valsartan.

# References

A list of the published evidence which has been reviewed in compiling the preceding section of *BESTMEDICINE*.

1   Martina B, Dieterle T, Sigle JP, Surber C, Battegay E. Effects of telmisartan and losartan on left ventricular mass in mild-to-moderate hypertension. A randomized, double-blind trial. *Cardiology* 2003; **99**: 169–70.

2   Lewis EJ. The role of angiotensin II receptor blockers in preventing the progression of renal disease in patients with type 2 diabetes. *Am J Hypertens* 2002; **15**: 123S–8S.

3   Kurikawa N, Suga M, Kuroda S, Yamada K, Ishikawa H. An angiotensin II type 1 receptor antagonist, olmesartan medoxomil, improves experimental liver fibrosis by suppression of proliferation and collagen synthesis in activated hepatic stellate cells. *Br J Pharmacol* 2003; **139**: 1085–94.

4   Puchler K, Laeis P, Stumpe KO. Blood pressure response, but not adverse event incidence, correlates with dose of angiotensin II antagonist. *J Hypertens Suppl* 2001; **19(Suppl 1)**: S41–8.

5   Giles TD, Robinson TD. Effects of olmesartan medoxomil on systolic blood pressure and pulse pressure in the management of hypertension. *Am J Hypertens* 2004; **17**: 690–5.

6   Millar-Craig MW, Bishop CN, Raftery EB. Circadian variation of blood-pressure. *Lancet* 1978; **1**: 795–7.

7   Kelly-Hayes M, Wolf PA, Kase CS *et al.* Temporal patterns of stroke onset. The Framingham Study. *Stroke* 1995; **26**: 1343–7.

8   Tofler GH, Muller JE, Stone PH *et al.* Modifiers of timing and possible triggers of acute myocardial infarction in the Thrombolysis in Myocardial Infarction Phase II (TIMI II) Study Group. *J Am Coll Cardiol* 1992; **20**: 1049–55.

9   Mead M. The need for 24-hour blood pressure control. *Br J Cardiol* 2003; **10**: 310–14.

10  The sixth report of the Joint National Committee on prevention, detection, evaluation, and treatment of high blood pressure. *Arch Intern Med* 1997; **157**: 2413–46.

11  Neutel JM, Elliott WJ, Izzo JL, Chen CL, Masonson HN. Antihypertensive efficacy of olmesartan medoxomil, a new angiotensin II receptor antagonist, as assessed by ambulatory blood pressure measurements. *J Clin Hypertens (Greenwich)* 2002; **4**: 325–31.

12  Ball KJ, Williams PA, Stumpe KO. Relative efficacy of an angiotensin II antagonist compared with other antihypertensive agents. Olmesartan medoxomil versus antihypertensives. *J Hypertens Suppl* 2001; **19(Suppl 1)**: S49–56.

13  Oparil S, Williams D, Chrysant SG, Marbury TC, Neutel J. Comparative efficacy of olmesartan, losartan, valsartan, and irbesartan in the control of essential hypertension. *J Clin Hypertens (Greenwich)* 2001; **3**: 283–91.

14  Brunner HR, Stumpe KO, Januszewicz A. Antihypertensive efficacy of olmesartan medoxomil and candesartan cilexetil assessed by 24-hour ambulatory blood pressure monitoring in patients with essential hypertension. *Clin Drug Invest* 2003; **23**: 419–30.

15  Chrysant SG, Marbury TC, Robinson TD. Antihypertensive efficacy and safety of olmesartan medoxomil compared with amlodipine for mild-to-moderate hypertension. *J Hum Hypertens* 2003; **17**: 425–32.

16  Chrysant SG, Weber MA, Wang AC, Hinman DJ. Evaluation of antihypertensive therapy with the combination of olmesartan medoxomil and hydrochlorothiazide. *Am J Hypertens* 2004; **17**: 252–9.

17  Neutel JM, Smith DH, Weber MA, Wang AC, Masonson HN. Use of an olmesartan medoxomil-based treatment algorithm for hypertension control. *J Clin Hypertens (Greenwich)* 2004; **6**: 168–74.

18  Brown MJ, Cruickshank JK, Dominiczak AF *et al.* Better blood pressure control: how to combine drugs. *J Hum Hypertens* 2003; **17**: 81–6.

19  Chobanian AV, Bakris GL, Black HR *et al.* The Seventh Report of the Joint National Committee on Prevention, Detection, Evaluation, and Treatment of High Blood Pressure: the JNC 7 report. *JAMA* 2003; **289**: 2560–72.

20  Williams B, Poulter NR, Brown MJ *et al.* Guidelines for management of hypertension: report of the fourth working party of the British Hypertension Society, 2004-BHS IV. *J Hum Hypertens* 2004; **18**: 139–85.

21  Ichikawa S, Takayama Y. Long-term effects of olmesartan, an angiotensin II receptor antagonist, on blood pressure and the renin-angiotensin-aldosterone system in hypertensive patients. *Hypertens Res* 2001; **24**: 641–6.

22  Miyazaki M, Takai S. Anti-atherosclerotic efficacy of olmesartan. *J Hum Hypertens* 2002; **16(Suppl 2)**: S7–12.

23  Ferrario CM. Use of angiotensin II receptor blockers in animal models of atherosclerosis. *Am J Hypertens* 2002; **15**: 9S–13S.

24  Nangaku M, Miyata T, Sada T *et al.* Anti-hypertensive agents inhibit *in vivo* the formation of advanced glycation end products and improve renal damage in a type 2 diabetic nephropathy rat model. *J Am Soc Nephrol* 2003; **14**: 1212–22.

25  Mizuno M, Sada T, Kato M, Koike H. Renoprotective effects of blockade of angiotensin II AT1 receptors in an animal model of type 2 diabetes. *Hypertens Res* 2002; **25**: 271–8.

**26** Fliser D, Buchholz K, Haller H. Antiinflammatory effects of angiotensin II subtype 1 receptor blockade in hypertensive patients with microinflammation. *Circulation* 2004; **110**: 1103–7.

**27** Simons WR. Comparative cost effectiveness of angiotensin II receptor blockers in a US managed care setting: olmesartan medoxomil compared with losartan, valsartan, and irbesartan. *Pharmacoeconomics* 2003; **21**: 61–74.

## Acknowledgements

Figure 1 is adapted from Puchler *et al.*, 2001.[4]
Figure 2 is adapted from Neutel *et al.*, 2002.[11]
Figure 3 is adapted from Oparil *et al.*, 2001.[13]
Figure 4 is adapted from Chrysant *et al.*, 2004.[16]

# 9. Drug review – Telmisartan (Micardis®)

*Dr Richard Clark*
*CSF Medical Communications Ltd*

## Summary

Hypertension can be treated effectively with a variety of drug therapies. Frequently, however, combinations of these agents are required for blood pressures to be controlled to published guideline targets.[1] Telmisartan, an <u>angiotensin II receptor antagonist,</u> has proved to be effective in controlling hypertension in a large number of patients with hypertension when used either as a <u>monotherapy</u> or in combination with the <u>thiazide diuretic,</u> hydrochlorothiazide (HCTZ). Telmisartan, in common with other angiotensin II receptor antagonists, blocks the effects of <u>angiotensin II</u> by competitively binding to angiotensin II type 1 ($AT_1$) receptors. It has a longer plasma half-life than other angiotensin II receptor antagonists, which may account for its effective control of blood pressure over a 24-hour period. This has implications for the control of the early morning surge in blood pressure and thus may help to prevent excess <u>mortality</u> and <u>morbidity</u> (e.g. <u>myocardial infarction [MI]</u> or strokes) occurring between 6 am and noon. Clinical trials have shown that telmisartan, with or without HCTZ, has a good tolerability and safety profile, and is better tolerated than <u>angiotensin-converting enzyme (ACE) inhibitors</u> and the <u>β-blocker,</u> atenolol.

## Introduction

Angiotensin II plays a major role in <u>cardiovascular homeostasis</u> and, being a potent <u>vasoconstrictor,</u> is thought to be a major determinant of blood pressure, and thus is implicated in hypertension. Drugs that modify the <u>renin–angiotensin system,</u> such as the ACE inhibitors and <u>angiotensin II receptor antagonists,</u> have now become well-accepted treatments for hypertension. However, ACE is not a very specific <u>enzyme</u> because of other pathways of angiotensin II. ACE inhibitor treatment can also lead to an accumulation of <u>bradykinin</u> – a vasodilator but also an inflammatory mediator – that can lead to side-effects such as cough.

Angiotensin II receptor antagonists are more specific than ACE inhibitors. For example, they block the effects of angiotensin II generated by pathways other than the renin–angiotensin–aldosterone system (e.g. by the enzyme chymase) by binding to the $AT_1$ receptor. This specificity for the $AT_1$ receptor translates clinically into a more favourable side-effect profile.

In addition to its vasoconstrictor effects, angiotensin II mediates vascular hypertrophy and the development of atherosclerosis by stimulating the growth of vascular smooth muscle cells. Angiotensin II is also involved in the development of left ventricular hypertrophy (LVH) – a major risk factor for cardiovascular morbidity and mortality – and also plays a role in the progression of renal disease. Antihypertensive therapies that block the effects of angiotensin II have been shown to induce regression of LVH and to improve renal haemodynamics in patients with renal disease.[2,3]

Telmisartan is a non-peptide drug that binds selectively to $AT_1$ receptors, thus blocking the action of angiotensin II. Telmisartan is licensed in the UK for the treatment of hypertension.

This section focuses on the clinical efficacy and safety of telmisartan and discusses the evidence that has accumulated for the drug in the context of data obtained from studies with other antihypertensive agents including other angiotensin II receptor antagonists, ACE inhibitors, calcium-channel blockers, β-blockers and the thiazide diuretic, HCTZ.

## Clinical efficacy

### Dose-ranging studies

 Dose-ranging studies are particularly important to ensure that the optimum dose of a drug can be determined in order that benefit can be realised with the least risk of side-effects.

Whilst it is important to establish an appropriate drug dose range, as a class the angiotensin II receptor antagonists appear to exhibit relatively flat dose–response curves.[4] However, this may be an anomaly associated with investigations into a fairly narrow range of drug doses near the top of the dose–response curve. Indeed, it is possible to establish a conventional dose–response relationship for telmisartan when an appropriate range of doses is used.[4] Patients with mild-to-moderate hypertension (n=274) were given telmisartan, 20, 40, 80, 120 or 160 mg, or placebo, once daily for 4 weeks, in a randomised, double-blind, parallel-group study.[4] A clear dose–response relationship was apparent, with all doses in excess of the 20 mg dose reducing blood pressure compared with placebo ($p < 0.05$). Furthermore, further reductions in blood pressure were obtained in patients receiving telmisartan, 80 mg, compared with those receiving telmisartan, 40 mg ($p < 0.05$). However, doses above 80 mg did not elicit further decreases in diastolic blood pressure. These data support prescribing practice in that telmisartan is normally introduced at 40 mg/day and increased to a maximum dose of 80 mg/day in non-responders.

### Placebo-controlled and open-label trials

A number of placebo-controlled trials have been performed, which have demonstrated that treatment with telmisartan is superior to placebo at a range of doses, using standard clinic blood pressure measurements and ambulatory blood pressure monitoring (ABPM).[5–8] These trials are summarised in Table 1. Superior 'round-the-clock' control of blood pressure was observed for telmisartan but not with losartan or amlodipine in two of these studies.[6,7] The significance of this 24-hour control of blood pressure is discussed more fully in the following section.

## 24-hour control of blood pressure

Ideal attributes for an antihypertensive include the provision of 24-hour blood pressure control, attenuation of the early morning surge in blood pressure and the maintenance of normal circadian patterns of blood pressure.[4] Circadian variations in blood pressure occur such that blood pressure is at its lowest at 3 am, and starts to rise again during the early hours of the morning before waking, with the sharpest increase between 6 am and 9 am.[9] Cerebral haemorrhage and MI may be precipitated by rapid increases in blood pressure, such as those that occur in the morning in normotensive or hypertensive patients. Significantly, most strokes occur between 8 am and noon and most MIs occur between 6 am and noon.[10,11] Furthermore, cardiovascular risk is related to patients' overall blood pressure load – the magnitude of blood pressure elevation and the duration of raised blood pressure.[12] Although the current emphasis in treatment guidelines is to 'treat to target blood pressure', the need for effective 24-hour blood pressure control should not be neglected. Indeed, the sixth annual report of the Joint National Committee (JNC-VI) stated that optimal drug formulations should provide 24-hour efficacy with a once-daily dose, with at least 50% of the peak effect remaining at the end of 24 hours.[13] Thus, an effective antihypertensive should provide consistent and smooth reductions in blood pressure over 24 hours, reducing the risk of blood pressure variability.

> Optimal drug formulations should provide 24-hour efficacy with a once-daily dose, with at least 50% of the peak effect remaining at the end of 24 hours.

The best way to measure 24-hour blood pressure control is by the use of ABPM, which has been employed in several studies that compare telmisartan with other antihypertensive agents. In fact, ABPM seems to have a greater predictive value for target-organ damage in hypertensive patients than standard clinic blood pressure measurements.[14,15]

A meta-analysis of ABPM data from five clinical trials of angiotensin II receptor antagonists has recently been published.[16] This drew upon large, multicentre trials, two with a double-blind placebo-controlled design and three with a prospective, randomised, open-label, blinded endpoint design. Despite these differences in study design, the investigators concluded it was valid to pool the results based on their own validation methods. Patients (n=1566) treated with once-daily placebo, telmisartan, 40 mg or 80 mg, losartan, 50 mg, valsartan, 80 mg, and amlodipine, 5 mg, were included in the meta-analysis. An examination of blood pressure control during the morning period (6.00–11.59 am), demonstrated that both doses of telmisartan provided good blood pressure control (Figure 1). Telmisartan, 80 mg, provided superior diastolic (DBP) and systolic blood pressure (SBP) reductions than losartan, 50 mg, or valsartan, 80 mg (all comparisons $p<0.0125$), and greater SBP reductions than telmisartan, 40 mg ($p<0.0125$).

**Table 1.** Summary of placebo-controlled telmisartan trials in patients with mild-to-moderate hypertension.[5–8]

| Drug regimen | Patients | Outcomes |
| --- | --- | --- |
| Telmisartan, 40, 80 or 120 mg/day, or enalapril, 20 mg/day, or placebo 4-week, randomised, double-blind, double-dummy, parallel-group trial[5] | n=207 | • All doses of telmisartan and enalapril reduced BP compared with placebo treatment ($p \leq 0.01$). <br> • Telmisartan, 40, 80 or 120 mg, and enalapril, 20 mg, reduced supine DBP by 10.0, 15.5, 12.5 and 10.2 mmHg, respectively (from baseline). <br> • There was no significant dose-related increase in response rates, or significant differences in DBP between the telmisartan and enalapril groups. <br> • Higher DBP and SBP trough/peak ratios were obtained in patients receiving telmisartan than enalapril ($\geq 85$ *vs* 65% and $>80$ *vs* 76%, respectively; no *p*-value reported). <br> • The overall incidence of adverse events was not significantly different between those receiving telmisartan, 40, 80 or 120 mg, enalapril, 20 mg, or placebo (25, 17, 29, 31 and 28%, respectively; $p \geq 0.05$). |
| Telmisartan, 40 or 80 mg/day, or losartan, 50 mg/day, or placebo 6-week, randomised, double-blind, double-dummy, parallel-group trial[6] | n=223 | • ABPM at 6 weeks showed that all active treatments produced reductions from baseline in 24-hour mean SBP and DBP compared with placebo ($p<0.01$). <br> • During the 18–24-hour period after dosing, the ABPM reductions in SBP and DBP with telmisartan, 40 or 80 mg (10.7/6.8 mmHg and 12.2/7.1 mmHg, respectively), were greater than those observed for losartan 6.0/3.7 mmHg ($p<0.05$). <br> • Telmisartan, 80 mg, produced greater reductions in SBP and DBP than losartan during all monitored periods of the 24-hour ABPM ($p<0.05$). <br> • The overall incidence of adverse effects was similar in all active treatment groups. |

ABPM, ambulatory blood pressure monitoring; BP, blood pressure; DBP, diastolic blood pressure; HCTZ, hydrochlorothiazide; SBP, systolic blood pressure.

A further <u>meta-analysis</u> of ABPM data has compared telmisartan and losartan for the reduction of mean DBP during the last 6 hours of the 24-hour dosing interval.[17] Data were extracted from two randomised, <u>double-blind</u>, <u>double-dummy</u>, titration-to-response studies conducted in patients with mild-to-moderate hypertension (n=720). All patients received telmisartan, 40 mg/day, or losartan, 50 mg/day, with dose titration after 4 weeks to telmisartan, 80 mg/day, or losartan, 100 mg/day, respectively, if seated <u>trough</u> DBP was at least 90 mmHg.

## Table 1. Continued

| Drug regimen | Patients | Outcomes |
| --- | --- | --- |
| Telmisartan, 40–120 mg/day, or amlodipine, 5–10 mg/day, or placebo 12-week, randomised, double-blind, parallel-group trial[7] | n=232 | • Active treatments were titrated upwards according to patient response and normal clinic BP measurements showed that telmisartan and amlodipine treatments reduced supine BP by a similar extent (SBP: 16.5 vs 17.4 mmHg, respectively; DBP: 11.6 vs 11.6 mmHg, respectively; both $p<0.001$ vs placebo).<br>• Telmisartan and amlodipine treatment reduced mean systolic and diastolic ABPM ($p<0.001$).<br>• Telmisartan reduced DBP by a greater extent than amlodipine during the night-time interval (10 pm–6 am) and the final 4 hours of the dosing interval ($p<0.05$).<br>• There was a similar incidence of overall adverse events in the active treatment and placebo groups. However, oedema was more common in the amlodipine than the telmisartan or placebo groups (22, 5 and 6% respectively; $p=0.001$). |
| Telmisartan, 20, 40, 80 or 160 mg/day, or HCTZ, 6.25, 12.5 or 25 mg/day, or 12 pairwise combinations of telmisartan–HCTZ, or placebo 8-week, double-blind, double-dummy, parallel-group trial[8] | n=818 | • Combination or monotherapy was more effective than placebo ($p<0.01$), and treatment with telmisartan, 40 or 80 mg, plus HCTZ, 12.5 mg, was more effective than the respective monotherapies in reducing SBP and DBP.<br>• In general, the occurrence of adverse effects was similar in those receiving active treatments or placebo. |

ABPM, ambulatory blood pressure monitoring; BP, blood pressure; DBP, diastolic blood pressure; HCTZ, hydrochlorothiazide; SBP, systolic blood pressure.

ABPM was performed at baseline and at the end of the trial. Titration to the higher dose was required in 60 and 70% of telmisartan- and losartan-treated patients, respectively ($p=0.01$). Telmisartan produced greater reductions in DBP and SBP than losartan during the last 6 hours of the 24-hour dosing interval (6.6 vs 5.1 and 9.9 vs 7.8 mmHg, respectively; $p<0.01$ and $p=0.01$, respectively).

A 6-week, randomised, double-blind, double-dummy, parallel-group study evaluated ABPM in patients with mild-to-moderate hypertension (n=223) receiving telmisartan, 40 or 80 mg/day, losartan, 50 mg/day, or placebo.[6] All active treatments provided significant reductions in patients' mean 24-hour SBP or DBP ($p<0.05$). Plots showing 24-hour ABPM show clear separation between patients receiving placebo and active treatments (Figure 2). During the 18–24-hour period after dosing, the reductions in SBP and DBP with telmisartan, 40 mg (10.7 and

Telmisartan produced greater reductions in DBP and SBP than losartan during the last 6 hours of the 24-hour dosing interval.

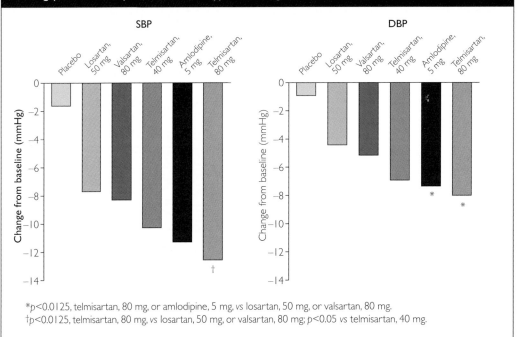

**Figure 1.** Mean reduction in systolic blood pressure (SBP) and diastolic blood pressure (DBP) during the morning (6.00–11.59 am) with various antihypertensive agents.[16]

*$p<0.0125$, telmisartan, 80 mg, or amlodipine, 5 mg, vs losartan, 50 mg, or valsartan, 80 mg.
†$p<0.0125$, telmisartan, 80 mg, vs losartan, 50 mg, or valsartan, 80 mg; $p<0.05$ vs telmisartan, 40 mg.

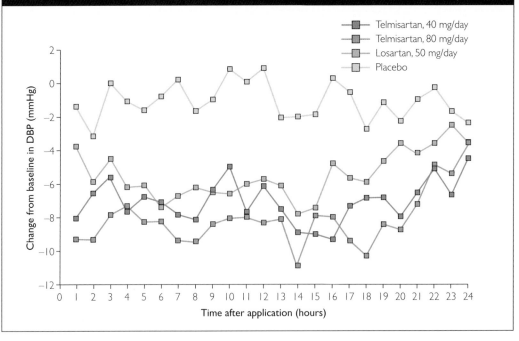

**Figure 2.** Ambulatory blood pressure monitoring plot of the mean change from baseline in diastolic blood pressure (DBP) at week 6 of a randomised, double-blind, double-dummy, parallel-group study in patients with mild-to-moderate hypertension.[6]

6.8 mmHg, respectively), and telmisartan, 80 mg (12.2 and 7.1 mmHg, respectively), were significantly greater than those observed with losartan (6.0 and 3.7 mmHg, respectively; $p<0.05$). In addition, telmisartan, 80 mg, provided greater reductions in both SBP and DBP than losartan throughout the 24-hour period ($p<0.05$). Telmisartan, 40 mg, produced greater reductions in SBP and DBP during the night-time (10.01 pm–5.59 am) and the morning (6.00–11.59 am) periods than losartan (all $p<0.05$). Interestingly, the 3.7 and 2.2 mmHg reductions in SBP and DBP, respectively, observed during the 18–24-hour post-dosing period in the losartan group were not significantly different from the reductions observed with placebo. This study clearly demonstrates that telmisartan has superior antihypertensive efficacy to losartan particularly in the last 6 hours of the 24-hour interval. Thus, all other factors being equal, telmisartan with its long-lasting antihypertensive efficacy should be preferred over other angiotensin II receptor antagonists such as losartan that lose their efficacy at the end of the dosing interval.[18]

ABPM has also been used to compare blood pressure control afforded by telmisartan and the ACE inhibitor enalapril in a 12-week, prospective, randomised, open-label, blinded-endpoint trial.[19] Patients (n=522) with mild-to-moderate hypertension received telmisartan, 40 mg, or enalapril, 10 mg, both given once daily, with titration to 80 and 20 mg once daily, respectively, if required to control a patient's DBP to below 90 mmHg. Telmisartan and enalapril produced similar reductions in SBP and DBP over all the ABPM periods evaluated (last 6 hours, 24 hours, daytime and night-time). However, a greater reduction in seated trough DBP was observed in patients treated with telmisartan than with enalapril (–9.69 *vs* –7.67 mmHg, respectively; $p<0.01$). In addition, more patients receiving telmisartan than enalapril achieved a seated DBP response (59 *vs* 50%, respectively; $p<0.05$), defined as DBP under 90 mmHg or at least a 10 mmHg reduction. Compared with telmisartan, enalapril was associated with a higher incidence of cough and hypotension (8.9 *vs* 0.8% and 3.9 *vs* 1.1%, respectively; no *p*-values reported). Thus, telmisartan provides 24-hour blood pressure control that is at least as effective as that provided by the ACE inhibitor enalapril, and appears to have a more favourable side-effect profile.

In summary, these studies have demonstrated that telmisartan provides excellent 24-hour control of blood pressure, which is particularly important to reduce patients' overall blood pressure load and should also help to prevent the excess of cardiovascular events that are associated with the 'morning surge' of blood pressure.

Telmisartan provides excellent 24-hour control of blood pressure which should help to prevent the excess of cardiovascular events that are associated with the 'morning surge' of blood pressure.

## Telmisartan *vs* other angiotensin II receptor antagonists

### Telmisartan *vs* losartan

Only a few trials have directly compared telmisartan with other angiotensin II receptor antagonists. Superior long-lasting control of blood pressure has been demonstrated for telmisartan over losartan in a randomised, double-blind trial in 223 patients with mild-to-moderate hypertension, as discussed in the previous section.[6]

Fixed-dose combinations of telmisartan (40 or 80 mg/day) in combination with 12.5 mg/day HCTZ, have been compared with losartan, 50 mg/day plus HCTZ, 12.5 mg/day, in patients with mild-to-moderate hypertension (n=597).[20] Telmisartan, 80 mg/day, plus HCTZ, 12.5 mg/day, lowered 24-hour DBP by 2.3 mmHg more than the losartan–HCTZ combination ($p<0.001$). Moreover, during the last 6 hours of the dosing interval, both the 40 and 80 mg/day doses of telmisartan in combination with HCTZ reduced ambulatory blood pressure by 1.8 and 2.5 mmHg more than those receiving the losartan–HCTZ combination ($p<0.05$ and $p<0.001$, respectively). Both telmisartan–HCTZ combinations lowered SBP by a greater extent than the losartan–HCTZ combination over the 24-hour dosing interval and over the last 6 hours of the dosing interval ($p<0.05$ in favour of both telmisartan–HCTZ combinations). All treatments were well tolerated and treatment-related adverse events occurred in 10, 7 and 5% of patients receiving telmisartan, 40 mg/day plus HCTZ, 80 mg/day plus HCTZ, and losartan plus HCTZ, respectively (no *p*-values reported). Thus, in summary, telmisartan is a more effective antihypertensive agent than losartan at the doses investigated, in patients with mild-to-moderate hypertension, particularly during the last few hours of the dosing interval, and is also well tolerated.

> Telmisartan is a more effective antihypertensive agent than losartan in patients with mild-to-moderate hypertension, particularly during the last few hours of the dosing interval, and is also well tolerated.

### Telmisartan *vs* valsartan

A number of recently published trials have compared the relative antihypertensive efficacy of telmisartan and valsartan.[21,22] These studies have superseded earlier studies that compared non-equivalent doses of both agents, and which reported greater blood-pressure lowering efficacy for telmisartan.[23]

A randomised, double-blind, parallel-group, forced-titration study evaluated the antihypertensive effects of telmisartan (40 mg/day for 2 weeks, titrated to 80 mg/day for 4–6 weeks) and valsartan (80 mg/day for 2 weeks, titrated to 160 mg/day for 4–6 weeks) in controlling early morning blood pressure in patients with mild-to-moderate hypertension (n=490).[21] At the end of the study, ABPM measurements were determined after the final dose of active medication. Telmisartan was shown to reduce both SBP and DBP, as determined by ABPM, over the final 6 hours of the dosing interval by a greater extent than valsartan (–11.0/–7.6 mmHg *vs* –8.7/–5.8 mmHg; $p=0.02$ for SBP and $p=0.01$ for DBP, in favour of telmisartan). Reductions in mean 24-hour blood pressure were also greater with telmisartan than with valsartan, though this difference was not statistically significant (–10.3/–6.9 mmHg *vs* –8.7/–5.9 mmHg; *p*=0.06 for SBP and *p*=0.06 for DBP). Both agents were shown to be well tolerated in this study, with a similar incidence of adverse events in both treatment groups.[21] Thus, in conclusion, telmisartan reduced early morning SBP and DBP by a greater extent than valsartan.

In contrast, in a smaller, randomised, open-label, parallel-group study (n=70), which compared telmisartan and valsartan given at their maximum recommended daily doses (telmisartan, 80 mg/day, and valsartan, 160 mg/day) for 3 months, valsartan was shown to be more effective in lowering blood pressure over 24 hours, despite its shorter elimination half-life (7 hours *vs* 24 hours with telmisartan).[22] Thus, whilst both drugs significantly reduced the 24-hour mean blood pressure as determined by ABPM, valsartan reduced SBP and DBP by a greater extent than telmisartan (–18.6/–12.1 mmHg *vs* –10.8/–8.4 mmHg; *p*<0.001). Twenty-four-hour pulse pressure was also significantly reduced with valsartan, but not telmisartan. However, the trough/peak ratio and smoothness index for SBP was reported to be higher for telmisartan than for valsartan, although both parameters for DBP were similar.

Given the conflicting nature of these studies, further large-scale, head-to-head comparative trials appear to be warranted to determine the relative antihypertensive effects of telmisartan and valsartan.

## Telmisartan vs ACE inhibitors

### Telmisartan vs enalapril

Several studies have compared telmisartan with enalapril in various patient populations: patients with mild-to-moderate hypertension, severe hypertension, and in elderly patients with mild-to-moderate hypertension.[19,24,25] These studies are summarised in Table 2 and show that telmisartan is at least as effective as enalapril in patients with mild-to-moderate or severe hypertension, with or without combined HCTZ or amlodipine therapy. Furthermore, treatment with telmisartan was associated with a lower incidence of cough than enalapril.

### Telmisartan vs lisinopril

Telmisartan has been compared with lisinopril as monotherapy and in combination with HCTZ in a 1-year, randomised, double-blind, double-dummy, parallel-group, dose-titration study in 578 patients with mild-to-moderate hypertension.[26] Initially, patients received either telmisartan, 40 mg/day, or lisinopril, 10 mg/day. Doses were then titrated to 80 and then 160 mg/day in the case of telmisartan, or 20 and then 40 mg/day with lisinopril, respectively, as required to control DBP (<90 mmHg). Thereafter, HCTZ 12.5–25 mg/day could be added to either regimen to maintain the control of DBP. Similar proportions of patients had their blood pressure controlled with telmisartan and lisinopril monotherapy (67 and 63%, respectively). At the end of the

> Telmisartan is at least as effective as enalapril in patients with mild-to-moderate or severe hypertension, and is associated with a lower incidence of cough.

**Table 2.** Summary of trials comparing telmisartan and enalapril in patients with hypertension.[19,24,25]

| Drug regimen | Patients | Outcomes |
|---|---|---|
| Telmisartan, 40–80 mg/day, or enalapril, 10–20 mg/day 12-week, prospective, randomised, open-label, blinded-endpoint, parallel-group trial[19] | Patients (n=522) with mild-to-moderate hypertension | • Telmisartan and enalapril reduced SBP and DBP by a similar extent over all ABPM periods (24 hours, daytime, night-time and last 6 hours of dosing). <br> • Telmisartan had a greater effect on mean seated trough DBP than enalapril (−2.2 mmHg, $p<0.01$). <br> • A greater proportion of patients achieved a seated DBP response (<90 mmHg and/or a ≥10 mmHg reduction from baseline) with telmisartan than with enalapril (59 vs 50%, $p<0.05$). <br> • Enalapril was associated with a higher incidence of cough (8.9 vs 0.8% and hypotension (3.9 vs 1.1%). |
| Telmisartan, 80–160 mg/day, or enalapril, 20–40 mg/day, as monotherapy, or plus HCTZ, 25 mg/day, ±amlodipine, 5 mg/day 8-week, randomised, open-label trial[24] | Patients (n=86) with severe hypertension | • At initial monotherapeutic doses (telmisartan, 80 mg, and enalapril, 20 mg), 3.6 and 0% of patients respectively were controlled (DBP <90 mmHg). <br> • Doubling the dose of monotherapy (telmisartan, 160 mg and enalapril, 40 mg) increased control rates to 7.5 and 0%, respectively. <br> • Addition of HCTZ to telmisartan, 160 mg, and enalapril, 40 mg, increased control rates to 33.9 and 20.8%, respectively. <br> • Adding amlodipine, 5 mg, to this regimen increased control rates to 55.2 and 34.8%, respectively. <br> • There were no significant differences in safety and tolerability between the telmisartan and enalapril treatment regimens. |
| Telmisartan, 20–80 mg/day, or enalapril, 5–20 mg/day, both plus HCTZ, 12.5–25 mg/day, if required 26-week, randomised, double-blind, parallel-group trial[25] | Elderly patients (n=278)[a] with mild-to-moderate hypertension | • Telmisartan and enalapril regimens reduced supine DBP by 12.8 and 11.4 mmHg, respectively ($p=0.074$) and supine SBP by 22.1 and 20.1 mmHg ($p=0.350$). <br> • Similar proportions of patients responded (DBP <90 mmHg) to telmisartan and enalapril regimens (63 and 62%, respectively). <br> • Both treatments were effective in lowering BP over the 24-hour dosing interval, as judged by ABPM. <br> • Both treatments were well tolerated, though the incidence of treatment-related cough was twice as high in the enalapril group (16 vs 7%). |

[a]65 years of age or older.

ABPM, ambulatory blood pressure monitoring; BP, blood pressure; DBP, diastolic blood pressure; HCTZ, hydrochlorothiazide; SBP, systolic blood pressure.

study, supine DBP was controlled in 83 and 87% of patients receiving telmisartan and lisinopril, respectively. Fewer treatment-related side-effects occurred in patients given telmisartan than lisinopril (28 *vs* 40%, respectively; *p*=0.001). In particular, fewer patients who received telmisartan experienced treatment-related cough (3 *vs* 7%, respectively; *p*=0.018) and cough led to discontinuation less often with telmisartan than with lisinopril treatment (0.3 *vs* 3.1%, respectively; *p*=0.007).

A randomised, open-label, crossover study compared telmisartan, 80 mg, with lisinopril, 20 mg, in previously untreated patients with essential hypertension (n=32) and used both normal clinic blood pressure monitoring and ABPM.[27] No significant difference in SBP or DBP, or pulse pressure, was detected between the two treatments. Furthermore, no significant differences in trough/peak ratio and smoothness index (measuring the duration and the homogeneity of the antihypertensive effect, respectively) were found between the treatments.

In conclusion, telmisartan has a similar antihypertensive efficacy as lisinopril, as measured by clinic and ABPM methods, and a similar long duration and homogeneity of antihypertensive action over 24 hours. However, telmisartan is associated with fewer treatment-related side-effects than lisinopril.

> Telmisartan has a similar antihypertensive efficacy as lisinopril, but is associated with fewer treatment-related side-effects.

## Telmisartan *vs* perindopril

The antihypertensive efficacy of telmisartan and perindopril has been compared using self-blood pressure measurement (SBPM) and automated office blood pressure measurement in a prospective, randomised, open-label, parallel-group study in patients with mild-to-moderate hypertension.[28] Patients (n=441) received telmisartan, 40 mg, or perindopril, 4 mg, for 6 weeks, and those whose clinic DBP remained higher or equal to 90 mmHg had their dose of telmisartan or perindopril doubled for the remaining 6 weeks of the study. A greater reduction in trough DBP occurred in patients receiving telmisartan compared with those given perindopril (6.6 *vs* 5.1 mmHg, respectively; *p*=0.018), and similar results were obtained for clinic blood pressure results. The requirement to double the dose of antihypertensive was less frequent in the telmisartan group than in the perindopril group (41 *vs* 55%, respectively; *p*=0.005). The overall incidence of adverse events was comparable (34 *vs* 32%, respectively; no *p-value* reported), and most were mild-to-moderate in intensity and transient in nature. However, the incidence of cough was less frequent in patients receiving telmisartan than those given perindopril (<1 *vs* 5%, respectively; *p*=0.007). Thus, telmisartan is more effective, and associated with a lower incidence of cough, than perindopril at the doses administered in this study.

> Telmisartan is more effective, and associated with a lower incidence of cough, than perindopril.

## Telmisartan vs β-blockers

### Telmisartan vs atenolol

One study has compared the efficacy and tolerability of telmisartan and atenolol, in combination with HCTZ, as necessary, for the treatment of mild-to-moderate hypertension in 533 patients.[29] This 26-week, randomised, double-blind, double-dummy, parallel-group, titration-to-response study compared doses of telmisartan, 40 mg/day titrated up to 120 mg/day, with atenolol, 50 mg/day titrated up to 100 mg/day, as necessary to achieve DBP control (≤90 mmHg or decrease from baseline of ≥10 mmHg). Open-label HCTZ, 12.5–25 mg, was added as required. A full morning mean supine DBP response (≤90 mmHg and/or a reduction from baseline of ≥10 mmHg) was observed in similar proportions of patients in the telmisartan and atenolol groups (84 and 78%, respectively; $p>0.05$). A reduction in baseline SBP of at least 10 mmHg was achieved in more patients receiving telmisartan than atenolol (80 vs 68%, respectively; $p=0.003$). There was no significant difference between the telmisartan and atenolol groups in the overall incidence of adverse events (53 vs 61%, respectively; $p>0.05$), or significant difference between any individual adverse events between treatments. Furthermore, both treatments were well tolerated with most adverse events being of mild or moderate severity. Thus, telmisartan appears to be at least as effective as atenolol for the treatment of hypertension.

> Telmisartan appears to be at least as effective as atenolol for the treatment of hypertension.

## Telmisartan vs calcium-channel blockers

### Telmisartan vs amlodipine

A 12-week, randomised, double-blind, parallel-group trial has compared telmisartan with the calcium-channel blocker, amlodipine, and placebo.[7] Patients with mild-to-moderate hypertension (n=232) were given placebo or telmisartan, 40 mg/day, or amlodipine, 5 mg/day, with doses of telmisartan and amlodipine increased by up to 120 mg and 10 mg/day, respectively, if required, to control DBP below 90 mmHg. Both conventional clinic blood pressures and ABPM were used. Clinic blood pressure monitoring detected no difference between the telmisartan and amlodipine groups, with both agents reducing supine blood pressure by a similar extent (SBP: 16.5 vs 17.4 mmHg, respectively; DBP: 11.6 vs 11.6 mmHg, respectively; both $p<0.001$ vs placebo). Furthermore, telmisartan and amlodipine treatments both reduced mean 24-hour systolic and diastolic ABPM (both $p<0.001$ vs placebo; Figure 3). When individual intervals were investigated with ABPM, telmisartan was found to reduce DBP by a greater extent than amlodipine during the night-time (10 pm–6 am) and final 4 hours of the dosing interval ($p<0.05$; Figure 3). Furthermore, heart rates were lower in those treated with telmisartan than those given amlodipine during the final 4 hours of the dosing period (–4.0 vs +0.5 beats/minute, respectively; $p=0.003$). Generally, both telmisartan and amlodipine were well tolerated in this study, but drug-related oedema occurred more

> Telmisartan was found to reduce DBP by a greater extent than amlodipine during the night-time (10 pm–6 am) and final 4 hours of the dosing interval.

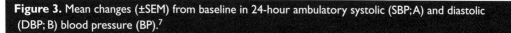

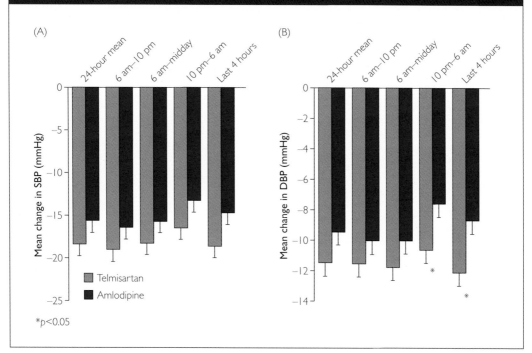

**Figure 3.** Mean changes (±SEM) from baseline in 24-hour ambulatory systolic (SBP; A) and diastolic (DBP; B) blood pressure (BP).[7]

commonly in those receiving amlodipine than those given telmisartan ($p$=0.001) or placebo ($p$=0.03).

In summary, telmisartan and amlodipine provided equivalent reductions in clinic blood pressure, but telmisartan was better tolerated. Telmisartan also imparted greater reductions than amlodipine in ambulatory blood pressure during the night-time and last 4 hours of the dosing interval.

## Combination with other hypertensive agents

Several trials have investigated combinations of telmisartan with other hypertensive agents, principally HCTZ. Some of these studies have been evaluated in previous sections of this review. For example, a telmisartan–HCTZ combination has been shown to be superior to losartan–HCTZ for the control of hypertension over the last 6 hours of the dosing period.[20] However, the studies that have principally focused on telmisartan combination therapy are summarised in Table 3.[30–32] These studies generally demonstrate that the antihypertensive potency of telmisartan–HCTZ combinations is superior to that obtained by telmisartan monotherapy. Furthermore, the telmisartan–HCTZ combination is also generally well tolerated.[33] As the majority of patients with hypertension require more than one agent to achieve their target blood pressure, and the combination of telmisartan with HCTZ fits

The antihypertensive potency of telmisartan–HCTZ combinations is superior to that obtained by telmisartan monotherapy.

**Table 3.** Summary of trials comparing telmisartan as monotherapy and combination therapy with other hypertensive agents in patients with mild-to-moderate hypertension.[30–32]

| Drug regimen | Patients | Outcomes |
|---|---|---|
| Telmisartan, 40 mg/day, with or without HCTZ, 12.5 mg/day 8-week, prospective, randomised, double-blind, parallel-group trial[30] | Patients (n=327) who had not responded[a] to telmisartan, 40 mg/day | • The telmisartan–HCTZ combination lowered both DBP and SBP by an additional 3.5 mmHg over telmisartan monotherapy (both $p<0.01$). <br>• DBP was reduced to <90 mmHg in more patients receiving the combination than those receiving monotherapy (65 vs 40%, respectively; $p<0.05$). <br>• SBP decreased by at least 10 mmHg in 64% of patients receiving telmisartan–HCTZ and 43% receiving telmisartan monotherapy ($p<0.05$). <br>• Both the combination and monotherapy were well tolerated, with no significant differences between treatment groups. |
| Telmisartan, 40–80 mg/day, plus HCTZ, 12.5–25 mg/day, plus another hypertensive, as required, to achieve DBP control[a] 4-year, open-label extension trial[31] | n=888 | • At the end of the study 65% were receiving telmisartan alone, 11.9 and 11.4% were receiving telmisartan plus HCTZ, 12.5 and 25 mg/day, respectively, and 11.6% were taking telmisartan plus another hypertensive ± HCTZ. <br>• Overall, 84% of patients achieved a DBP <90 mmHg. <br>• All treatments were generally well tolerated, with most adverse events mild or moderate in intensity and unrelated to the study drugs. |
| Telmisartan, 80 mg/day, with or without HCTZ, 12.5–25 mg/day, or another antihypertensive, as required, to achieve DBP control[a] 1-year, open-label extension trial[32] | n=489 | • At the end of the study, the proportion of patients with DBP <90 mmHg was: telmisartan, 80 mg/day (70%), telmisartan, 80 mg/day plus HCTZ, 12.5 mg/day (56%), telmisartan, 80 mg/day plus HCTZ, 25 mg/day (55%), telmisartan, 80 mg/day plus other hypertensive ±HCTZ (65%). <br>• Progressively greater reductions in BP occurred with the sequential addition of HCTZ and other antihypertensives, though adding HCTZ, 12.5 mg/day, to telmisartan, 80 mg/day was particularly effective. |

[a]DBP <90 mmHg.
BP, blood pressure; DBP, diastolic blood pressure; HCTZ, hydrochlorothiazide; SBP, systolic blood pressure.

with step 2 of the British Society of Hypertension guidelines for combining antihypertensive drugs, this seems to be an ideal drug combination.[1]

## General practice-based studies

A study based in the primary-care community has provided valuable information about the use of telmisartan in this setting.[34] GPs recruited 2705 patients who were either untreated at the time of study entry with uncontrolled blood pressure (≥140/90 mmHg; n=1957), treated but uncontrolled on current therapy (n=685) or treated and controlled on current <u>monotherapy</u> but with unacceptable side-effects (n=63). Previous antihypertensive therapy was discontinued and treatment with telmisartan, 40 mg/day, initiated and increased to 80 mg/day if blood pressure remained at 130/85 mmHg or higher. In total, treatment lasted 6 weeks, with the greatest reductions occurring in previously untreated patients (Figure 4). Significant reductions from <u>baseline</u> in SBP and DBP occurred for the all-patient group, the previously untreated group and the previously treated but uncontrolled group ($p<0.001$; Figure 4). However, small rises in BP occurred in the treated and blood pressure controlled group (Figure 4). Interestingly, significant mean reductions in SBP and DBP occurred when switching from monotherapy with <u>diuretics</u>, β-blockers, other <u>angiotensin II receptor antagonists</u>, ACE inhibitors or <u>calcium-channel blockers</u> to telmisartan ($p<0.001$ for all comparisons).

Prescribing data collected by the Doctors' Independent Network (DIN) based on a panel of 100 UK-based GP practices (encompassing 400 doctors and 850,000 patients) have been used to evaluate the

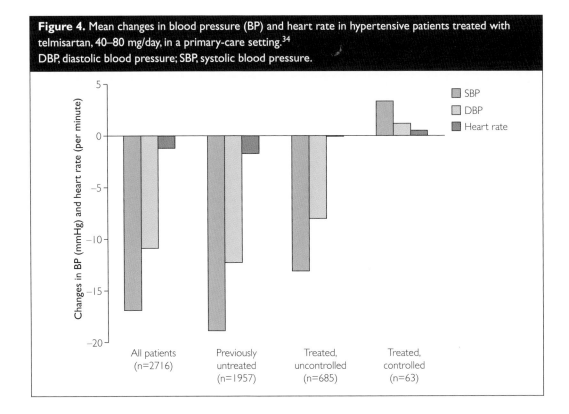

**Figure 4.** Mean changes in blood pressure (BP) and heart rate in hypertensive patients treated with telmisartan, 40–80 mg/day, in a primary-care setting.[34]
DBP, diastolic blood pressure; SBP, systolic blood pressure.

proportion of patients initiated on telmisartan, 40 mg, who required their dose to be titrated to 80 mg during the first year of therapy. These data indicate that 80.3% of patients remained on the 40 mg dose during the period December 2001 to December 2002, and did not require titration to a higher dose. The DIN-LINK database is maintained by the independent company CompuFile (Woking, Surrey; *www.compufile.co.uk/overview_reports.htm*).

## Special patient populations

### Diabetic patients

A double-blind, placebo-controlled study of 119 patients with type 2 diabetes and mild essential hypertension (DBP: 91–104 mmHg) evaluated the relative antihypertensive efficacy of telmisartan and eprosartan, and also determined the effects of both agents upon glucose homeostasis and plasma lipid profiles.[35] Patients were randomised to 12 months' treatment with eprosartan 600 mg, telmisartan, 40 mg, or placebo, administered once daily. Telmisartan and eprosartan both reduced seated trough SBP compared with baseline (mean reductions: –8 and –7 mmHg, respectively; $p<0.01$ *vs* baseline). Likewise, seated trough DBP was also significantly reduced by both agents. However, the DBP-lowering effect of telmisartan was more profound than eprosartan (–8 and –4 mmHg for telmisartan and eprosartan, respectively; $p<0.05$). Interestingly, the plasma lipid profile was also significantly improved with telmisartan, but not with eprosartan. Thus, improvements from baseline were observed in terms of total cholesterol ($p<0.01$), low density lipoprotein cholesterol ($p<0.01$) and triglyceride levels ($p<0.05$) after telmisartan treatment. However, neither agent had any effect on body mass index or glucose metabolism. In conclusion, this study demonstrates that in this mildly hypertensive diabetic patient population, telmisartan provides more profound reductions in DBP than eprosartan with the additional benefit of favourable modifications to the atherogenic lipid profile.

> Telmisartan provides more profound reductions in DBP than eprosartan with the additional benefit of favourable modifications to the atherogenic lipid profile.

A further study has compared telmisartan with the calcium-channel blocker, nifedipine (gastrointestinal therapeutic system [GITS]) in an equivalent patient population to that described in the previous study.[36] A total of 116 patients with adequate glycaemic control at baseline were randomised to 12 months' treatment with telmisartan, 40 mg/day, or nifedipine, 20 mg/day. Both treatments elicited significant reductions from baseline in seated trough SBP (7 and 10 mmHg, for telmisartan and nifedipine, respectively; both $p<0.01$ *vs* baseline) and DBP (–8 and 9 mmHg, respectively; both $p<0.01$ *vs* baseline), but had no effect on body mass index or glucose metabolism. However, consistent with the previous study, telmisartan treatment was associated with significant reductions in both total cholesterol (–9%) and low density lipoprotein cholesterol (–11.5%) compared with nifedipine (–2 and –1.5%, respectively; both comparisons $p<0.01$ in favour of telmisartan). Thus, whilst both telmisartan and nifedipine reduced blood pressure by a similar extent, telmisartan was associated with significant improvements in the plasma lipid profile, relative to nifedipine.

## Patients with diabetic nephropathy

ACE inhibitors are known to prevent the progression of microalbuminuria to overt proteinuria and are considered to be the first-line treatment choice for nephropathy in diabetic patient populations. As such, it is of significant clinical interest to compare the relative efficacy of an angiotensin II receptor antagonist with an established ACE inhibitor regimen in diabetic nephropathy. The recently published DETAIL study (Diabetics Exposed to Telmisartan and Enalapril) was a long-term, prospective evaluation of the relative renoprotective effects of telmisartan and the ACE inhibitor, enalapril, in patients with type 2 diabetes and early nephropathy.[37] A total of 250 patients were randomised to telmisartan (80 mg/day) or enalapril (20 mg/day) treatment for 5 years. Change in glomerular filtration rate (as a marker of renal function) after 5 years' treatment was the primary endpoint and was determined in both treatment groups. This analysis revealed that telmisartan was not inferior to enalapril in providing long-term renoprotection in this diabetic patient population with early signs of nephropathy. Further studies, however, are required to evaluate the relative effects of telmisartan and other ACE inhibitors in patients with more advanced diabetic nephropathy.

# Safety and tolerability

Pooled tolerability data from 5363 patients receiving telmisartan in 27 studies, including 1554 patients who received telmisartan for over 1 year, demonstrated that telmisartan is associated with relatively few side-effects, most of which are mild in intensity and transient in nature.[38] Furthermore, fewer discontinuations due to adverse events occurred in patients taking telmisartan than in patients receiving placebo (2.8 *vs* 6.1%). Moreover, 1334 patients receiving telmisartan monotherapy (20–160 mg/day) and 414 patients taking telmisartan in combination with HCTZ, had a similar overall incidence of adverse events to those receiving placebo.[38]

The most common adverse events in patients receiving telmisartan, 20–160 mg/day, are shown in Figure 5. Back pain, diarrhoea, and upper-respiratory tract infections are more common in patients treated with telmisartan, though the incidence of headache is more common in those given placebo (statistical analyses not reported).

A large, open-label, post-marketing surveillance study conducted in Germany has evaluated the safety and tolerability of telmisartan (40–80 mg/day) given to patients (n=19,870) with essential hypertension over a period of 6 months.[39] Overall, adverse events were reported in 1.9% of patients, whilst global tolerability (as reported by physicians) was considered to be very good, in 74.7% of patients. There were no reported adverse effects of telmisartan treatment upon metabolic

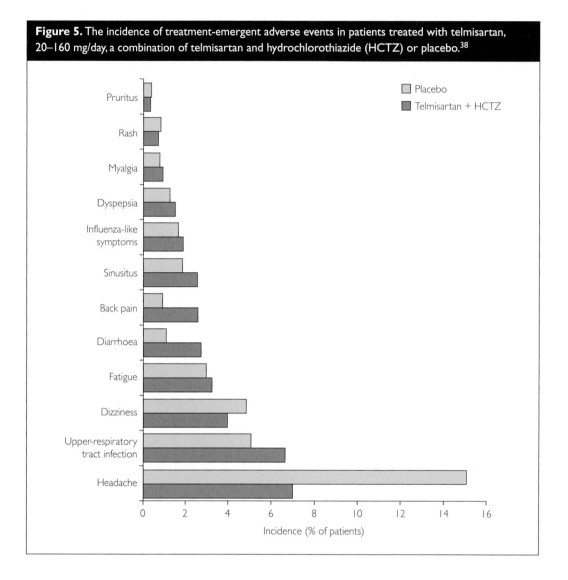

**Figure 5.** The incidence of treatment-emergent adverse events in patients treated with telmisartan, 20–160 mg/day, a combination of telmisartan and hydrochlorothiazide (HCTZ) or placebo.[38]

parameters such as plasma cholesterol and triglycerides or glucose levels, whilst there were also no effects upon serum creatinine or potassium. Moreover, telmisartan was well tolerated across a broad range of patient subgroups stratified by age, gender, concomitant disease status, and previous or present additional antihypertensive medication. Finally, this analysis reported mean reductions in SBP and DBP of 30 and 16 mmHg, respectively, with 76% of patients considered to be responders to treatment. Again, these blood pressure-lowering effects were consistent in the different subpopulations of patients described previously.

In terms of <u>drug interactions</u>, telmisartan has been reported to increase the plasma concentration of digoxin when both agents are co-administered.[40] The manufacturer of telmisartan therefore recommends that plasma digoxin levels should be monitored in such cases.[40]

## Pharmacoeconomics

There is a paucity of pharmacoeconomic data for telmisartan. A cost-effectiveness (decision–analytic) model has been used to explore therapeutic options for the treatment of patients with mild-to-moderate hypertension, incorporating costs of drugs, physician visits and treatment for <u>adverse events</u>.[41] This study found that telmisartan was the second-least expensive first-line therapy (after HCTZ) at US$2392 over 15 months (HCTZ, US$2057; atenolol, US$2426; enalapril, US$2838; amlodipine, US$3018). However, further pharmacoenomic evaluations, particularly from a UK perspective, are clearly required.

# Key points

● Telmisartan is a highly selective 'insurmountable' $AT_1$ receptor antagonist, dissociating very slowly once bound to its receptor, and has a longer plasma half-life than the other angiotensin II receptor antagonists. Each of these factors probably contribute to its long duration of action.

● Dose-ranging studies support the use of an initial dose of 40 mg/day titrating to 80 mg/day where appropriate.

● An ideal antihypertensive drug controls blood pressure over a 24-hour period with a once-daily dose and attenuates the early morning surge in blood pressure, which is associated with excess cardiovascular morbidity and mortality.

● Telmisartan provides superior blood pressure control over 24 hours compared with many other antihypertensives, including other angiotensin II receptor antagonists, particularly over the last 4–6 hours of the dosing interval, due to its long duration of action.

● Telmisartan is at least as effective as the ACE inhibitors enalapril, lisinopril and perindopril for the reduction of hypertension, but is better tolerated.

● Similar or superior reductions in blood pressure parameters were associated with telmisartan compared with the β-blocker atenolol, and the calcium-channel blocker amlodipine. Furthermore, drug-related oedema occurred more commonly in patients receiving amlodipine. Thus, telmisartan is at least as effective as these agents, and appears to be better tolerated than amlodipine.

● Combinations of telmisartan and HCTZ are well tolerated and provide greater efficacy than telmisartan monotherapy.

● Pooled tolerability data from 5363 patients receiving telmisartan showed that telmisartan, with or without HCTZ, is associated with relatively few side-effects, most of which are mild in intensity and transient in nature.

● Pharmacoeconomic data have shown telmisartan to be less expensive than treatment with atenolol, enalapril and amlodipine in patients with mild-to-moderate hypertension, although further cost-effectiveness data are required.

# References

A list of the published evidence which has been reviewed in compiling the preceding section of *BESTMEDICINE*.

1 Brown MJ, Cruickshank JK, Dominiczak AF *et al*. Better blood pressure control: how to combine drugs. *J Hum Hypertens* 2003; **17**: 81–6.

2 Martina B, Dieterle T, Sigle JP, Surber C, Battegay E. Effects of telmisartan and losartan on left ventricular mass in mild-to-moderate hypertension. A randomized, double-blind trial. *Cardiology* 2003; **99**: 169–70.

3 Cupisti A, Rizza GM, D'Alessandro C, Morelli E, Barsotti G. Effect of telmisartan on the proteinuria and circadian blood pressure profile in chronic renal patients. *Biomed Pharmacother* 2003; **57**: 169–72.

4 Meredith PA. Optimal dosing characteristics of the angiotensin II receptor antagonist telmisartan. *Am J Cardiol* 1999; **84**: 7K–12K.

5 Smith DH, Matzek KM, Kempthorne-Rawson J. Dose response and safety of telmisartan in patients with mild-to-moderate hypertension. *J Clin Pharmacol* 2000; **40**: 1380–90.

6 Mallion J, Siche J, Lacourciere Y. ABPM comparison of the antihypertensive profiles of the selective angiotensin II receptor antagonists telmisartan and losartan in patients with mild-to-moderate hypertension. *J Hum Hypertens* 1999; **13**: 657–64.

7 Lacourciere Y, Lenis J, Orchard R *et al*. A comparison of the efficacy and duration of action of the angiotensin II receptor blocker telmisartan to amlodipine. *Blood Press Monit* 1998; **3**: 295–302.

8 McGill JB, Reilly PA. Telmisartan plus hydrochlorothiazide versus telmisartan or hydrochlorothiazide monotherapy in patients with mild-to-moderate hypertension: a multicenter, randomized, double-blind, placebo-controlled, parallel-group trial. *Clin Ther* 2001; **23**: 833–50.

9 Millar-Craig MW, Bishop CN, Raftery EB. Circadian variation of blood-pressure. *Lancet* 1978; **1**: 795–7.

10 Kelly-Hayes M, Wolf PA, Kase CS *et al*. Temporal patterns of stroke onset. The Framingham Study. *Stroke* 1995; **26**: 1343–7.

11 Tofler GH, Muller JE, Stone PH *et al*. Modifiers of timing and possible triggers of acute myocardial infarction in the Thrombolysis in Myocardial Infarction Phase II (TIMI II) Study Group. *J Am Coll Cardiol* 1992; **20**: 1049–55.

12 Mead M. The need for 24-hour blood pressure control. *Br J Cardiol* 2003; **10**: 310–14.

13 The sixth report of the Joint National Committee on prevention, detection, evaluation, and treatment of high blood pressure. *Arch Intern Med* 1997; **157**: 2413–46.

14 Mancia G. Clinical benefits of consistent reduction in the daily blood pressure of hypertensive patients. *J Clin Hypertens (Greenwich)* 2002; **4(Suppl 1)**: 9–14.

15 Meredith PA. A chronotherapeutic approach to effective blood pressure management. *J Clin Hypertens (Greenwich)* 2002; **4**: 15–19.

16 Neutel J, Smith DH. Evaluation of angiotensin II receptor blockers for 24-hour blood pressure control: meta-analysis of a clinical database. *J Clin Hypertens (Greenwich)* 2003; **5**: 58–63.

17 Smith DH, Cramer MJ, Neutel JM, Hettiarachchi R, Koval S. Comparison of telmisartan versus losartan: meta-analysis of titration-to-response studies. *Blood Press Monit* 2003; **8**: 111–17.

18 Messerli FH. ...and losartan was no better than placebo. *J Hum Hypertens* 1999; **13**: 649–50.

19 Amerena J, Pappas S, Ouellet JP, Williams L, O'Shaughnessy D. ABPM comparison of the anti-hypertensive profiles of telmisartan and enalapril in patients with mild-to-moderate essential hypertension. *J Int Med Res* 2002; **30**: 543–52.

20 Lacourciere Y, Gil-Extremera B, Mueller O, Byrne M, Williams L. Efficacy and tolerability of fixed-dose combinations of telmisartan plus HCTZ compared with losartan plus HCTZ in patients with essential hypertension. *Int J Clin Pract* 2003; **57**: 273–9.

21 White WB, Lacourciere Y, Davidai G. Effects of the angiotensin II receptor blockers telmisartan versus valsartan on the circadian variation of blood pressure: impact on the early morning period. *Am J Hypertens* 2004; **17**: 347–53.

22 Calvo C, Hermida RC, Ayala DE, Ruilope LM. Effects of telmisartan 80 mg and valsartan 160 mg on ambulatory blood pressure in patients with essential hypertension. *J Hypertens* 2004; **22**: 837–46.

23 Bakris G. Comparison of telmisartan vs. valsartan in the treatment of mild to moderate hypertension using ambulatory blood pressure monitoring. *J Clin Hypertens (Greenwich)* 2002; **4**: 26–31.

24 Neutel JM, Smith DH, Reilly PA. The efficacy and safety of telmisartan compared to enalapril in patients with severe hypertension. *Int J Clin Pract* 1999; **53**: 175–8.

25 Karlberg BE, Lins LE, Hermansson K. Efficacy and safety of telmisartan, a selective AT1 receptor antagonist, compared with enalapril in elderly patients with primary hypertension. TEES Study Group. *J Hypertens* 1999; **17**: 293–302.

26 Neutel JM, Frishman WH, Oparil S, Papademitriou V, Guthrie G. Comparison of telmisartan with lisinopril in patients with mild-to-moderate hypertension. *Am J Ther* 1999; **6**: 161–6.

27 Stergiou GS, Efstathiou SP, Roussias LG, Mountokalakis TD. Blood pressure- and pulse pressure-lowering effects, trough:peak ratio and smoothness index of telmisartan compared with lisinopril. *J Cardiovasc Pharmacol* 2003; **42**: 491–6.

28 Ragot S, Ezzaher A, Meunier A *et al*. Comparison of trough effect of telmisartan *vs* perindopril using self blood pressure measurement: EVERESTE study. *J Hum Hypertens* 2002; **16**: 865–73.

29  Freytag F, Schelling A, Meinicke T, Deichsel G. Comparison of 26-week efficacy and tolerability of telmisartan and atenolol, in combination with hydrochlorothiazide as required, in the treatment of mild-to-moderate hypertension: a randomized, multicenter study. *Clin Ther* 2001; **23**: 108–23.

30  Lacourciere Y, Martin K. Comparison of a fixed-dose combination of 40 mg telmisartan plus 12.5 mg hydrochlorothiazide with 40 mg telmisartan in the control of mild to moderate hypertension. *Am J Ther* 2002; **9**: 111–17.

31  Freytag F, Holwerda NJ, Karlberg BE, Meinicke TW, Schumacher H. Long-term exposure to telmisartan as monotherapy or combination therapy: efficacy and safety. *Blood Press* 2002; **11**: 173–81.

32  Neutel JM, Klein C, Meinicke TW, Schumacher H. Long-term efficacy and tolerability of telmisartan as monotherapy and in combination with other antihypertensive medications. *Blood Press* 2002; **11**: 302–9.

33  Fenton C, Keating GM, Scott LJ. Telmisartan/ hydrochlorothiazide: in the treatment of essential hypertension. *Drugs* 2003; **63**: 2013–26.

34  Giles TD, Bakris GL, Smith DH, Davidai G, Weber MA. Defining the antihypertensive properties of the angiotensin receptor blocker telmisartan by a practice-based clinical trial. *Am J Hypertens* 2003; **16**: 460–6.

35  Derosa G, Ragonesi PD, Mugellini A, Ciccarelli L, Fogari R. Effects of telmisartan compared with eprosartan on blood pressure control, glucose metabolism and lipid profile in hypertensive, type 2 diabetic patients: a randomized, double-blind, placebo-controlled 12-month study. *Hypertens Res* 2004; **27**: 457–64.

36  Derosa G, Cicero AF, Bertone G *et al.* Comparison of the effects of telmisartan and nifedipine gastrointestinal therapeutic system on blood pressure control, glucose metabolism, and the lipid profile in patients with type 2 diabetes mellitus and mild hypertension: a 12-month, randomized, double-blind study. *Clin Ther* 2004; **26**: 1228–36.

37  Barnett AH, Bain SC, Bouter P *et al.* Angiotensin-receptor blockade versus converting-enzyme inhibition in type 2 diabetes and nephropathy. *N Engl J Med* 2004; **351**: 1952–61.

38  Sharpe M, Jarvis B, Goa KL. Telmisartan: a review of its use in hypertension. *Drugs* 2001; **61**: 1501–9.

39  Michel MC, Bohner H, Koster J, Schafers R, Heemann U. Safety of telmisartan in patients with arterial hypertension: an open-label observational study. *Drug Saf* 2004; **27**: 335–44.

40  Boehringer Ingelheim International. Micardis® (telmisartan). *Summary of product characteristics.* January 2004.

41  Richter A, Gondek K, Ostrowski C, Dombeck M, Lamb S. Mild-to-moderate uncomplicated hypertension: further analysis of a cost-effectiveness study of five drugs. *Manag Care Interface* 2001; **14**: 61–9.

## Acknowledgements

Figure 2 is adapted from Neutel *et al.*, 2003.[16]
Figure 3 is adapted from Mallion *et al.*, 1999.[6]
Figure 4 is adapted from Lacourciere *et al.*, 1998.[7]
Figure 5 is adapted from Giles *et al.*, 2003.[34]
Figure 6 is adapted from Sharpe *et al.*, 2001.[38]

# 10. Drug review – Valsartan (Diovan®)

*Dr Richard Clark*
*CSF Medical Communications Ltd*

## Summary

Valsartan is a member of the class of agents termed <u>angiotensin II receptor antagonists</u>. Like the other members of this class, valsartan is an effective antihypertensive agent and has an excellent <u>safety and tolerability</u> profile. On the balance of available evidence, valsartan appears to be superior to losartan in terms of its antihypertensive action. However, it is difficult to draw similar conclusions when valsartan is compared with other angiotensin II receptor <u>antagonists</u> such as telmisartan or irbesartan based on the available clinical data. Comparative trials have shown that valsartan is as effective as <u>angiotensin-converting enzyme (ACE) inhibitors</u>, <u>calcium-channel blockers</u> and β-blockers, and is generally better tolerated. When valsartan is combined with hydrochlorothiazide (HCTZ), valsartan is particularly effective and is generally well tolerated. Whilst not the principal focus of this review, a series of large-scale, clinical outcomes studies have demonstrated that valsartan may offer <u>mortality</u> and <u>morbidity</u> benefits across a variety of diverse patient populations. Indeed, data from one of these studies – VALIANT (Valsartan in <u>Acute Myocardial Infarction [MI]</u> Trial) – has formed the basis for the recent approval of valsartan in the UK for use in a post-MI setting.

## Introduction

The peptide hormone <u>angiotensin II</u> has a central role in the regulation of blood pressure, fluid and <u>electrolyte</u> homeostasis. It is formed from its precursor, <u>angiotensin I</u>, by the <u>proteolytic action</u> of ACE. Although the treatment of hypertension has benefited from the development of ACE inhibitors, this class of agents has certain weaknesses. These include an inherent lack of specificity, as ACE affects other biochemical pathways such as the degradation of <u>bradykinin</u>. Thus, treatment with ACE inhibitors can cause an accumulation of bradykinin, and as bradykinin is an inflammatory mediator, ACE inhibitor therapy can lead to side-effects including cough.

Two main types of angiotensin II receptor subtypes – angiotensin II type-1 and type-2 receptors ($AT_1$ and $AT_2$, respectively) – have been identified. $AT_1$ is responsible for most of the well-known actions of angiotensin II, including vasoconstriction, aldosterone release and vascular hypertrophy, whereas the pathophysiological role of $AT_2$ receptors is not well characterised.[1] The development of specific non-peptide, orally active angiotensin II receptor antagonists to displace angiotensin II selectively from $AT_1$ receptors was a major breakthrough in the management of hypertension. This class of agents is not associated with bradykinin-mediated adverse events, such as cough, and have generally good tolerability profiles.

This section focuses on the clinical efficacy, tolerability and safety of valsartan, a non-peptide angiotensin II receptor antagonist used in the treatment of hypertension. The accumulated evidence for the use of this agent will be discussed in the context of data obtained from studies with other antihypertensive medications.

## Clinical efficacy and tolerability

### Placebo-controlled and dose-ranging studies

The efficacy and tolerability of a range of valsartan doses have been explored in a number of trials, and valsartan has been compared with placebo in some of these studies (Table 1).[2–5] A pooled analysis of nine randomised, double-blind, placebo-controlled trials in 4067 patients with hypertension, showed that all doses of valsartan, 10–320 mg/day, were more effective in reducing systolic (SBP) or diastolic blood pressure (DBP) than placebo ($p<0.05$).[6] A study in 736 patients that evaluated doses of valsartan from 20–320 mg/day showed that although the 80, 160 and 320 mg doses of valsartan were more effective than placebo and were generally well tolerated, more patients experienced dizziness in the 320 mg group than with lower doses.[2] Thus, the usual starting dose of valsartan, 80 mg once daily, seems optimal in most cases, with subsequent titration to 160 mg once daily also effective where required.[2,4,6] Another trial showed that valsartan was as effective as enalapril, and that both were more effective than placebo for the treatment of mild-to-moderate hypertension.[3]

### Valsartan vs other angiotensin II receptor antagonists

The efficacy of a range of doses of angiotensin II receptor antagonists have been compared in a number of clinical trials with clinic and/or ambulatory blood pressure as the main outcome measures (Table 2).[7–14] In two large-scale, flexible-dose trials, valsartan was shown to be at least as effective as losartan in reducing SBP or DBP (Table 2).[7,8] Furthermore, valsartan was shown to be superior to losartan such that a greater proportion of valsartan-treated patients were classified by the

*Dose-ranging studies are particularly important to ensure that the optimum dose of a drug can be determined in order that benefit can be realised with the least risk of side-effects.*

**Table 1.** Summary of trials comparing valsartan with placebo and/or dose-ranging studies in patients with hypertension.[2–5]

| Drug regimen | Patients | Outcomes |
| --- | --- | --- |
| Valsartan, 20, 80, 160, 320 mg/day, or placebo 8-week, randomised, double-blind, parallel-group study[2] | n=736 DBP 95–115 mmHg | • All doses of valsartan reduced DBP and SBP at 8 weeks from baseline ($p<0.001$). <br> • Compared with patients receiving placebo, there were reductions in DBP of 3.4, 5.2, 5.3 and 6.5 mmHg for the valsartan, 20, 80, 160 and 320 mg groups, respectively (all $p<0.001$). <br> • Compared with patients receiving placebo, there were reductions in SBP of 5.0, 7.3, 7.6 and 9.3 mmHg for the valsartan, 20, 80, 160 and 320 mg groups, respectively (all $p\leq0.002$). <br> • The proportion of patients classed as responders[a] was greater in those receiving valsartan, 80, 160 and 320 mg, than in the placebo group (43, 44, 52 and 21%, respectively; $p<0.001$). There was no significant difference in response rate between the 20 mg group and those receiving placebo (28 vs 21%, respectively; $p=0.149$). <br> • Valsartan was generally well tolerated with a placebo-like tolerability profile regardless of dose. The percentage of patients reporting adverse events in the valsartan, 20, 80, 160, 320 mg/day, or placebo groups was 50, 47, 44, 47 and 44%, respectively. |
| Valsartan, 80 mg/day, enalapril, 20 mg/day, or placebo 8-week, randomised, double-blind, parallel-group study[3] | n=348 DBP 95–115 mmHg | • Reductions in SBP from baseline for valsartan, enalapril and placebo groups were 12.4, 13.1 and 5.7 mmHg, respectively, and DBP reductions from baseline were 9.5, 9.4 and 4.5 mmHg, respectively. <br> • Valsartan and enalapril both reduced SBP ($p=0.004$ and $p=0.013$, respectively) and DBP ($p<0.001$ and $p=0.003$, respectively) compared with those patients given placebo. <br> • There was no significant difference between valsartan and enalapril in SBP and DBP reductions ($p=0.924$ and $p=0.436$, respectively) or in response rates (54 vs 58%, respectively; $p=0.628$). |

[a]DBP of <90 mmHg, or decrease from baseline of ≥10 mmHg.
DBP, diastolic blood pressure; SBP, systolic blood pressure.

## Table 1. Continued

| Drug regimen | Patients | Outcomes |
|---|---|---|
| Valsartan, 10, 40, 80, 160, 320 mg/day, or placebo 4-week, randomised, double-blind, parallel-group study[4] | n=122 DBP 95–115 mmHg | • Valsartan, 10, 40, 80 or 160 mg/day, reduced SBP by 3.6, 7.0, 11.1, 11.9 mmHg, and DBP by 4.9, 6.5, 8.2, 9.1 mmHg, respectively (all $p<0.001$ vs baseline). <br>• A positive dose–response relationship was observed: response rates[a] (24, 33, 46, 54 and 16% for valsartan, 10, 40, 80, 160 mg/day and placebo groups, respectively). <br>• The overall incidence of adverse events was not related to the dose of valsartan (44% with placebo vs 44, 36, 22 and 21% for valsartan, 10, 40, 80 and 160 mg, respectively). |
| Valsartan, 80–160 mg/day 8-week, single-blind, single-arm flexible-dose study[5] | n=256 DBP 95–115 mmHg | • The response rate to valsartan, 80 mg, was 45.4%, and of those patients not responding to this dose, 36.3% responded to valsartan, 160 mg. <br>• Ambulatory blood pressure monitoring showed consistent and smooth reductions in SBP and DBP over 24 and 32 hours after receiving valsartan, showing that once-daily dosing is appropriate. |

[a]DBP of <90 mmHg, or decrease from baseline of ≥10 mmHg.
DBP, diastolic blood pressure; SBP, systolic blood pressure.

> It appears reasonable to conclude that valsartan provides superior blood pressure control compared with losartan.

investigators as responders (61.6 vs 54.5%, respectively; $p=0.021$) (Table 2).[8] Three smaller randomised clinical trials have also evaluated the comparative antihypertensive efficacy of valsartan and losartan and have provided further evidence of a superior antihypertensive effect for valsartan.[15–17] Thus, for example, 24-hour, daytime and night-time ambulatory blood pressure readings were significantly lower with valsartan ($p<0.01$), whilst valsartan was also shown to exert a more homogeneous antihypertensive effect than losartan.[15] On the balance of the available data, therefore, it appears reasonable to conclude that valsartan provides superior blood pressure control compared with losartan.

Several trials have compared valsartan with irbesartan or telmisartan, but used fixed doses which may not be pharmacologically equivalent.[9,10,12–14] As patients should be treated to target blood pressure levels, it is important to titrate medication to effect. Thus, the rather artificial scenario in which fixed doses are compared is of limited practical value unless the entire range of approved doses are compared within fixed-dose trials. The differences between angiotensin II receptor antagonists may be largely explained by differences in dosing schedules.[18] Thus, it is particularly difficult to draw meaningful

**Table 2.** Summary of studies comparing valsartan with other angiotensin II receptor antagonists in patients with hypertension.[7–14]

| Drug regimen | Patients | Outcomes |
|---|---|---|
| Valsartan, 80–160 mg/day, or losartan, 50–100 mg/day 12-week, randomised, double-blind, parallel-group study[7] | n=495 DBP 95–115 mmHg | • There was no significant difference in efficacy between valsartan and losartan treatments.<br>• Mean reductions in trough DBP in the valsartan and losartan groups were 10.1 and 9.9 mmHg, respectively ($p=0.683$).<br>• The percentage of responders[a] was 59 vs 57%, respectively, for the valsartan and losartan groups ($p=0.827$).<br>• Valsartan and losartan reduced SBP by 11.9 and 10.6 mmHg, respectively ($p=0.388$). |
| Valsartan, 80–160 mg/day, losartan, 50–100 mg/day, or placebo 8-week, randomised, double blind, parallel-group study[8] | n=1369 DBP 95–115 mmHg | • Valsartan and losartan reduced DBP by 10.5 and 9.7 mmHg (both $p<0.001$ vs placebo), a difference (0.8 mmHg) that did not achieve significance (no $p$-value reported).<br>• More patients were classed as responders[a] in the valsartan than the losartan group (61.6 vs 54.5%, respectively; $p=0.021$).<br>• Valsartan and losartan were similarly well tolerated (one or more adverse event reported by 31.6, 29.3 and 32.0% of patients in the valsartan, losartan and placebo groups, respectively). |
| Valsartan, 80 mg/day, or irbesartan, 150 mg/day 8-week, randomised, double blind, parallel-group study[9] | n=426 DBP 95–110 mmHg | • Valsartan was less effective than irbesartan in reducing trough systolic ABP (7.5 vs 11.6 mmHg, respectively; $p<0.01$) and diastolic ABP (4.8 vs 6.7 mmHg, respectively; $p=0.035$).<br>• Inferior reductions in mean 24-hour ABP were obtained with valsartan than irbesartan (systolic: 7.8 vs 10.2 mmHg, respectively; $p<0.01$; diastolic: 4.8 vs 6.4 mmHg, respectively; $p=0.023$).<br>• The percentage of responders[a] in the valsartan and irbesartan groups were 44.3 and 63.9%, respectively ($p<0.001$).<br>• It is important to note that the doses of valsartan and irbesartan used in this trial may not be pharmacologically equivalent (see main text). |

[a]DBP of <90 mmHg, or decrease from baseline of ≥10 mmHg.
[b]Mean 24-hour DBP of <80 mmHg, or reduction from baseline of ≥10 mmHg.
ABP, ambulatory blood pressure; DBP, diastolic blood pressure; SBP, systolic blood pressure.

| Table 2. Continued | | |
| --- | --- | --- |
| Drug regimen | Patients | Outcomes |
| Valsartan, 80 mg/day, or irbesartan, 150 mg/day 8-week, randomised, open-label, crossover study[10] | n=40 DBP 95–115 mmHg | • Both valsartan and irbesartan reduced 24-hour, daytime and night-time ABP (both $p<0.001$ vs placebo wash-out period). • No significant differences were found between valsartan and irbesartan, including 24-hour systolic or diastolic ABP (−10.5 vs −10.5mmHg and −9.7 vs −9.5 mmHg, respectively; no p-values reported). • Clinic SBP/DBP decreases for valsartan and irbesartan (8.9/7.2 mmHg and 9.1/7.5 mmHg, respectively) were not significantly different between groups (no p-value reported). |
| Valsartan, 80–160 mg/day, or telmisartan, 40–80 mg/day 8-week, randomised, double-blind, parallel-group, forced-titration trial[11] | n=490 DBP 95–110 mmHg | • There was no significant difference in 24-hour ABP reductions between valsartan and telmisartan treatments (systolic ABP: 10.6 vs 11.8 mmHg, respectively [$p=0.18$]; diastolic ABP: 7.0 vs 7.9 mmHg, respectively [$p=0.16$]). • However, greater reductions in morning (6 am to noon) systolic ABP (12.0 vs 9.7 mmHg) and diastolic ABP (8.0 vs 6.6 mmHg) were obtained with telmisartan than valsartan ($p=0.03$ and $p=0.05$, respectively). • Greater reductions in the 6-hour interval before dosing for systolic ABP (11.0 vs 8.7 mmHg) and diastolic ABP (7.6 vs 5.8 mmHg) were obtained with telmisartan than valsartan ($p=0.02$ and $p=0.01$, respectively). |

[a]DBP of <90 mmHg, or decrease from baseline of ≥10 mmHg.
[b]Mean 24-hour DBP of <80 mmHg, or reduction from baseline of ≥10 mmHg.
ABP, ambulatory blood pressure; DBP, diastolic blood pressure; SBP, systolic blood pressure.

comparisons between valsartan and telmisartan or irbesartan based on the available clinical data as this information does not represent the normal clinical situation for patients with hypertension.

## Valsartan vs ACE inhibitors

Valsartan has been compared with the ACE inhibitors, enalapril, lisinopril or captopril in a number of randomised trials (Table 3).[19–24] Essentially, valsartan is at least as effective as ACE inhibitors in reducing SBP and DBP in a range of patients with hypertension, including the elderly.[19–24] The main difference between valsartan and ACE inhibitors is that valsartan is better tolerated, particularly with respect to the incidence of dry cough. However, the tolerability profiles of both drug

> Valsartan is better tolerated than ACE inhibitors, particularly with respect to the incidence of dry cough.

**Table 2.** Continued

| Drug regimen | Patients | Outcomes |
|---|---|---|
| Valsartan, 80 mg/day, or telmisartan, 80 mg/day 8-week, randomised, open-label, blinded endpoint trial[12] | n=214 DBP 95–114 mmHg | • Greater systolic or diastolic ABP reductions were obtained with telmisartan than valsartan in the 24-hour, morning or daytime periods (all $p<0.05$).<br>• However, the response rate[b] was not significantly different between the valsartan and telmisartan groups (49 vs 57%, respectively; $p=0.09$). |
| Valsartan, 160 mg/day, or telmisartan, 80 mg/day 12-week, randomised, open-label, parallel-group trial[13] | n=70 DBP 90–109 mmHg | • Valsartan was associated with greater reductions than telmisartan in 24-hour systolic ABP (18.6 vs 10.8 mmHg, respectively; $p<0.001$) and diastolic ABP (12.1 vs 8.4 mmHg, respectively; $p=0.014$).<br>• Valsartan reduced the systolic ABP by more than telmisartan throughout the entire 24-hour period; average reductions in diastolic DBP in the last 6 hours of the dosing interval were greater for valsartan than telmisartan (10.6 vs 7.6 mmHg, respectively; $p=0.006$).<br>• Valsartan, but not telmisartan, reduced 24-hour mean pulse pressure by 6.5 mmHg from baseline ($p<0.001$). However, the reduction from baseline in pulse pressure was not significant in the telmisartan group (no values/$p$-value reported). |
| Valsartan, 80 mg/day, irbesartan, 150 mg/day, losartan, 50 mg/day, or olmesartan, 20 mg/day 8-week, randomised, double-blind, parallel-group study[14] | n=588 DBP 100–115 mmHg | • The reductions in clinic DBP were greater with olmesartan (11.5 mmHg) than irbesartan (9.9 mmHg; $p=0.0412$), losartan (8.2 mmHg; $p=0.0002$), or valsartan (7.9 mmHg; $p<0.0001$).<br>• The reductions in SBP were not significantly different between olmesartan, irbesartan, losartan or valsartan treatments (11.3, 11.0, 9.5, 8.4 mmHg, respectively; $p>0.05$).<br>• The reduction in mean 24-hour DBP with olmesartan was greater than with losartan and valsartan (8.5 vs 6.2 and 5.6 mmHg, respectively; $p<0.05$ for both comparisons), but not irbesartan (7.4 mmHg, $p>0.05$).<br>• The reduction in mean 24-hour SBP with olmesartan was greater than for losartan and valsartan (12.5 vs 9.0 and 8.1 mmHg, respectively; $p<0.05$ for both comparisons), but not irbesartan (11.3 mmHg, $p>0.05$).<br>• All treatments were generally well tolerated, with treatment-related adverse events occurring in 11, 14, 12 and 13% of patients in the irbesartan, losartan, olmesartan and valsartan groups, respectively. |

[a]DBP of <90 mmHg, or decrease from baseline of ≥10 mmHg.
[b]Mean 24-hour DBP of <80 mmHg, or reduction from baseline of ≥10 mmHg.
ABP, ambulatory blood pressure; DBP, diastolic blood pressure; SBP, systolic blood pressure.

**Table 3.** Summary of trials comparing valsartan with angiotensin-converting enzyme (ACE) inhibitors in patients with hypertension.[19–24]

| Drug regimen | Patients | Outcomes |
|---|---|---|
| Valsartan, 80 mg/day, or enalapril, 20 mg/day, for 8 weeks, ±HCTZ, 12.5 mg/day, as required thereafter 12-week, randomised, double-blind, study[19] | n=189 DBP 95–120 mmHg | • Valsartan and enalapril monotherapy were equally effective in reducing SBP (17.2 vs 17.7 mmHg, respectively; $p=0.307$), and DBP (13.2 vs 12.0 mmHg, respectively; $p=0.475$).<br>• A similar proportion of patients responded[a] to valsartan and enalapril monotherapy (60.6 and 52.6%, respectively; $p=0.267$).<br>• Both treatments were well tolerated, with three patients receiving enalapril and one receiving valsartan discontinuing treatment due to cough. |
| Valsartan, 160 mg/day, or enalapril, 20 mg/day 16-week, randomised, open-label, blinded-endpoint, parallel-group study[20] | n=144 Aged 61–80 years DBP 95–110 mmHg | • A greater reduction in SBP/DBP was obtained with valsartan than enalapril (18.6/13.7 vs 15.6/10.9 mmHg, respectively; $p<0.01$).<br>• Valsartan improved elements of cognitive function, particularly episodic memory: word list memory score increased by 11.8% ($p<0.05$ vs baseline and $p<0.01$ vs enalapril) and word list recall score increased by 18.7% ($p<0.05$ vs baseline and $p<0.01$ vs enalapril).<br>• Enalapril did not improve cognitive function. |
| Valsartan, 80 mg/day, or enalapril, 20 mg/day, for 4 weeks ±indapamide, 1.25 mg/day, as required thereafter 8-week, randomised, open-, label, parallel-group study[21] | n=142 Colombians at altitudes of 2600, 1538 or 100 metres above sea level DBP 95–115 mmHg | • Valsartan and enalapril monotherapy (at 4 weeks) and ±indapamide (at 8 weeks) reduced SBP by a similar extent (14 vs 13.5 mmHg, respectively; $p=0.665$; 15.5 vs 16.0, respectively; $p=0.399$).<br>• Valsartan and enalapril monotherapy (at 4 weeks) and ±indapamide (at 8 weeks) reduced DBP by a similar extent (10.6 vs 10.9 mmHg, respectively; $p=0.516$; 12.6 vs 12.1, respectively; $p=0.739$).<br>• The treatment effects were independent of altitude, as analysed by ANOVA, with similar blood pressure reductions noted in the cities of Bogotá (2600 metres), Medellín (1538 metres) and Barranquilla (100 metres).<br>• Both treatments were generally well tolerated, with dry cough more frequently reported in the enalapril than the valsartan group (12.1 vs 3.4% of all adverse events, respectively; $p<0.05$). |

[a]DBP of <90 mmHg, or decrease from baseline of ≥10 mmHg.

ANOVA, analysis of variance; DBP, diastolic blood pressure; HCTZ, hydrochlorothiazide; SBP, systolic blood pressure.

**Table 3.** Continued

| Drug regimen | Patients | Outcomes |
|---|---|---|
| Valsartan, 80–160 mg/day, or lisinopril, 10–20 mg/day, or placebo 12-week, randomised, double-blind, flexible-dose study[22] | n=734 DBP 95–115 mmHg | • Treatment with valsartan, lisinopril or placebo reduced DBP from baseline by 8.29, 9.97 and 3.04 mmHg, respectively ($p<0.001$ for either active treatment vs placebo). There was no significant difference between valsartan and lisinopril in terms of DBP reductions ($p>0.05$). Similar results were obtained for SBP (no data reported). <br>• The incidence of drug-related adverse events was lower in the valsartan than the lisinopril group (22.8 and 27.8%, respectively; no $p$-value reported). <br>• A lower frequency of drug-related cough was reported for the valsartan than the lisinopril group (1.1 vs 8.0% respectively; no $p$-value reported). |
| Valsartan, 40–80 mg/day, or lisinopril, 2.5–20 mg/day, ±HCTZ, 12.5–25 mg/day, as required 1-year, randomised, double-blind, parallel-group, flexible-dose study[23] | n=501 DBP 96–115 mmHg Aged ≥65 years | • There was no significant difference in response rates[a] between valsartan and lisinopril groups (with or without HCTZ) at 12 weeks (both 80%; $p=0.925$) or at 52 weeks (81 and 87%; $p=0.148$). <br>• Fewer patients receiving valsartan than lisinopril experienced drug-related cough (7.5 vs 17.4%, respectively; no $p$-value reported). <br>• Discontinuation due to adverse events or laboratory abnormalities occurred in 11.7 and 18.6% of patients receiving valsartan and lisinopril, respectively (no $p$-value reported). |
| Valsartan, 80 mg/day, or captopril, 50 mg/day 8-week, randomised, open-label, parallel-group study[24] | n=197 DBP 95–115 mmHg | • Valsartan and captopril lowered SBP/DBP by a similar degree (21.8/12.5 vs 18.4/12.2, respectively; no $p$-value reported). <br>• The proportion of patients responding to treatment was similar for valsartan and captopril treatment groups (69 vs 71%, respectively; no $p$-value reported). <br>• Both medications were generally well tolerated, but no patients in the valsartan group reported adverse events whereas in the captopril group dry cough, headache and nausea/vomiting were reported by 22, 1 and 2%, respectively. |

[a]DBP of <90 mmHg, or a decrease from baseline of ≥10 mmHg.
DBP, diastolic blood pressure; HCTZ, hydrochlorothiazide; SBP, systolic blood pressure.

classes is generally good. Interestingly, valsartan, 160 mg/day, is not only more effective in reducing blood pressure than enalapril, 20 mg/day, in an elderly population, but also improves elements of cognitive function.[20] Thus, valsartan increased the word list memory score by 11.8% and the word list recall score by 18.7% (both parameters $p<0.05$ *vs* baseline and $p<0.01$ *vs* enalapril), though there was no effect of valsartan on other cognitive function assessments such as verbal fluency, the Boston naming test and word list recognition. In contrast, enalapril did not improve cognitive function as assessed by any of these tests.[20]

### Valsartan vs calcium-channel blockers

The effects of valsartan treatment for hypertension have been compared with the calcium-channel blocker amlodipine in a variety of patient populations. Patients with mild-to-moderate hypertension (DBP >95 and <120 mmHg) were randomised to receive valsartan, 80 mg/day, or amlodipine, 5 mg/day, for 8 weeks.[25] If blood pressure was not adequately controlled (DBP >95 mmHg), amlodipine, 5 mg/day, could be added to both treatment groups after 8 weeks for the remaining 4 weeks of the study. Similar mean reductions in SBP and DBP were observed for the valsartan and amlodipine monotherapy groups at 8 weeks (13.1 *vs* 14.8 mmHg and 11.5 *vs* 11.1 mmHg, respectively; $p=0.82$ and $p=0.68$, respectively). Furthermore, the response rates at 8 weeks were also similar (66.7 and 60.2% in the valsartan and amlodipine groups, respectively; $p=0.39$). Further reductions in SBP and DBP blood pressure occurred during the last 4 weeks of the study, during which time some patients received additional amlodipine, but these reductions were comparable between the valsartan and amlodipine groups (16.5 *vs* 19.3 mmHg and 13.5 *vs* 14.8 mmHg, respectively; no *p*-values reported). Although both treatments were generally well tolerated, the treatment-related incidence of oedema was higher with amlodipine than with valsartan. Thus, oedema occurred in 2.4, 3.6 and 14.3% of patients receiving valsartan, 80 mg, and amlodipine, 5 mg and 10 mg, respectively (no *p*-values reported). There were no incidences of oedema in the valsartan–amlodipine (5 mg) group.

Long-term blood pressure trends and cardiovascular outcomes in patients at high cardiovascular risk have been investigated in the Valsartan Antihypertensive Long-term Use Evaluation (VALUE) study.[26,27] The blood pressure trends from the VALUE study are discussed here whilst the cardiovascular outcomes of patients enrolled into this study are discussed in subsequent sections of this review (see the Morbidity/Mortality Benefits section of the article).

The VALUE study was a randomised, double-blind, parallel-group trial that compared treatment with valsartan, 80–160 mg/day, with amlodipine, 5–10 mg/day, both titrated as required, with patients receiving additional treatment with HCTZ, 12.5–25 mg/day, and thereafter any other supplemental antihypertensives, in order to control blood pressure to target (<140/90 mmHg). An analysis of the long-term blood pressure trends in treated patients in the VALUE study has recently been published.[26] After 12 months of any antihypertensive treatment, SBPs and DBPs were reduced to 141.2 and 82.9 mmHg, respectively (both $p<0.0001$ vs baseline), with blood pressure decreasing further to 139.1/80.0 mmHg by 24 months ($p<0.0001$ vs 12 months) and 138.0/79.0 mmHg at 30 months ($p<0.0001$ vs 24 months). At 24 months, 39.7% of patients were receiving valsartan or amlodipine monotherapy, 26.6% were receiving HCTZ supplemental therapy, 15.1% other add-on drugs and 4.3% protocol drugs in non-standard doses. Thus, the antihypertensive regimens employed in the VALUE study provide excellent long-term blood pressure reductions, which surpass those reported in many other clinical trials. When the blood pressure lowering-effects of valsartan and amlodipine were compared directly in the VALUE study, it was noted that amlodipine provided a more pronounced response, particularly during the initial 6 months of treatment.[27] The difference between the two treatment groups at 1 month was 4.0/2.1 mmHg (difference between groups $p<0.001$). However, after 6 months' treatment, the differences between the two treatments were reduced, with an average difference of 2.0/1.6 mmHg between the groups. By the end of the study 56% and 62% of patients in the valsartan and amlodipine groups, respectively, had achieved their target blood pressure of <140/90 mmHg.

More recently, a 12-week randomised, double-blind trial has directly compared the relative blood pressure-lowering efficacies of valsartan (40–80 mg/day) and amlodipine (5–10 mg/day) when given as monotherapy to patients (n=246) with mild-to-moderate hypertension.[28] A 4-week placebo wash-out period ensured that no patient was receiving any additional antihypertensive agent during randomisation. Blood pressure was monitored throughout the study using a variety of measurements, including office, ambulatory and home measurements. Reductions in 24-hour trough SBP were more pronounced with the amlodipine regimen than with valsartan. Thus, SBP was reduced by 17.8 and 14.6 mmHg, respectively in the two groups ($p=0.025$). However, differences between the two treatments were not significant with regard to the primary endpoint of this study, DBP (−12.7 and −10.9 mmHg, respectively; $p=0.06$). Ambulatory blood pressure was also reduced by a significantly greater extent with amlodipine than with valsartan (SBP/DBP: −13.0/−10.8 vs −7.2/−4.9 for amlodipine vs valsartan, respectively; $p<0.05$). In addition, the slope of the morning surge in DBP was less steep with amlodipine than with valsartan, 48 hours after the lose dose, indicating a longer duration of action for amlodipine. However, the superior blood-pressure control associated with amlodipine was at the expense of a higher incidence of ankle oedema (15.3 vs 2.5%).

The efficacy and safety of valsartan and amlodipine have also been compared in 421 elderly patients (mean age 69 years) with isolated systolic hypertension (SBP 160–220 mmHg).[29] This 24-week, randomised, double-blind, parallel-group trial compared valsartan, 80–160 mg/day, with amlodipine, 5–10 mg/day, with additional

The antihypertensive regimens employed in the VALUE study provide excellent long-term blood pressure reductions, which surpass those reported in many other clinical trials.

HCTZ, 12.5 mg/day, for both groups after week 16 if blood pressure was uncontrolled. Similar reductions in SBP were observed in the valsartan and amlodipine groups at 16 weeks (30.7 vs 32.2 mmHg, respectively; both $p<0.001$ vs baseline) and at 24 weeks (33.4 vs 33.5 mmHg, respectively; $p<0.001$ vs baseline) (Figure 1). Overall, adverse events were observed in 20.2 and 31.9% of patients receiving valsartan and amlodipine, respectively ($p<0.003$), and peripheral oedema rates of 4.8 and 26.8%, respectively ($p<0.001$) were reported. Thus, valsartan has similar efficacy but better tolerability than amlodipine in elderly patients with isolated systolic hypertension. A substudy of this trial investigated 24-hour ambulatory blood pressure in 164 patients.[30] There were no significant differences in mean 24-hour, daytime and night-time systolic ambulatory blood pressure between the valsartan and amlodipine treatments ($p>0.05$). However, amongst 138 responders (mean 24-hour blood pressure and peak blood pressure levels on treatment were lower than baseline values) valsartan had a greater antihypertensive effect than amlodipine over a 24-hour period (18.3 vs 15.0 mmHg, respectively; $p=0.02$) and during daytime hours (20.4 vs 16.6 mmHg, respectively; $p=0.02$). Thus, valsartan is at least as effective as amlodipine (and more so in those responding to treatment) in reducing isolated systolic hypertension in the elderly, and is also better tolerated.

> Valsartan is at least as effective as amlodipine (and more so in those responding to treatment) in reducing isolated systolic hypertension in the elderly, and is also better tolerated.

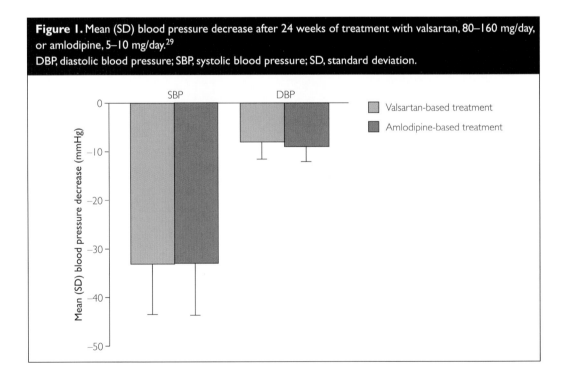

**Figure 1.** Mean (SD) blood pressure decrease after 24 weeks of treatment with valsartan, 80–160 mg/day, or amlodipine, 5–10 mg/day.[29]
DBP, diastolic blood pressure; SBP, systolic blood pressure; SD, standard deviation.

## Valsartan vs β-blockers

The efficacy and tolerability of valsartan and the β-blocker, atenolol, have been compared for the treatment of patients (n=103) with severe primary hypertension (mean DBP of at least 110 mmHg and less than 120 mmHg).[31] Patients participating in this double-blind trial were randomised to receive treatment for 6 weeks with either valsartan, 160 mg/day, or atenolol, 100 mg/day, and supplemental HCTZ, 25 mg/day, and verapamil, 240 mg/day, were given if required. There was no significant difference between the efficacy of valsartan and atenolol treatments: DBP was reduced by 19.9 and 20.7 mmHg and SBP by 30.7 and 26.5 mmHg, respectively ($p$=0.819 and $p$=0.161 for valsartan vs atenolol). Moreover, the response rates (DBP reduced to less than 90 mmHg or by at least 10 mmHg) in the valsartan and atenolol groups were similar (85.1 and 86.1%, respectively; $p$=0.887). The proportion of patients in the valsartan and atenolol groups requiring additional HCTZ was 83.6 and 97.2%, respectively, and 64.2 and 58.3%, respectively, also required verapamil (no statistical analysis performed). Both treatments were generally well tolerated, with a comparable incidence of adverse events in the valsartan and atenolol groups (38.8 and 50%, respectively). Thus, valsartan is equally effective and at least as well tolerated as atenolol for the treatment of severe primary hypertension.

> Valsartan is equally effective and at least as well tolerated as atenolol for the treatment of severe primary hypertension.

## Comparison or combination with HCTZ

Effective blood pressure control is often not achieved with antihypertensive monotherapy, so combination treatment may be required. Effective combinations consist of agents with different primary modes of action, such as valsartan and the thiazide diuretic, HCTZ.[32] A double-blind, parallel-group study assessed valsartan and HCTZ monotherapy and combinations of valsartan and HCTZ.[33] Hypertensive patients (n=871) were randomised to receive valsartan, 80 or 160 mg/day, HCTZ, 12.5 or 25 mg/day, combination therapy (at the aforementioned four doses) or placebo. All combination treatments produced greater reductions in SBP and DBP than the corresponding monotherapies, and this was reflected in the response rates (Figure 2). Combination treatment was well tolerated, as were the monotherapies, though the higher doses of the combination produced a slightly greater incidence of dizziness compared with valsartan monotherapy (no $p$-value reported).

> All combination treatments produced greater reductions in SBP and DBP than the corresponding monotherapies.

Other smaller trials have compared the valsartan and HCTZ combination with the respective monotherapies.[34,35] An 8-week, randomised, double-blind trial in 217 patients with hypertension poorly controlled after 4 weeks' treatment with HCTZ, 12.5 mg/day, showed that treatment with valsartan, 80 mg, plus HCTZ, 12.5 mg, was more effective than monotherapy with HCTZ, 12.5 or 25 mg/day.[34] Combination treatment reduced DBP by 11.3 mmHg compared with 2.9 and 5.7 mmHg in the HCTZ, 12.5 and 25 mg/day monotherapy groups, respectively ($p$<0.001 for combination treatment vs either monotherapy). The tolerability of study medication was comparable in

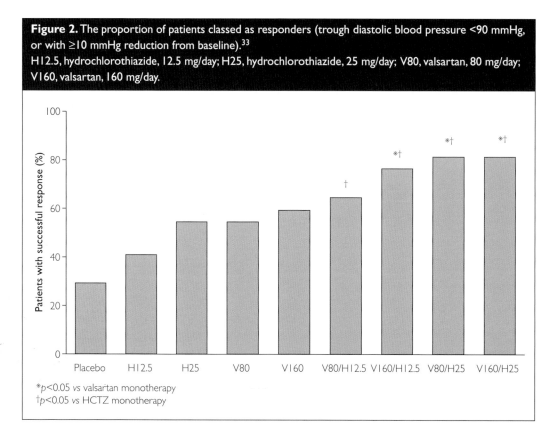

**Figure 2.** The proportion of patients classed as responders (trough diastolic blood pressure <90 mmHg, or with ≥10 mmHg reduction from baseline).[33]
H12.5, hydrochlorothiazide, 12.5 mg/day; H25, hydrochlorothiazide, 25 mg/day; V80, valsartan, 80 mg/day; V160, valsartan, 160 mg/day.

*p<0.05 vs valsartan monotherapy
†p<0.05 vs HCTZ monotherapy

all three groups. Another double-blind, parallel-group trial compared the efficacy and safety of 8 weeks' treatment with valsartan, 160 mg/day, plus HCTZ, 12.5 or 25 mg/day, with valsartan, 160 mg/day monotherapy.[35] The patients recruited for this study had blood pressure that was inadequately controlled after 4 weeks' treatment with valsartan, 160 mg/day. The greatest reductions in blood pressure were obtained with valsartan, 160 mg/day, plus HCTZ, 25 mg/day (Figure 3). Moreover, this group had a greater proportion of responders (68%) than the valsartan, 160 mg/day group (49%; p<0.001) or the valsartan, 160 mg/day, plus HCTZ, 12.5 mg/day group (62%; p<0.01). All treatments were generally well tolerated and the incidence of adverse events was very low and similar between treatment groups.

Pulse pressure (defined as SBP minus DBP) is thought to be an important indicator of cardiovascular risk, particularly in middle-aged and elderly populations.[36] Thus, a randomised, double-blind, parallel-group study of patients (n=2002) with hypertension investigated 8 weeks' treatment with valsartan, 160 mg/day, with or without HCTZ, 12.5 or 25 mg/day.[36] Valsartan monotherapy reduced pulse pressure by 4.7 mmHg, whilst valsartan plus HCTZ, 12.5 or 25 mg/day, reduced pulse pressure by 6.7 and 7.5 mmHg, respectively (p<0.05 and p<0.001 vs valsartan monotherapy, respectively). Therefore, combination treatment with valsartan/HCTZ provides an additional dose-related

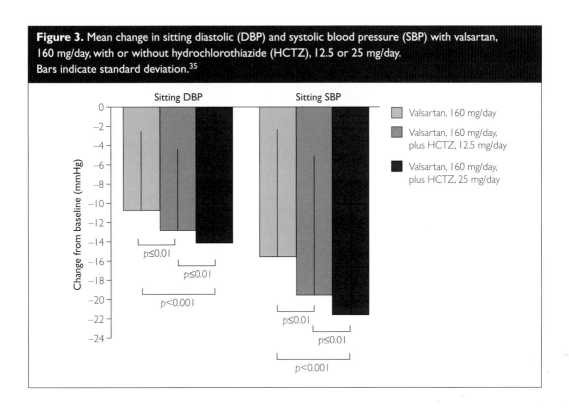

**Figure 3.** Mean change in sitting diastolic (DBP) and systolic blood pressure (SBP) with valsartan, 160 mg/day, with or without hydrochlorothiazide (HCTZ), 12.5 or 25 mg/day. Bars indicate standard deviation.[35]

reduction in pulse pressure over that achieved with valsartan monotherapy.

## Efficacy in general practice

The efficacy and tolerability of valsartan, alone or as part of a combination regimen, has been evaluated by a 6-month, open-label, post-marketing surveillance study of patients with hypertension in general practice (n=7256).[37] A total of 3855 (53%) of patients were given valsartan as monotherapy (mostly as 80 mg/day), 1162 (16%) also received the thiazide-related compound, chlortalidone, at a dose of 12.5 mg/day, 347 (4.8%) received valsartan plus other antihypertensive agents, and the remainder were not evaluable due to inadequate records. SBP and DBP were reduced significantly from baseline, and by a similar degree, in the valsartan monotherapy and valsartan plus chlortalidone groups at 8 weeks (25.6/17.3 vs 24.6/15.4 mmHg, respectively; no p-value reported). Overall tolerability was high, with 98.5 and 97.7% of patients in the valsartan monotherapy and valsartan plus chlortalidone groups evaluated as having excellent or good tolerability ratings by the study investigators.

A German post-marketing surveillance study evaluated the efficacy and tolerability of 6 months' valsartan monotherapy in 26,488 patients (trial 1) and that of a fixed combination of valsartan and HCTZ given to 28,440 patients over 3 months (trial 2).[38] Sixty-one per cent of patients in trial 1 received only valsartan therapy without any need for additional antihypertensive medication. In patients receiving the valsartan–HCTZ combination, this figure increased to 75.8%. Valsartan, either alone or in combination with HCTZ, provided marked reductions in both SBP and DBP (–29.5/–15.6 mmHg, respectively, for valsartan monotherapy; –27.3/–14.7 mmHg for valsartan–HCTZ combination therapy). Both treatment regimens were well tolerated with 97.5 and 99.3% of patients reporting no adverse events in trials 1 and 2, respectively.

Thus, these large post-marketing surveillance studies indicate that valsartan (either alone or combined with other antihypertensive agents) provides excellent blood-pressure lowering efficacy and good tolerability in patients presenting in general practice.

## Elderly patient populations

Valsartan demonstrated good efficacy and excellent tolerability profiles in elderly populations in a randomised, open-label, blinded-endpoint, parallel-group study (in comparison with enalapril) in patients aged 61–80 years, and in a randomised, double-blind, parallel-group, flexible-dose study (in comparison with lisinopril) in those aged at least 65 years of age (see the Valsartan *vs* ACE Inhibitors section of this article).[20,23] Valsartan has also demonstrated efficacy in a population of 146 patients of at least 65 years of age (mean age 73 years) with systolic hypertension.[39] In this double-blind, parallel-group trial, patients were randomised to receive either valsartan, 80 mg or placebo, for 4 weeks, after which time the valsartan group were force-titrated to a 160 mg/day dose for a further 4 weeks whilst those in the placebo group continued to receive placebo. Reductions of SBP were greater in the valsartan than the placebo group (19.2 *vs* 8.8 mmHg, respectively; $p<0.001$). Furthermore, the tolerability for valsartan was comparable with that for placebo, with adverse events occurring in 42.5 and 38.4% of patients, respectively.

Increased arterial stiffness is the major cause of increased pulse pressure, and both of these factors are known to be independent risk factors for cardiovascular disease in the elderly.[40] The effect of various antihypertensives has been investigated in patients (n=76) aged at least 65 years of age with hypertension in an open-label trial.[40] Patients were randomised to receive valsartan, 80 mg/day, temocapril, 2–4 mg/day (an ACE inhibitor), cilnidipine, 10 mg/day (a calcium-channel blocker), or nifedipine, 20 mg/day, for 3 months. Valsartan had a greater effect on reducing brachial-ankle pulse wave velocity (baPWV) than temocapril, cilnidipine or nifedipine (all $p<0.01$). Reductions in pulse pressure were similar for the valsartan, temocapril and cilnidipine groups (29.6, 25.7, 28.0 mmHg, respectively, $p<0.01$ *vs* baseline), but was not significantly reduced from baseline in the nifedipine group (9.9 mmHg; $p>0.05$).

## Patients with type 2 diabetes mellitus

Valsartan may have beneficial effects in patients with type 2 diabetes that are independent of its antihypertensive effects. Patients with type 2 diabetes and microalbuminuria, with or without hypertension (n=332), were randomly assigned to receive valsartan, 80 mg/day, or amlodipine, 50 mg/day, for 24 weeks, in the Microalbuminuria Reduction with Valsartan (MARVAL) study.[41] Dose-doubling and, if required, additional treatment with bendroflumethiazide and doxazosin, were used to achieve target blood pressure (135/85 mmHg). The primary outcome was the percentage change in elevated urine albumin excretion rate (UAER). At the end of the trial UAER was 56 and 92% of baseline levels with valsartan and amlodipine treatments, respectively (*p*<0.001 valsartan *vs* amlodipine). Valsartan lowered UAER similarly in both the hypertensive and normotensive groups, with more patients reverting to normoalbuminuria with valsartan than amlodipine (29.9 *vs* 14.5%, respectively; *p*=0.001). Similar reductions in UAER to those reported in this trial have been found in normotensive and hypertensive patients (n=122) with type 2 diabetes treated with valsartan or captopril for 1 year compared with placebo-treated patients.[42] Thus, valsartan appears to be effective in lowering microalbuminuria independently of its antihypertensive effects in patients with type 2 diabetes.

> Valsartan seems to be effective in lowering microalbuminuria independently of its antihypertensive effects in patients with type 2 diabetes.

## 24-hour control of blood pressure

The 24-hour control of blood pressure with valsartan, although good, appears to be less effective than the angiotensin II receptor antagonists irbesartan and telmisartan, but superior to amlodipine (see the Valsartan *vs* Angiotensin II Receptor Antagonists and the Valsartan *vs* Calcium-Channel Blockers sections of this article).[9,11,30] A further study has investigated the administration time-dependent effects of valsartan on ambulatory blood pressure.[43] Hypertensive patients were randomised to receive valsartan, 160 mg/day, either on awakening or at bed-time, for 3 months. Mean SBP and DBP reductions were similar whether given in the morning or at bed-time (17.0 *vs* 14.6 and 11.3 *vs* 11.4 mmHg, respectively; *p*>0.174 for treatment–time effect).

The 24-hour antihypertensive effect of various doses of valsartan has been explored in a double-blind, placebo-controlled study.[44] Patients (n=217) were randomised to receive valsartan, 20, 80, 160 or 320 mg/day, or placebo, for 8 weeks. This trial showed that doses of valsartan of 80 mg/day, or greater, reduced systolic and diastolic ambulatory blood pressure compared with placebo during both daytime and night-time periods. Moreover, the circadian pattern of blood pressure was preserved and was similar to that observed at baseline, but shifted into the normotensive range. Thus, valsartan doses of 80 mg/day, or greater, provided effective 24-hour control of blood pressure without the loss of diurnal variation. The Food and Drug Administration (FDA) in the US have since approved the 320 mg dose of valsartan as the maximum recommended dose.

> Valsartan doses of 80 mg/day, or greater, provided effective 24-hour control of blood pressure without the loss of diurnal variation.

A subgroup of patients in an 8-week placebo-controlled study of valsartan were evaluated using ambulatory blood pressure monitoring for a further 24 hours at the end of the study.[5] Half (n=10) of these patients skipped one dose of the study drug and were monitored for a further 24 hours. Data from this analysis indicated that consistent blood pressure reductions were achieved with valsartan over a 24-hour period and these reductions were maintained for up to 32 hours in those who had missed a dose of study medication.

## Patient compliance

Patient treatment compliance with valsartan, amlodipine or lisinopril has been evaluated in a retrospective observational study of 142,954 patients.[45] More patients receiving valsartan persisted with their treatment 12 months beyond the date of their first prescription, compared with those taking amlodipine or lisinopril (63, 53 and 50%, respectively; $p<0.001$ for both comparisons). Moreover, the crude and adjusted compliance rates were also greater for those taking valsartan than amlodipine or lisinopril, as reflected by the adjusted mean medication possession ratio (75, 67 and 65%, respectively; $p<0.0001$ for both comparisons). Thus, patients are more likely to comply and persist with their treatment in the long term with valsartan than amlodipine or lisinopril treatment.

## Morbidity/mortality benefits

Although the principal objective of this review is to consider the use of valsartan within its primary licensed indication of hypertension, data from a number of significant trials have recently been published which have evaluated the efficacy of valsartan in terms of cardiovascular outcomes. The results from three studies – the Valsartan Heart Failure Trial (ValHEFT), the VALUE trial and the VALIANT trial – will be considered briefly in this section.[27,46,47]

In ValHEFT, patients (n=5010) with New York Heart Association (NYHA) class II, III or IV heart failure, were randomly assigned to receive valsartan, 40 mg twice daily, or placebo, in addition to their standard therapy for heart failure. The dose of valsartan was doubled every 2 weeks until a dose of 160 mg, twice daily, was reached.[a]

The primary study endpoints were all-cause mortality and the combined endpoint of mortality and morbidity (incidence of cardiac arrest with resuscitation, hospitalisation for heart failure, or intravenous inotropic or vasodilator therapy for at least 4 hours). Mortality rates were similar in the valsartan and placebo groups (19.7 vs 19.4%, respectively; $p=0.80$). However, there was a difference between the valsartan and placebo groups for the combined endpoint of all-cause mortality and morbidity (28.8 vs 32.1%, respectively; $p=0.009$) (Figure 4). This difference was predominantly driven by a reduction in the number of hospitalisations for heart failure in the valsartan than the placebo group (13.9 vs 18.5%, respectively; $p=0.00001$). When a subgroup analysis was performed on the 8% of patients who did not receive an ACE inhibitor as the background treatment for heart failure, an even more profound relative risk reduction in the combined endpoint was observed with

---

[a]Valsartan is not currently licensed in the UK for this indication.

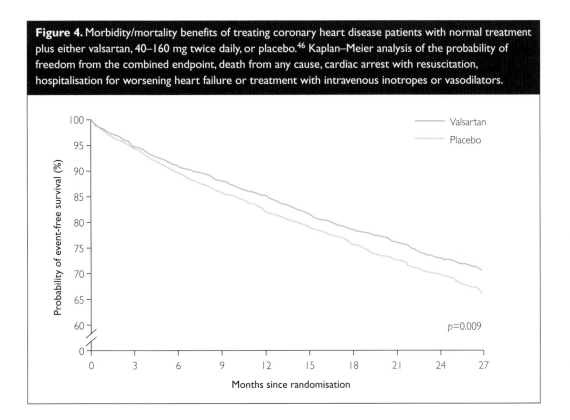

**Figure 4.** Morbidity/mortality benefits of treating coronary heart disease patients with normal treatment plus either valsartan, 40–160 mg twice daily, or placebo.[46] Kaplan–Meier analysis of the probability of freedom from the combined endpoint, death from any cause, cardiac arrest with resuscitation, hospitalisation for worsening heart failure or treatment with intravenous inotropes or vasodilators.

valsartan treatment (relative risk reduction, 44.5%; $p=0.0002$ *vs* placebo). In conclusion, there appears to be <u>morbidity</u> but not <u>mortality</u> benefits in adding valsartan treatment to standard care for heart-failure patients.

The VALUE study evaluated whether a valsartan-based treatment regimen would provide more benefit in terms of reducing <u>cardiovascular</u> morbidity and mortality than an amlodipine treatment regimen for the same level of blood pressure control in hypertensive patients at high risk of cardiovascular events.[27] The study was prospectively designed to evaluate blood pressure reductions over the course of treatment. These data have been reviewed in an earlier section of this article together with further detail regarding the study design (see Valsartan *vs* <u>Calcium-Channel Blockers</u>).[26] The primary <u>endpoint</u> (a composite of cardiac mortality and morbidity) occurred in equal proportions of patients in the valsartan (10.6%) and the amlodipine groups (10.4%; hazard ratio 1.04, $p=0.49$; Table 4). The <u>Kaplan–Meier curves</u> separated during the initial 6 months of treatment, but converged and overlapped towards the end of the study. There were also notable differences between the groups with regard to the timing of the occurrence of the primary endpoint. Thus, during the first 6 months of treatment when amlodipine provided more marked reductions in blood pressure (see Valsartan *vs* Calcium-Channel Blockers), the odds ratio for the occurrence of the primary endpoint favoured amlodipine treatment. However, differences in the

There may be morbidity, but not mortality benefits in adding valsartan treatment to standard care for heart-failure patients.

**Table 4.** Clinical endpoints in the Valsartan Antihypertensive Long-term use Evaluation (VALUE) study.[27]

| Endpoint | Incidence of event (%) | | | |
| --- | --- | --- | --- | --- |
| | Valsartan (n=7649) | Amlodipine (n=7596) | Hazard ratio | p-value |
| **Primary endpoint** | | | | |
| Composite endpoint (cardiac mortality and morbidity) | 10.6 | 10.4 | 1.04 | 0.49 |
| Cardiac mortality | 4.0 | 4.0 | 1.01 | 0.90 |
| Cardiac morbidity | 7.7 | 7.6 | 1.02 | 0.71 |
| **Secondary endpoint** | | | | |
| Myocardial infarction | 11.4 | 9.6 | 1.19 | 0.02 |
| Heart failure | 11.0 | 12.4 | 0.89 | 0.12 |
| Stroke | 10.0 | 8.7 | 1.15 | 0.08 |
| All-cause mortality | 25.6 | 24.8 | 0.45 | 1.04 |
| New-onset diabetes | 13.1 | 16.4 | 0.77[a] | <0.0001 |

[a]Odds ratio for occurrence of new onset diabetes (incidence rates based on patients without diabetes at baseline).

odds ratios were attenuated over the following months with continuing treatment. In terms of secondary endpoints, treatment with amlodipine was associated with a significantly lower incidence of MI (9.6 *vs* 11.4%; *p*=0.02), although the rate of fatal events was equivalent in both groups. The difference in event rates between the treatment groups may reflect the more significant blood pressure reductions observed with amlodipine within the early phase of the study. However, there appeared to be fewer cases of heart failure in the valsartan group, although the difference between the treatment arms did not reach significance (11.0 *vs* 12.4%). Moreover, for heart failure hospitalisations, there was a trend in favour of valsartan treatment over the final 4 years of the study. Notably, there was 23% higher incidence of new-onset diabetes in patients treated with the amlodipine-based regimen compared with a valsartan-based approach (16.4 *vs* 13.1%; odds ratio 0.77; *p*<0.0001), and suggests a potentially positive effect of valsartan treatment on long-term glucose metabolism. In terms of tolerability, valsartan was associated with significantly fewer treatment discontinuations as a consequence of adverse events than amlodipine. Oedema occurred twice as frequently with amlodipine as with valsartan.

A series of *post hoc* analyses of patient data derived from the VALUE study attempted to adjust for differences in blood pressure reductions between the two treatment arms by using a statistical technique of serial median matching.[48] After 6 months' treatment (the point at which the titration schedules were completed to achieve blood pressure control), 5006 pairs of patient data matched exactly for SBP, age, sex and the presence or absence of comorbid coronary disease, stroke or diabetes were obtained. Combined cardiac events, MI, stroke and mortality were virtually identical in the two cohorts, although hospitalisation for heart failure was significantly lower with valsartan. Furthermore, achieving blood pressure control (SBP <140 mmHg) within 6 months was associated with significant benefits for cardiac outcomes compared with non-responders, regardless of the treatment regimen the patients received. Thus, the risk of a cardiac event was reduced by 24%, that of stroke by 40% and the risk of all-cause mortality reduced by 21% with valsartan-based treatment. This finding indicates the value of early and successful intervention with antihypertensive regimens in this patient population.

The VALIANT study compared mortality rates in patients with MI complicated by left ventricular systolic dysfunction, heart failure, or both, who were assigned treatment with either valsartan, the ACE inhibitor, captopril, or a combination of both agents.[47] ACE inhibitors such as captopril have previously been shown in large clinical trials to reduce mortality and cardiovascular events in such a patient population. In the VALIANT study, a total of 14,703 patients were randomised (0.5–10 days after MI) to treatment with valsartan monotherapy (n=4909), captopril monotherapy (n=4909), or the valsartan–captopril combination (n=4885). Doses of each study drug were titrated over four steps to a maximum of 160 mg, twice daily for valsartan, and a maximum of 50 mg, three-times daily for captopril. The maximum doses in the combination arm of the trial were 80 mg twice daily and 50 mg three-times daily for valsartan and captopril, respectively. The primary endpoint of the study was death from any cause and the median follow-up was 24.7 months. The mortality endpoint occurred at an equivalent frequency in the valsartan (19.9%) and captopril (19.5%) groups (hazard ratio: 1.00; $p$=0.98). Further statistical analyses revealed that valsartan was not inferior to captopril with regard to mortality and the composite endpoint of fatal and non-fatal cardiovascular events. Although the combination regimen was also not inferior to captopril in terms of mortality (mortality rates: 19.3 $vs$ 19.5%, respectively; hazard ratio: 0.98; $p$=0.73), it was associated with a higher incidence of adverse events. Thus, valsartan appears to be at least as effective as a proven ACE inhibitor regimen in reducing mortality and cardiovascular morbidity in patients who are at a high risk of future cardiovascular events after an initial MI. Despite offering the potential of full inhibition of the renin–angiotensin system, the combination of both agents offered no additional mortality or morbidity benefits compared with ACE inhibitor monotherapy and was associated with a higher incidence of adverse events. The findings of the VALIANT study have formed the basis for the recent approval of valsartan in the UK to improve survival following MI in clinically stable patients with signs, symptoms or radiological evidence of left ventricular failure and/or with left ventricular systolic dysfunction post MI. Valsartan is the first angiotensin II receptor antagonist to be licensed for such an indication.

Valsartan is at least as effective as a proven ACE inhibitor regimen in reducing mortality and cardiovascular morbidity in patients who are at a high risk of future cardiovascular events after an initial MI.

## Safety and tolerability

Valsartan has an excellent safety and tolerability profile. The numerous clinical trials comparing valsartan and placebo for the treatment of hypertension have shown that valsartan has a placebo-like tolerability profile, both with regard to the incidence and the severity of adverse events.[2,3,5] Moreover, the incidence of adverse events seems to be independent of valsartan dose.[4] A pooled analysis of data from placebo-controlled trials of valsartan, 40–160 mg/day, involving 3204 patients show that the most common side-effects (i.e. those occurring in more than 1% of patients) were headache, dizziness and fatigue (Figure 5).[49] The incidence of headache, though the most common adverse event associated with valsartan treatment, is consistently numerically lower than in patients receiving placebo.[2,3,49] Moreover, the incidence of adverse events irrespective of the relationship with trial medication, showed that patients given valsartan had a numerically lower incidence of headache or total adverse events than those receiving placebo (0.9 *vs* 3.1 and 6.3 *vs* 10.6 adverse events per person, respectively).[5] Although other antihypertensive agents such as ACE inhibitors and calcium-channel blockers are also associated with good tolerability profiles, the incidence of cough is lower in patients treated with valsartan than the ACE inhibitors enalapril, lisinopril and captopril.[21–24] Furthermore, the treatment-related incidence of oedema was higher in patients given amlodipine than valsartan (2.4, 3.6 and 14.3% of patients receiving valsartan, 80 mg, and amlodipine, 5 mg and 10 mg, respectively [no *p*-values reported]). There were no incidences of oedema in patients

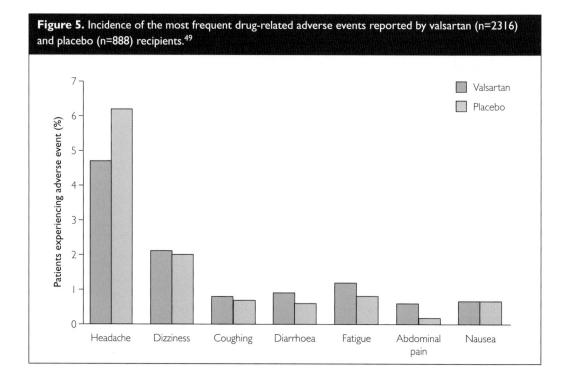

**Figure 5.** Incidence of the most frequent drug-related adverse events reported by valsartan (n=2316) and placebo (n=888) recipients.[49]

given the valsartan–amlodipine (5 mg) combination.[25] The overall incidence of <u>adverse events</u> associated with valsartan were lower than with amlodipine treatment (20.2 and 31.9%, respectively; $p<0.003$) and valsartan was also associated with a lower rate of <u>peripheral oedema</u> (4.8 and 26.8%, respectively; $p<0.001$).[28]

The incidence of laboratory abnormalities was lower in valsartan than ACE inhibitor recipients, with a greater than 100% increase in <u>bilirubin levels</u> occurring in 6.0 and 12.9% of patients receiving valsartan and ACE inhibitors, respectively (no <u>p-value</u> reported).[49] Similarly, 0.8 $vs$ 1.6% experienced a greater than 50% increase in <u>serum creatinine</u> levels, and 4.4 $vs$ 6.4% experienced a greater than 20% increase in <u>serum potassium</u> levels in valsartan and ACE inhibitor recipients, respectively (no $p$-values reported).[49]

The <u>safety and tolerability</u> of valsartan in combinations with HCTZ has been evaluated in several trials involving a total of 2159 patients.[50] Of these, 2066 received valsartan/HCTZ (all combinations of valsartan, 80 and 160 mg/day, with HCTZ, 12.5 and 25 mg/day).[50] The overall incidence of adverse events with valsartan/HCTZ was similar to that for <u>placebo</u>, with the most common adverse events in the valsartan group being headache, dizziness and <u>nasopharyngitis</u> (including <u>pharyngitis</u> plus <u>rhinitis</u>), occurring in 5.1, 3.9 and 2.7% of patients, respectively.

## Pharmacoeconomics

The 8-year health and economic outcomes of treatment with valsartan and the <u>calcium-channel blocker</u> amlodipine have been estimated using a <u>Markov model</u> in patients with type 2 diabetes and <u>microalbuminuria</u>.[51] This was based on the clinical <u>endpoints</u> from the 6-month randomised trial, MARVAL.[41] Patients treated with valsartan were predicted to have US$32,412 lower medical costs per patient than those treated with amlodipine ($92,058 $vs$ $124,470, respectively; $p<0.01$) over an 8-year period. Moreover, patients treated with valsartan gained 7 months per patient of quality-adjusted survival relative to those treated with amlodipine (77 $vs$ 70 months, respectively; $p<0.01$). However, one should always be cautious when predicting long-term results, even from quite lengthy (in this case, 6-month) trials.

The cost-effectiveness of <u>angiotensin II receptor antagonists</u> has been assessed in a US managed-care setting, based on a randomised, double-blind, parallel-group trial of irbesartan, 150 mg/day, losartan, 50 mg/day, olmesartan, 20 mg/day, and valsartan, 80 mg/day.[14,52] However, the trial on which this analysis was based was an 8-week, fixed-dose trial at the recommended normal starting doses of these medications. Thus, it seems extremely unlikely that this study could accurately predict long-term (i.e. 1–5 year) pharmacoeconomic data, as most patients will need <u>titration</u> to achieve and maintain a target blood pressure, and may require supplemental antihypertensives too. This is unlikely to occur in 8 weeks' treatment. Therefore, the estimations from this trial will not be considered further as part of this review.

Patients treated with valsartan were predicted to have US$32,412 lower medical costs per patient than those treated with amlodipine ($92,058 $vs$ $124,470, respectively) over an 8-year period.

## Key points

● Valsartan is an <u>angiotensin II receptor antagonist</u> that is highly selective for the AT$_1$ receptor subtype.

● The usual starting dose of valsartan, 80 mg once daily, seems optimal in most cases, with subsequent titration to 160 mg once daily, if required. However, patients with moderate-to-severe <u>renal</u> impairment or those undergoing <u>haemodialysis</u> should receive a lower initial dose of 40 mg/day.

● On the balance of available data valsartan is probably superior to losartan in terms of its antihypertensive effects. However, it is difficult to compare valsartan and other angiotensin II receptor <u>antagonists</u> based on the available data.

● Valsartan is at least as effective as the ACE inhibitors, enalapril, lisinopril or captopril, and is generally better tolerated.

● In general, valsartan appears to be as effective as the <u>calcium-channel blocker</u>, amlodipine, and is better tolerated in some trials, with a lower rate of oedema and/or total number of <u>adverse events</u>.

● Combining valsartan with HCTZ can produce an antihypertensive effect that is more effective than either agent used as <u>monotherapy</u>, and is as generally well tolerated.

● Valsartan is particularly effective in elderly and diabetic populations, and may have a beneficial effect in diabetic patients that is independent of its antihypertensive activity.

● Doses of valsartan of at least 80 mg/day provide effective 24-hour control of blood pressure without the loss of <u>diurnal variation</u>.

- Valsartan has been shown to exert significant beneficial effects in terms of <u>cardiovascular</u> <u>mortality</u> and morbidity in patients with heart failure (ValHEFT), in patients with hypertension at high-risk of future cardiovascular events (VALUE) and in patients with recent MI complicated by left ventricular systolic dysfunction and/or heart failure (VALIANT).

- Valsartan has an excellent <u>safety and tolerability</u> profile, with the most common associated side-effects being headache, dizziness and fatigue.

# References

A list of the published evidence which has been reviewed in compiling the preceding section of *BESTMEDICINE*.

1　Criscione L, de Gasparo M, Buhlmayer P *et al.* Pharmacological profile of valsartan: a potent, orally active, nonpeptide antagonist of the angiotensin II AT1-receptor subtype. *Br J Pharmacol* 1993; **110**: 761–71.

2　Oparil S, Dyke S, Harris F *et al.* The efficacy and safety of valsartan compared with placebo in the treatment of patients with essential hypertension. *Clin Ther* 1996; **18**: 797–810.

3　Holwerda NJ, Fogari R, Angeli P *et al.* Valsartan, a new angiotensin II antagonist for the treatment of essential hypertension: efficacy and safety compared with placebo and enalapril. *J Hypertens* 1996; **14**: 1147–51.

4　Pool JL, Glazer R, Chiang YT, Gatlin M. Dose-response efficacy of valsartan, a new angiotensin II receptor blocker. *J Hum Hypertens* 1999; **13**: 275–81.

5　Lasko BH, Laplante A, Hebert D, Bonnefis-Boyer S. Canadian valsartan study in patients with mild-to-moderate hypertension. *Blood Press Monit* 2001; **6**: 91–9.

6　Pool J, Oparil S, Hedner T *et al.* Dose-responsive antihypertensive efficacy of valsartan, a new angiotensin II-receptor blocker. *Clin Ther* 1998; **20**: 1106–14.

7　Elliott WJ, Calhoun DA, DeLucca PT *et al.* Losartan versus valsartan in the treatment of patients with mild to moderate essential hypertension: data from a multicenter, randomized, double-blind, 12-week trial. *Clin Ther* 2001; **23**: 1166–79.

8　Hedner T, Oparil S, Rasmussen K *et al.* A comparison of the angiotensin II antagonists valsartan and losartan in the treatment of essential hypertension. *Am J Hypertens* 1999; **12**: 414–17.

9　Mancia G, Korlipara K, van Rossum P, Villa G, Silvert B. An ambulatory blood pressure monitoring study of the comparative antihypertensive efficacy of two angiotensin II receptor antagonists, irbesartan and valsartan. *Blood Press Monit* 2002; **7**: 135–42.

10　Malacco E, Piazza S, Meroni R, Milanesi A. Comparison of valsartan and irbesartan in the treatment of mild-to-moderate hypertension: a randomised, open-label, crossover study. *Curr Ther Res* 2000; **61**: 789–97.

11　White WB, Lacourciere Y, Davidai G. Effects of the angiotensin II receptor blockers telmisartan versus valsartan on the circadian variation of blood pressure: impact on the early morning period. *Am J Hypertens* 2004; **17**: 347–53.

12　Bakris G. Comparison of telmisartan *vs* valsartan in the treatment of mild-to-moderate hypertension using ambulatory blood pressure monitoring. *J Clin Hypertens (Greenwich)* 2002; **4**: 26–31.

13　Calvo C, Hermida RC, Ayala DE, Ruilope LM. Effects of telmisartan 80 mg and valsartan 160 mg on ambulatory blood pressure in patients with essential hypertension. *J Hypertens* 2004; **22**: 837–46.

14　Oparil S, Williams D, Chrysant SG, Marbury TC, Neutel J. Comparative efficacy of olmesartan, losartan, valsartan, and irbesartan in the control of essential hypertension. *J Clin Hypertens (Greenwich)* 2001; **3**: 283–91.

15　Fogari R, Zoppi A, Mugellini A *et al.* Comparative efficacy of losartan and valsartan in mild-to-moderate hypertension: results of 24-hour ambulatory blood pressure monitoring. *Curr Ther Res* 1999; **60**: 195–206.

16　Fogari R, Mugellini A, Zoppi A *et al.* A double-blind, crossover study of the antihypertensive efficacy of angiotensin II-receptor antagonists and their activation of the renin-angiotensin system. *Curr Ther Res* 2000; **61**: 669–79.

17　Fogari R, Mugellini A, Zoppi A *et al.* Efficacy of losartan, valsartan, and telmisartan in patients with mild-to-moderate hypertension: a double-blind, placebo-controlled, crossover study using ambulatory blood pressure monitoring. *Curr Ther Res* 2002; **63**: 1–14.

18　Maillard MP, Wurzner G, Nussberger J *et al.* Comparative angiotensin II receptor blockade in healthy volunteers: the importance of dosing. *Clin Pharmacol Ther* 2002; **71**: 68–76.

19　Mallion JM, Boutelant S, Chabaux P *et al.* Valsartan, a new angiotensin II antagonist; blood pressure reduction in essential hypertension compared with an angiotensin converting enzyme inhibitor, enalapril. *Blood Press Monit* 1997; **2**: 179–84.

20　Fogari R, Mugellini A, Zoppi A *et al.* Effects of valsartan compared with enalapril on blood pressure and cognitive function in elderly patients with essential hypertension. *Eur J Clin Pharmacol* 2004; **59**: 863–8.

21　Botero R, Matiz H, Maria E *et al.* Efficacy and safety of valsartan compared with enalapril at different altitudes. *Int J Cardiol* 2000; **72**: 247–54.

22　Black HR, Graff A, Shute D *et al.* Valsartan, a new angiotensin II antagonist for the treatment of essential hypertension: efficacy, tolerability and safety compared to an angiotensin-converting enzyme inhibitor, lisinopril. *J Hum Hypertens* 1997; **11**: 483–9.

23　Bremner AD, Baur M, Oddou-Stock P, Bodin F. Valsartan: long-term efficacy and tolerability compared to lisinopril in elderly patients with essential hypertension. *Clin Exp Hypertens* 1997; **19**: 1263–85.

24　Prabowo P, Arwanto A, Soemantri D *et al.* A comparison of valsartan and captopril in patients with essential hypertension in Indonesia. *Int J Clin Pract* 1999; **53**: 268–72.

25　Corea L, Cardoni O, Fogari R *et al.* Valsartan, a new angiotensin II antagonist for the treatment of essential hypertension: a comparative study of the efficacy and safety against amlodipine. *Clin Pharmacol Ther* 1996; **60**: 341–6.

26 Julius S, Kjeldsen SE, Brunner H *et al.* VALUE trial: Long-term blood pressure trends in 13,449 patients with hypertension and high cardiovascular risk. *Am J Hypertens* 2003; **16**: 544–8.

27 Julius S, Kjeldsen SE, Weber M *et al.* Outcomes in hypertensive patients at high cardiovascular risk treated with regimens based on valsartan or amlodipine: the VALUE randomised trial. *Lancet* 2004; **363**: 2022–31.

28 Radauceanu A, Boivin JM, Bernaud C, Fay R, Zannad F. Differential time effect profiles of amlodipine, as compared to valsartan, revealed by ambulatory blood pressure monitoring, self blood pressure measurements and dose omission protocol. *Fundam Clin Pharmacol* 2004; **18**: 483–91.

29 Malacco E, Vari N, Capuano V *et al.* A randomized, double-blind, active-controlled, parallel-group comparison of valsartan and amlodipine in the treatment of isolated systolic hypertension in elderly patients: the Val-Syst study. *Clin Ther* 2003; **25**: 2765–80.

30 Palatini P, Mugellini A, Spagnuolo V *et al.* Comparison of the effects on 24-h ambulatory blood pressure of valsartan and amlodipine, alone or in combination with a low-dose diuretic, in elderly patients with isolated systolic hypertension (Val-syst Study). *Blood Press Monit* 2004; **9**: 91–7.

31 Cifkova R, Peleska J, Hradec J *et al.* Valsartan and atenolol in patients with severe essential hypertension. *J Hum Hypertens* 1998; **12**: 563–7.

32 Verheijen I, Fierens FL, Debacker JP, Vauquelin G, Vanderheyden PM. Interaction between the partially insurmountable antagonist valsartan and human recombinant angiotensin II type-1 receptors. *Fundam Clin Pharmacol* 2000; **14**: 577–85.

33 Benz JR, Black HR, Graff A *et al.* Valsartan and hydrochlorothiazide in patients with essential hypertension. A multiple dose, double-blind, placebo controlled trial comparing combination therapy with monotherapy. *J Hum Hypertens* 1998; **12**: 861–6.

34 Schmidt A, Adam SA, Kolloch R, Weidinger G, Handrock R. Antihypertensive effects of valsartan/hydrochlorothiazide combination in essential hypertension. *Blood Press* 2001; **10**: 230–7.

35 Mallion JM, Carretta R, Trenkwalder P *et al.* Valsartan/hydrochlorothiazide is effective in hypertensive patients inadequately controlled by valsartan monotherapy. *Blood Press Suppl* 2003; **Suppl 1**: 36–43.

36 Carretta R, Trenkwalder P, Martinez F *et al.* Pulse pressure responses in patients treated with Valsartan and hydrochlorothiazide combination therapy. *J Int Med Res* 2003; **31**: 370–7.

37 Madi JC, Oigman W, Franco R, Armaganijan D. Valsartan alone and as part of combination therapy in general practice in Brazil. *Int J Clin Pract* 2001; **55**: 520–3.

38 Scholze J, Probst G, Bertsch K. Valsartan alone and in combination with hydrochlorothiazide in general practice. *Clin Drug Invest* 2000; **20**: 1–7.

39 Neutel JM, Bedigian MP. Efficacy of valsartan in patients aged > or =65 years with systolic hypertension. *Clin Ther* 2000; **22**: 961–9.

40 Takami T, Shigemasa M. Efficacy of various antihypertensive agents as evaluated by indices of vascular stiffness in elderly hypertensive patients. *Hypertens Res* 2003; **26**: 609–14.

41 Viberti G, Wheeldon NM. Microalbuminuria reduction with valsartan in patients with type 2 diabetes mellitus: a blood pressure-independent effect. *Circulation* 2002; **106**: 672–8.

42 Muirhead N, Feagan BF, Mahon J *et al.* The effects of valsartan and captopril on reducing microalbuminuria in patients with type 2 diabetes mellitus: a placebo-controlled trial. *Curr Ther Res* 1999; **60**: 650–60.

43 Hermida RC, Calvo C, Ayala DE *et al.* Administration time-dependent effects of valsartan on ambulatory blood pressure in hypertensive subjects. *Hypertension* 2003; **42**: 283–90.

44 Neutel J, Weber M, Pool J *et al.* Valsartan, a new angiotensin II antagonist: antihypertensive effects over 24 hours. *Clin Ther* 1997; **19**: 447–58.

45 Wogen J, Kreilick CA, Livornese RC, Yokoyama K, Frech F. Patient adherence with amlodipine, lisinopril, or valsartan therapy in a usual-care setting. *J Manag Care Pharm* 2003; **9**: 424–9.

46 Cohn JN, Tognoni G. A randomized trial of the angiotensin-receptor blocker valsartan in chronic heart failure. *N Engl J Med* 2001; **345**: 1667–75.

47 Pfeffer MA, McMurray JJ, Velazquez EJ *et al.* Valsartan, captopril, or both in myocardial infarction complicated by heart failure, left ventricular dysfunction, or both. *N Engl J Med* 2003; **3 49**: 1893–906.

48 Weber MA, Julius S, Kjeldsen SE *et al.* Blood pressure dependent and independent effects of antihypertensive treatment on clinical events in the VALUE Trial. *Lancet* 2004; **363**: 2049–51.

49 Markham A, Goa KL. Valsartan. A review of its pharmacology and therapeutic use in essential hypertension. *Drugs* 1997; **54**: 299–311.

50 Novartis Pharmaceuticals UK Ltd. Co-Diovan® (valsartan/hydrochlorothiazide combination). *Summary of product characteristics.* July 2004.

51 Smith DG, Nguyen AB, Peak CN, Frech FH. Markov modeling analysis of health and economic outcomes of therapy with valsartan versus amlodipine in patients with type 2 diabetes and microalbuminuria. *J Manag Care Pharm* 2004; **10**: 26–32.

52 Simons WR. Comparative cost effectiveness of angiotensin II receptor blockers in a US managed care setting: olmesartan medoxomil compared with losartan, valsartan, and irbesartan. *Pharmacoeconomics* 2003; **21**: 61–74.

# Acknowledgements

Figure 1 is adapted from Malacco *et al.*, 2003.[29]

Figure 2 is adapted from Benz *et al.*, 1998.[33]

Figure 3 is adapted from Mallion *et al.*, 2003.[35]

Figure 4 is adapted from Cohn and Tognoni, 2001.[46]

Figure 5 is adapted from Markham and Goa, 1997.[49]

# PATIENT NOTES
*Dr Mark Davis*

> *The patient and healthcare professional should decide together that drug treatment is needed.*

## When is blood pressure treatment prescribed?

When lifestyle changes have failed to bring high blood pressure under control, drug treatment will be needed. The majority of people with high blood pressure will require two or more drugs to control their blood pressure satisfactorily and this should be made clear to the individual and be understood from the start. It is also particularly important for the patient to understand that the need to take more than one type of blood pressure medication does not mean that their blood pressure is particularly severe or dangerous. The patient and healthcare professional should decide together that drug treatment is needed and which drugs are best suited to the individual needs of that patient.

## What treatment is available?

There are six main 'classes' of drug that are commonly used to treat hypertension and all of them have benefits and, to a variable degree, side-effects. On average, all these classes of medication are similarly effective at lowering blood pressure. However, in individuals there is a large variation in the effectiveness of the different drug classes, with some people responding better to a particular class of drug than others. This is likely to reflect the different causes of blood pressure in different people and to the different ways that people absorb, make use of, and dispose of, the drug within their bodies. Many attempts have been made to find ways of predicting which people will respond best to a particular drug class, though none have been very successful. The two notable exceptions to this are age and ethnicity. These factors have been incorporated into 'AB/CD' rule. Additionally some drugs combine usefully with other drug classes, the combination working particularly well together to produce additional blood pressure lowering.

## How is a particular drug or combination of drugs chosen?

The British Hypertension Society (BHS; *www.hyp.ac.uk/bhs*) have suggested the 'AB/CD' rule as a pragmatic way of deciding what drug combinations should be used in a given individual. This is an attempt to predict which drugs are likely to produce the greatest blood pressure-lowering effect and which combination of drugs is most likely to take the patient to their blood pressure target. This is based on the likelihood of certain groups of people having high or low levels of a substance called renin, which is involved in the renin–angiotensin system, and is an important factor in the development of high blood pressure. The 'A' (angiotensin-converting [ACE]-inhibitors and angiotensin receptor blockers [alternatively called angiotensin II receptor antagonists) and the 'B' (β-adrenoceptor blocking drugs or β-blockers) drugs inhibit this system, thereby resulting in a lowering of blood pressure. Therefore, people who tend to have high renin levels should usually use one of these drugs first. The people who fall into this group are likely to be younger and are not of African or Afro–Caribbean origin. Older people and those of African or Afro–Caribbean origin are likely to have lower renin levels and, therefore, in these individuals it is better to start with drugs whose main mode of action is not related to the renin–angiotensin system. Typically these included the 'C' (calcium-channel blockers) and the 'D' (diuretics) drugs which both have different mechanisms of action to each other. However, as the majority of people require a combination of drugs to get their blood pressure to their target level, the next rational step is to use a combination from the two distinct groups (e.g. A + D). If the blood pressure still fails to get to the target level a third drug may be required, and an ideal combination in this case would be A + C + D.

All things being equal it is the reduction in blood pressure that is important rather than any likely benefits additional to blood pressure lowering. However, other conditions that the patient may have will make certain choices of drug better than others. The BHS gives guidance on this matter and this is explained in detail in Table 3 of the following section. For instance, anyone who has angina and needs blood pressure treatment should consider either using a β-blocker or a rate-limiting calcium-channel blocker. Anyone with heart failure should take an ACE-inhibitor or an angiotensin-receptor blocker. Conversely, there are some conditions that mean that certain drugs should be avoided. For instance, anyone with asthma who needs a blood pressure-lowering drug should not be using a β-blocker.

## How do these drugs work and what are their side-effects?

### ACE inhibitors

These drugs block the production of angiotensin II within the renin–angiotensin system. This results in a dilatation (or widening) of the blood vessels leading to a drop in blood pressure. The main side-effect of these drugs is a dry and

*The majority of people require a combination of drugs to get their blood pressure to their target level.*

persistent cough, which occurs in about 10% of the people who take them.

## Angiotensin receptor blockers (ARBs) (or angiotensin II receptor antagonists)

This is the most recently introduced class of antihypertensive drugs. They have a selective action and block type 1 angiotensin II receptors ($AT_1$ receptors), leading to a reduction in blood pressure in a similar way to the ACE inhibitors. As such, they are likely to share the same beneficial effects and have the great advantage of not causing the dry cough associated with the ACE inhibitors. The evidence underlying the use of these agents is provided in detail in the individual drug review sections of this edition of *BESTMEDICINE*.

## β-blockers

Despite the fact that β-blockers have been in use for many years and have been extensively investigated, there is still some doubt as to the main mechanism by which they lower blood pressure. However, the effects of these drugs are believed to arise from a combination of their effect on the strength at which the heart pumps out blood and their effect on the renin–angiotensin system. In people at high risk of developing type 2 diabetes, the combination of β-blockers and diuretics may increase the likelihood of that person developing diabetes, and therefore, this combination should be avoided in these at-risk individuals. β-blockers can cause a variety of troublesome side-effects including fatigue, coldness of the extremities and sleep disturbances with nightmares, and they should be avoided by people with asthma.

## Calcium-channel blockers (CCBs)

This group of drugs causes the muscles within the blood vessels to relax resulting in a reduction in the pressure within the circulation. CCBs produce their most common side-effects as a direct result of this mode of action, which include ankle swelling and headache.

## Diuretics

There are a number of different types of diuretics and the way in which they work is complex. Their main action is to cause a loss of sodium through the kidney which results in a loss of water, thereby reducing the blood volume and consequently blood pressure. They are mostly well tolerated but they do have a variety of side-effects in some people.

*Angiotensin II receptor antagonists have a selective action and block type 1 angiotensin II receptors leading to a reduction in blood pressure.*

### α-blockers (α-adrenoceptor blocking drugs)

These are viewed by most healthcare professionals as 'second-line' drugs. However, they can produce good blood pressure reductions when added to other blood pressure treatments. They are generally well tolerated and are particularly useful for men with benign prostatic hypertrophy (an enlarged prostate gland).

## What happens if treatment fails to reduce blood pressure?

Not everyone can have their blood pressure controlled to target with a combination of drugs that they can tolerate. In some cases both the patient and their doctor have to admit defeat and take comfort from the fact that whatever blood pressure reduction they have achieved will result in a significant reduction of that person's cardiovascular risk. However, some people who still have poor blood pressure control on three or more drugs may require the opinion of a specialist to provide further advice.

*Not everyone can have their blood pressure controlled to target with a combination of drugs that they can tolerate.*

# 11. Improving practice

Dr Mark Davis, MB, ChB, MRCGP, DRCOG, DOcc Med
General Practitioner, Leeds, Secretary, Primary Care Cardiovascular Society

## Summary

Hypertension is a significant problem both in the UK and globally, and its management is a major part of GPs' daily workload. However, despite the fact that uncontrolled hypertension places patients at a greater risk of <u>cardiovascular disease (CVD)</u> and death, its management in primary care is still <u>suboptimal</u>, despite some improvements in recent years. A number of initiatives have been instigated which, it is hoped, will improve the management of the condition in the UK. These include the National Service Frameworks (NSFs) in England and the new General Medical Services (GMS) contract for GPs. In addition, the availability of new guidelines from the British Hypertension Society (BHS) for the management of hypertension in the UK offers us clear, simple and practical advice to improve the care of our patients. The BHS guidelines call for treatment initiation at certain thresholds determined by the magnitude of blood pressure elevation, the level of cardiovascular risk and the presence or absence of other <u>comorbidities</u> such as diabetes. In order for patients to achieve new and more stringent blood pressure targets, these guidelines indicate that multiple drug treatment (based on the AB/CD treatment algorithm) is likely to be necessary. The availability of the new GMS contract has driven the need for effective clinical audit, particularly with regard to our performance in the control of hypertension.

☛ *Remember that the author of the Improving Practice is addressing his healthcare professional colleagues rather than the 'lay' reader. This provides a fascinating insight into many of the challenges faced by doctors in the day-to-day practice of medicine (see Reader's Guide).*

## Disease burden

The World Health Organization (WHO) has identified hypertension as one of the most important preventable causes of premature <u>morbidity</u> and <u>mortality</u> in developed and developing countries. It affects about one billion people worldwide and is the most common treatable risk factor for CVD in patients over 50 years of age. If we accept that a blood pressure above 140/90 mmHg requires cardiovascular risk calculation as a minimum requirement, which may necessitate the initiation of treatment, there are an estimated 42% of people aged 35–64 years with a blood pressure above this level. When we consider patients over 60 years then 70% will have hypertension. The majority of this latter group of patients will have isolated systolic hypertension.

The ageing of the population in developing countries and the growing 'epidemic' of CVD in developing countries will ensure that by 2020, coronary heart disease (CHD) and stroke will respectively rank the first and fourth major causes of death and disability worldwide.

It is well recognised that people with hypertension frequently have a clustering of additional risk factors for CVD. These include dyslipidaemia, impaired glucose tolerance and central obesity which, in common with hypertension, are all features of the metabolic syndrome. As a result of this clustering of risk factors, the treatment of blood pressure in isolation will leave patients at an unacceptably high risk of cardiovascular complications and death. Consequently, we are now encouraged to calculate overall cardiovascular risk in patients with hypertension by identifying multiple risk factors and then intervening appropriately.

Meta-analyses of large-scale randomised controlled clinical trials have demonstrated that reductions in systolic blood pressure (SBP) of 10–14 mmHg and in diastolic blood pressure (DBP) of 5–6 mmHg lower the incidence of stroke by two-fifths and CHD by one-fifth. The evidence base for the benefits of intervention in patients with high blood pressure gives us an obligation to improve our management of hypertension, although the number of patients involved represents a continuing and significant challenge for primary-care professionals.

National surveys continue to expose the fact that there is still substantial under-diagnosis, under-treatment and poor rates of blood pressure control within the UK, although there are some signs that this situation is slowly improving.

## The challenges facing primary care

We are in the fortunate position of having access to a number of clear and practical guidelines for the management of hypertension. The BHS has recently published its fourth set of guidelines (Guidelines for Management of Hypertension: The Report of the Fourth Working Party of the British Hypertension Society 2004 [BHS IV]. *Journal of Human Hypertension* 2004; **18**: 139–85). A user-friendly version of these guidelines was also published in the *British Medical Journal* (*BMJ* 2004; **328**: 634–40). These guidelines are intended for GPs, practice nurses and generalists in hospital and I would commend them to you.

The principal objectives of these guidelines are:
- to promote the primary prevention of hypertension and cardiovascular disease by advocating changes to the diet and lifestyle of the whole population

- to increase the detection and treatment of undiagnosed hypertension by routine screening and to increase the awareness of hypertension amongst the public
- to ensure that patients taking antihypertensive drugs have their blood pressure controlled, as far as is possible, to optimal targets
- to reduce the risk of CVD in treated hypertensive patients by non-pharmacological methods and by the appropriate use of <u>statins</u> and aspirin where appropriate
- to increase the identification and treatment of patients with mild hypertension who are at high risk of CVD (e.g. elderly patients, patients with <u>ischaemic</u> heart disease, people with diabetes, people with <u>target-organ damage</u> or people with multiple risk factors)
- to promote continued adherence to drug treatment by optimising the use of drugs, minimising side-effects and increasing the information and choice given to patients.

New systems of healthcare delivery will be needed to ensure that these new guidelines are implemented effectively in primary care. We will not be successful unless multidisciplinary teams work in a systematic and structured way to advise, educate and support our patients. There will also need to be a move away from rigid clinic-based care towards greater use of remote centres such as pharmacies. There is clearly also a need for the extended role provided by nurse practitioners, pharmacists and other healthcare professionals if we are to build the foundations for a service that enables widespread and effective detection, monitoring and treatment of high blood pressure and its associated increased risk of CVD.

> New systems of healthcare delivery will be needed to ensure that these new guidelines are implemented effectively in primary care.

## Initiatives to improve hypertension management

Primary Care Trusts (PCTs) have an important role in supporting and enhancing primary care. They will also take the lead in the development of the new types of service delivery, as discussed in the previous section.

The Department of Health has provided the lead in the prevention of CVD through its NSFs in England (in particular the NSFs for CHD, diabetes and older people). There are also comparable initiatives in Scotland and Wales. The NSFs suggest that we prioritise our efforts by treating hypertension optimally in those at greatest risk. This includes those people with existing occlusive vascular disease and diabetes. They also support our efforts to identify those who have yet to exhibit manifest occlusive vascular disease but who, because of multiple risk factors, are at high risk of CVD.

The National Institute for Clinical Excellence (NICE) has recently published guidance on the management of essential hypertension. The NICE guidance is broadly supportive of the BHS guidelines. It is important to note, however, that the NICE guidelines focuses solely on the treatment of essential hypertension in uncomplicated patients and they do not consider blood pressure management in the many important

The new GMS contract, published in 2003, is an important step towards the development of primary care in the UK. Of the 550 clinical points available in the GMS contract, 129 relate directly to hypertension.

subgroups as outlined in the BHS IV guidance. Moreover, NICE does not give advice on when to use aspirin and statins to further reduce the CVD risk in individuals with high blood pressure. However, NICE does support the basic principle of risk assessment followed by treatment. NICE uses a different treatment algorithm to BHS IV, but in practice our patients will end up using similar drug combinations to control their blood pressure no matter which guidelines are implemented. The latest guidelines from the Joint British Societies on the prevention of CVD will be published during 2005.

The new GMS contract, published in 2003, is an important step towards the development of primary care in the UK. The quality framework has a significant leaning towards CVD prevention and management and, as such, the detection and management of hypertension features strongly. The payment consequent upon achieving the quality indicators should encourage practices to improve hypertension management and will reward them for delivering quality care. Of the 550 clinical points available in the GMS contract, 129 relate directly to hypertension. A further 15 points out of the 184 organisational points available also relate to hypertension.

## Practical advice to meet these challenges

Nobody working in primary care will underestimate the size of the challenge that we have been set. Practices will be able to identify those patients in whom blood pressure control is desirable by using the disease registers. Patients with existing CVD should be identifiable by using our CHD and stroke registers. They should be subject to regular review, and by using practice protocols and the templates that are readily available on our IT systems, it should be possible to Read-code all the actions that we take. Once these are Read-coded it is relatively straightforward to undertake a search and identify those whose blood pressure is not to target.

Patients with diabetes should also be added to our 'secondary prevention' remit. Evidence clearly suggests that diabetics are at particular risk from raised blood pressure and as such, the targets that are set for diabetics are particularly challenging. The thresholds and targets for intervention in hypertension taken from the BHS guidelines are set out in Table 1.

Many of our patients with hypertension will not yet be known to us. The new GMS contract encourages us to record blood pressure in patients aged over 45 years at a minimum of 5-year intervals. This is good practice and can be done opportunistically either by GPs or by nursing staff. It is also likely that an increasing number of pharmacists will offer blood pressure screening as part of their service, and if this information is transmitted to the practices, this will help us enormously in our task.

A management algorithm supported by the new BHS guidelines for patients with different levels of blood pressure is presented in Figure 1. This algorithm indicates that patients with a sustained blood pressure above 160/100 mmHg should receive treatment no matter what other risk factors

---

**Table 1.** Thresholds and treatment targets for antihypertensive drug treatment. Adapted from Williams *et al. BMJ* 2004; **328**: 634–40.

---

- Antihypertensive treatment should be initiated in patients with sustained SBP ≥160 mmHg or sustained DBP ≥100 mmHg despite non-pharmacological measures.
- Antihypertensive treatment should be initiated in patients with SBP 140–159 mmHg or sustained DBP 90–99 mmHg if target-organ damage is present, or there is evidence of CVD or diabetes, or where the 10-year CVD risk is ≥20%.
- For most patients, the recommended blood pressure target is ≤140/85 mmHg. In those with diabetes, renal impairment or established CVD, a lower target of ≤130/80 mmHg is recommended.
- When using ambulatory blood pressure readings, mean daytime pressures are preferable (this value should be approximately 10/5 mmHg lower than office blood pressure equivalent for thresholds and targets). Similar adjustments are required for averages of home blood pressure readings.

---

CVD, cardiovascular disease; DBP, diastolic blood pressure; SBP, systolic blood pressure.

---

are present. An SBP of 140–160 mmHg and a DBP of 90–100 mmHg warrant further risk assessment. A sustained blood pressure within these parameters would necessitate treatment if there is target-organ damage or CVD complications, or if the patient has diabetes or a 10-year risk of CVD above 20%. CVD complications or target organ damage include:

- stroke, transient ischaemic attack, dementia, carotid bruits
- left ventricular hypertrophy or left ventricular strain on electrocardiogram (ECG)
- heart failure
- myocardial infarction, angina, coronary artery bypass graft or angioplasty
- fundal haemorrhages or exudates, papilloedema
- proteinuria
- renal impairment (raised creatinine).

There are various validated ways of calculating cardiovascular risk but the most commonly used are those recommended in the Joint British Societies' guidelines. These have been updated and simplified and allow for calculation of CVD, rather than CHD risk, to reflect the importance of stroke prevention as well as CHD prevention. The BHS has published these new tables in its guidelines and it is hoped that they will soon be published in the form of a 'Factfile' by the British Heart Foundation. If patients with mild-to-moderate hypertension do not fulfil the above criteria then it is adequate to reassess their blood pressure and CVD risk annually. Blood pressures below 140/90 mmHg do not require intervention.

In our hypertensive patients we should also undertake the following routine investigations:

- urine strip tests for protein and blood
- serum creatinine and electrolytes

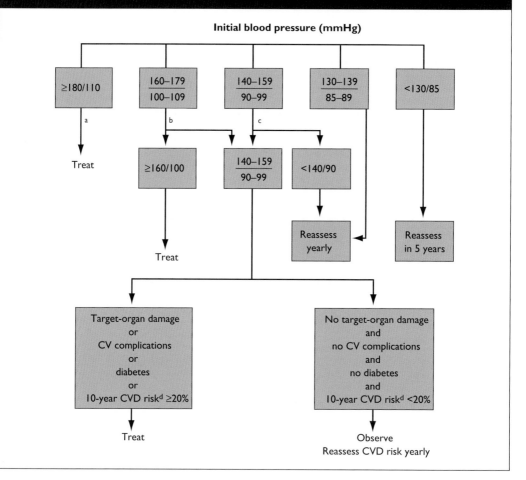

**Figure 1.** British Hypertension Society guidelines for the management of hypertension. Adapted from Williams *et al. BMJ* 2004; **328**: 634–40.
[a]Unless malignant phase of hypertensive emergency, confirm over 1–2 weeks then treat.
[b]If CV complications, target-organ damage, or diabetes are present, confirm over 3–4 weeks then treat; if absent remeasure weekly and treat if blood pressure persists at this level over 4–12 weeks.
[c]If CV complications, target-organ damage, or diabetes are present, confirm over 3–4 weeks then treat; if absent remeasure monthly and treat if this level is maintained and if estimated 10-year CVD risk is ≥20%.
[d]Assessed with risk chart for CVD.
CV, cardiovascular; CVD, cardiovascular disease.

- blood glucose levels (ideally fasting blood glucose)
- serum lipid profile (high density lipoprotein cholesterol [HDL-C] and total cholesterol at the very least; fasted for triglycerides)
- ECG.

As shown in Table 1, the target blood pressure for most of our patients is below 140/85 mmHg. For patients with diabetes, renal impairment or established CVD, a lower target of below 130/80 mmHg is recommended. It is accepted that even with optimal treatment, some patients will not be able to achieve these targets. Because of this, a minimum audit standard has been set which is under 150/90 mmHg in most patients and below 140/80 mmHg in those at the highest risk.

# Disease management

Advice on lifestyle modification should be provided to all patients who are being considered for pharmacological interventions. There is some evidence that lifestyle modification can prevent those with borderline or high–normal blood pressures becoming hypertensive and needing treatment. The lifestyle measures that have been shown to lower blood pressure and reduce the rise of blood pressure with age are shown in Table 2.

To succeed with lifestyle modification some members of the practice team will need to acquire the skills and enthusiasm that are required to achieve behaviour modification.

We know that certain lifestyle measures reduce the risk of CVD and these include smoking cessation and reducing the intake of total and saturated fats and their replacement with monounsaturated fats such as olive oil. To succeed with lifestyle modification some members of the practice team will need to acquire the skills and enthusiasm that are required to achieve behaviour modification. Considerable time will need to be spent with patients and other family members in order to give them the best advice as to how lifestyle change can be achieved.

## *Pharmacological interventions*

Meta-analyses of blood pressure lowering trials have confirmed that, in general, the main determinant of benefit from antihypertensive drugs is the magnitude of the blood pressure reduction that is achieved rather than the choice of therapy. Although there is only minimal evidence for differences between classes of drugs with regard to cardiovascular outcomes, there are a number of important caveats to this. For example, calcium-channel blocker-based therapy may be less protective than other agents with regard to the development of heart failure, although some small benefits for these agents have been reported with regard to stroke prevention. The Losartan Intervention For Endpoint Reduction in Hypertension (LIFE) study has demonstrated even larger benefits for

---

**Table 2.** Lifestyle measures to lower blood pressure. Adapted from Williams *et al. BMJ* 2004; **328**: 634–40.

- Maintenance of normal body weight (BMI 20–25 kg/m$^2$)
- Reduce salt intake to <100 mmol/day (equivalent to <6 g of NaCl or <2.4g of Na$^+$ per day)
- Limit alcohol consumption (males: ≤3 units/day; females: ≤2 units/day)
- Engage in regular aerobic physical exercise (e.g. brisk walking) for at least 30 minutes per day on most days of the week, and at least 3 days of the week
- Consume at least five portions of fresh fruit and vegetables daily
- Reduce the intake of total and saturated fat

BMI, body mass index.

angiotensin II receptor antagonist therapy over β-blocker therapy with regard to stroke prevention, despite broadly similar blood pressure reductions being achieved with both agents. Finally, in specific groups of patients, there can be compelling indications and compelling contra-indications to different drugs (Table 3).

Should none of these special considerations apply, I feel that our choice of drug therapy should follow the AB/CD algorithm suggested by the BHS (Figure 2). The theory underpinning this algorithm is that hypertension can be broadly classified as high renin or low renin, and is therefore best treated initially with one of the two categories of hypertensive drugs. This tends to be age and race dependent.

The classes of drugs within the AB/CD algorithm are:-
- (A) angiotensin-converting enzyme (ACE) inhibitors or angiotensin II receptor antagonists
- (B) β-blockers
- (C) calcium-channel blockers
- (D) diuretics.

Drugs in the A and B class inhibit the renin–angiotensin system, whilst those in the C and D classes do not. As you can see from the algorithm in Figure 2 those patients who are younger than 55 years and Caucasian should be started on A or B drugs. Patients over 55 years or of Afro-Caribbean origin should start on C or D drugs. As most people require more than one drug to control blood pressure it is usual that step 2 will be reached and this will involve the combination of an A or B drug with a C or D drug. The BHS recommends caution when using a B and D combination in patients at especially high risk of developing diabetes. This caution is justified given the availability of trial evidence which indicates that this combination results in an increased incidence of new-onset diabetes.

There is general agreement that the agent used ideally should be effective for 24 hours when taken as a once-daily dose. Unless it is necessary to lower blood pressure urgently, an interval of at least 4 weeks should be allowed to observe a full response before altering the treatment regimen.

Most drugs provide similar blood pressure reductions. The placebo-adjusted reductions for patients with blood pressures of about 160/95 mmHg are approximately 10/5 mmHg. Thus, to reach the revised targets, the vast majority of patients will require combination therapy.

It is likely that most of the management of hypertension within a practice setting will be carried out by nurses working to a practice protocol which should make it clear when patients need to be referred to a GP. Similarly GPs should be clear as to when they should consider referral for a specialist opinion. The BHS indications for specialist referral are summarised in Table 4.

As hypertension is only one of a number of risk factors that can co-exist in this patient population, the BHS also provides guidance on the use of statins and aspirin in both primary and secondary prevention patient populations.

**Table 3.** Indications, cautions and contra-indications for the major classes of antihypertensive agents. Adapted from Williams et al. BMJ 2004;**328**: 634–40.

| Drug class | Compelling indications | Possible indications | Cautions | Contra-indications |
|---|---|---|---|---|
| α-blockers | BPH | – | Postural hypertension<br>Heart failure[a] | Urinary incontinence |
| ACE inhibitors | Heart failure<br>Left ventricular dysfunction post-MI or established CHD<br>Type 1 diabetic nephropathy<br>Secondary stroke prevention[b] | Chronic renal disease[c]<br>Type 2 diabetic nephropathy<br>Proteinuric renal disease | Renal impairment[c]<br>Peripheral vascular disease[d] | Pregnancy<br>Renovascular disease[e] |
| AIIRAs | ACE inhibitor intolerance<br>Type 2 diabetic nephropathy<br>Hypertension with left ventricular hypertrophy<br>Heart failure in ACE inhibitor-intolerant patients<br>Post-MI | Left ventricular dysfunction post-MI<br>Intolerance of other antihypertensives<br>Proteinuric renal disease, chronic renal disease[c]<br>Heart failure | Renal impairment[c]<br>Peripheral vascular disease[d] | Pregnancy<br>Renovascular disease[e] |
| β-blockers | MI, angina | Heart failure[f]<br>Peripheral vascular | Heart failure[f]<br>Heart block disease<br>Diabetes (except with CHD) | Asthma or COPD |

[a] In heart failure when used as monotherapy.
[b] In combination with a thiazide or thiazide-like diuretic.
[c] ACE inhibitor or AIIRAs may be beneficial in chronic renal failure but should only be used with caution, close supervision and specialist advice when there is established and significant renal impairment.
[d] Caution with ACE inhibitor and AIIRAs in peripheral vascular disease because of its association with renovascular disease.
[e] ACE inhibitors and AIIRAs are sometimes used in patients with renovascular disease under specialist supervision.
[f] β-blockers are used increasingly to treat stable heart failure, but may worsen heart failure.
[g] Thiazides or thiazide-like diuretics may sometimes be necessary to control blood pressure in those with a history of gout, ideally in combination with allopurinol.
ACE, angiotensin-converting enzyme; AIIRA, angiotensin II receptor antagonist; BPH, benign prostatic hyperplasia; CHD, coronary heart disease; COPD, chronic obstructive pulmonary disease; ISH, isolated systolic hypertension; MI, myocardial infarction.

**Table 3.** Continued

| Drug class | Compelling indications | Possible indications | Cautions | Contra-indications |
|---|---|---|---|---|
| Calcium–channel blockers (dihydropyridine) | Elderly, ISH | Angina | – | – |
| Calcium–channel blockers (rate limiting) | Angina | Elderly | Combination with β-blockers | Heart block Heart failure |
| Thiazides/thiazide-like diuretics | Elderly, ISH Heart failure Secondary stroke prevention | – | – | Gout[g] |

[a]In heart failure when used as monotherapy.

[b]In combination with a thiazide or thiazide-like diuretic.

[c]ACE inhibitor or AIIRAs may be beneficial in chronic renal failure but should only be used with caution, close supervision and specialist advice when there is established and significant renal impairment.

[d]Caution with ACE inhibitor and AIIRAs in peripheral vascular disease because of its association with renovascular disease.

[e]ACE inhibitors and AIIRAs are sometimes used in patients with renovascular disease under specialist supervision.

[f]β-blockers are used increasingly to treat stable heart failure, but may worsen heart failure.

[g]Thiazides or thiazide-like diuretics may sometimes be necessary to control blood pressure in those with a history of gout, ideally in combination with allopurinol.

ACE, angiotensin-converting enzyme; AIIRA, angiotensin II receptor antagonist; BPH, benign prostatic hyperplasia; CHD, coronary heart disease; COPD, chronic obstructive pulmonary disease; ISH, isolated systolic hypertension; MI, myocardial infarction.

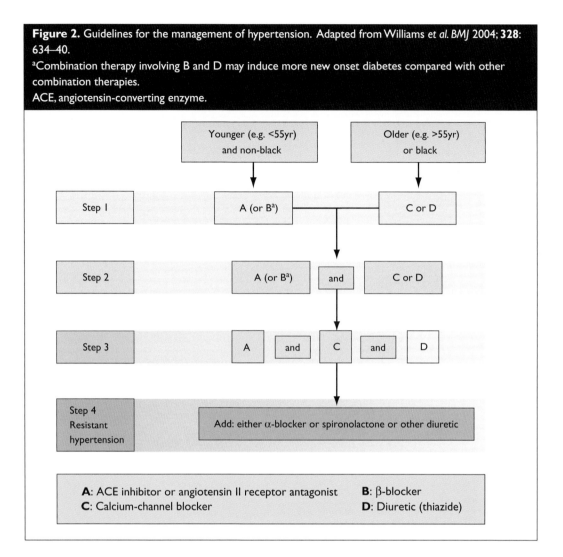

**Figure 2.** Guidelines for the management of hypertension. Adapted from Williams *et al. BMJ* 2004; **328**: 634–40.
[a]Combination therapy involving B and D may induce more new onset diabetes compared with other combination therapies.
ACE, angiotensin-converting enzyme.

## Patient involvement

An essential component of successful blood pressure management is to obtain the active participation of each individual. Patients with high blood pressure should be involved in the decision as to what lifestyle changes they need to take and whether drug therapy is appropriate. The likely risk reduction obtained as a consequence of antihypertensive treatment should be understood. They should also be aware of the likelihood that they will need to take two or three drugs to achieve sufficient reductions and be conscious of the possible side-effects that they may encounter. Wherever possible a written treatment plan should be drawn up and given to the patient.

With modern semi-automated blood pressure machines, it is possible to involve more patients in the measurement of their own blood pressure, which can save visits to a primary healthcare team. However, it is important to remember that the targets are based on 'clinic' blood

Patients with high blood pressure should be involved in the decision as to what lifestyle changes they need to take and whether drug therapy is appropriate.

**Table 4.** Indications for specialist referral. Adapted from Williams *et al. BMJ* 2004; **328**: 634–40.

**Urgent treatment required**
- Accelerated hypertension (severe hypertension and retinopathy [grade III-IV])
- Severe hypertension (>220/120 mmHg)
- Impending complications (e.g. transient ischaemic attack, left ventricular failure)

**Possible underlying cause**
- Any clue in history or examination of a secondary cause (e.g. hypokalaemia with increased or high–normal plasma sodium [Conn's syndrome])
- Elevated creatinine
- Proteinuria or haematuria
- Sudden onset or worsening of hypertension
- Resistance to multidrug regimen (at least three drugs)
- Young age (<20 years: any hypertension; <30 years: needing treatment)

**Therapeutic problems**
- Multiple drug intolerance
- Multiple drug contra-indications
- Persistent non-adherence or non-compliance

**Special situations**
- Unusual blood pressure variability
- White coat hypertension
- Hypertension in pregnancy

pressures and home measurements will usually be lower. A correction factor of 10/5 mmHg should be used when considering home results. Individual patients can obtain information directly from the Blood Pressure Association (*www.bpassoc.org.uk*).

## Clinical audit

The survival of practices in the age of performance management means that electronic audit is no longer optional.

It is now essential that interventions relating to blood pressure control are recorded electronically. The survival of practices in the age of performance management means that electronic audit is no longer optional. We need to ensure that the templates that we use are correctly Read-coded, thereby enabling the information to be retrieved easily from our systems. It seems likely that many practices will use the quality indicators as detailed in the new GMS contract as a basis for their audit. Programmes which interrogate our databases, such as the Population Manager in the EMIS system, will enable us to monitor our progress towards quality points whenever we wish to. Correct Read-coding will also enable individual practices to undertake more sophisticated searches should they so wish.

With regard to blood pressure control, it is important that we should try to achieve the targets as suggested by the BHS and not to use the audit standard as our therapeutic target. Self-evidently, should we attempt to hit the more challenging clinical targets, success in the GMS audit will be more likely and our patients will achieve greater benefit. Hypertension indicators in the GMS contract are outlined in Table 5. In due course, the results of comparable audits carried out by different practices within the PCT will be published and will form the basis of 'league tables'.

**Table 5.** Hypertension quality indicators in the new General Medical Services contract. Adapted from Williams *et al. J Hum Hypertens* 2004; **18**: 139–85.

|  | Points | Maximum threshold |
|---|---|---|
| **Secondary prevention in CHD** | | |
| *Ongoing management* | | |
| Percentage of patients with CHD whose notes have a record of BP in previous 15 months | 7 | 90% |
| Percentage of patients with CHD in whom last BP reading (within the last 15 months) is ≤150/90 mmHg | 19 | 70% |
| **Stroke or TIAs** | | |
| *Ongoing management* | | |
| Percentage of patients with TIA or stroke who have a record of BP in previous 15 months | 2 | 90% |
| Percentage of patients with a history of TIA or stroke in whom last BP reading (within the last 15 months) is ≤150/90 mmHg | 5 | 70% |
| **Hypertension** | | |
| *Records* | | |
| The practice can produce a register of patients with established hypertension | 9 | – |
| *Diagnosis and management* | | |
| Percentage of patients with hypertension whose notes record smoking status at least once | 10 | 90% |
| Percentage of patients with hypertension who smoke, whose notes contain a record that smoking cessation advice has been offered at least once | 10 | 90% |
| *Ongoing management* | | |
| Percentage of patients with hypertension in whom there is a record of BP in the past 9 months | 20 | 90% |
| Percentage of patients with hypertension in whom last BP reading (within the last 9 months) is ≤150/90 mmHg | 56 | 70% |
| **Diabetes mellitus** | | |
| *Ongoing management* | | |
| Percentage of patients with diabetes in whom there is a record of BP in the past 15 months | 3 | 90% |
| Percentage of patients with diabetes in whom last BP reading is ≤145/85 mmHg | 17 | 55% |
| **Records and information about patients** | | |
| The BP of patients aged 45 years and over is recorded in the preceding 5 years for at least 55% of patients | 10 | – |
| The BP of patients aged 45 years and over is recorded in the preceding 5 years for at least 75% of patients | 5 | – |

BP, blood pressure; CHD, coronary heart disease; TIA, transient ischaemic attack.

## Conclusion

It is in the interests of each practice, as well as in the interest of the population that it serves, that we make real progress in reducing blood pressure in our patient population and thereby reduce their cardiovascular risk. As more trial evidence emerges, it is likely that the current guidance will be modified further.

The detection and treatment of high blood pressure and its associated CVD risk will continue to be a key focus of healthcare policy in the UK. We should continue to assess the need for treatment on the basis of absolute risk. The ongoing reorganisation of healthcare within the UK and the emphasis on clinical audit, quality of care and improvements in the systems of care provides us with an excellent opportunity to deliver improved hypertension management and thereby reduce the burden of CVD for the population we serve.

The detection and treatment of high blood pressure and its associated CVD risk will continue to be a key focus of healthcare policy in the UK.

## Key points

- Hypertension is one of the most important and preventable causes of <u>morbidity</u> and <u>mortality</u> globally. Large numbers of patients are considered to be hypertensive in the UK.

- Individuals with hypertension are likely to have multiple risk factors for CVD, necessitating an assessment of overall <u>cardiovascular</u> risk and multiple drug intervention where indicated.

- Hypertension is <u>suboptimally</u> managed in primary care in the UK, although there are signs of improvement. Consequently, primary care faces a major challenge in improving the care of hypertensive patients.

- The new guidelines from the BHS provide us with clear and practical advice for the management of hypertension. However, new systems of healthcare delivery will be needed to allow this guidance to be implemented effectively. The entire community healthcare team including nurses and pharmacists will be at the forefront of this strategy.

- A number of other initiatives provide the lead in CVD disease management and emphasise the importance of effective hypertension management. These include the NSFs for CHD, diabetes and for Older People, and the new GMS contract.

- A major proportion of clinical points in the new GMS contract are related directly to the effective management of hypertension.

- Treatment is indicated when a patient has sustained and elevated blood pressure above 160/100 mmHg. This threshold is lower in patients with diabetes and evidence of vascular disease. Patients with milder hypertension require risk assessment, which will drive the decision to treat.

- The BHS guidelines adopt the AB/CD algorithm for treatment, and indicate that multiple-drug therapy is likely to achieve the more stringent blood pressure targets that have been set.

- Patients should be actively involved in the decisions regarding lifestyle changes and drug intervention.

- Clinical audit is now an essential part of primary care, driven by the quality standards in the new GMS contract. It is likely that the quality indicators in this framework will be adopted as the basis for clinical audit in practices across the UK.

# PATIENT NOTES
*Dr Mark Davis*

*There are still far too many people who are at an increased risk of cardiovascular disease.*

## Blood pressure lowering and cardiovascular risk management in practice

In recent years there have been major changes in the way family doctors and nurses deal with risk factors for cardiovascular disease. Over the past 30 years, we have also seen an encouraging reduction in the incidence of cardiovascular disease in the UK population. This has largely been due to the significant reduction in smoking in the population, but is also due to improvements in the detection and treatment of risk factors, particularly high blood pressure and raised cholesterol. However, there should be no room for complacency. Despite these improvements there are still far too many people who are at an increased risk of cardiovascular disease either as a result of a failure to diagnose hypertension, or because of inadequate treatment when it is actually diagnosed.

There are many reasons for this, but there seem to be three main barriers that we need to overcome to improve the management of hypertension in practice. These include issues which relate specifically to:
- healthcare professionals
- patients
- healthcare systems.

## Hypertension management in the UK

Healthcare professionals in the UK are highly trained and are motivated to do a good job. There are good guidelines available which provide helpful information for clinicians. These include those produced by the British Hypertension Society (BHS), the Joint British Societies and the National Institute for Clinical Excellence (NICE). The different guidelines are broadly compatible and any could be used to good effect. Despite this there is still some confusion about what constitutes 'best practice'. Further educational initiatives are required to make this 'best practice' an integral part of routine clinical care.

## The importance of patient education and the doctor–patient partnership

Our patients are the most important part of the hypertension jigsaw. Several studies have shown, to nobody's surprise, that many patients remain poorly informed about their condition. They either are unaware that they have high blood pressure, or if they do know about it they are poorly informed about the implications of the condition and the treatment they need. Some of the blame for this must lie with healthcare professionals who may not have given the necessary information.

If patients do not understand their condition or the interventions that are necessary to control their blood pressure, it is hardly surprising that 50% of patients who are given medication for high blood pressure are failing to take it after 1 year. Most people with high blood pressure will require more than one class of medication to control their blood pressure. Often they will be offered other tablets to reduce their cholesterol (e.g. the statins – see *BESTMEDICINE Lipid Disorders* CSF Medical Communications, Oxford: 2004) or to make their blood less 'sticky' (e.g. low-dose aspirin). The main reasons for 'non-adherence' (or 'non-compliance') with medication include:
- a lack of symptoms in the majority of patients
- emerging side-effects after treatment
- a lack of communication between doctor and patient.

*An effective partnership between the patient and the doctor and/or nurse is essential for the successful management of hypertension.*

An effective partnership between the patient and the doctor and/or nurse is, therefore, essential for the successful management of hypertension. Understandably, patients always have reservations about taking medication. In one study, for example, 80% of patients consciously balanced the reasons they had been given by the doctor for taking the medication against the reservations they had about drug treatment. Involving patients in self-management programmes has been shown to improve confidence and promotes better medicine taking. All of this is common sense but the information we have must be acted upon if we are to continue to reduce the harm that is caused by persistent high blood pressure.

## How is the health service reacting to improve practice in hypertension?

The NHS needs to make structural changes and adopt different ways of working when it comes to hypertension and other cardiovascular risk factors. The Department of Health has invested a huge amount of effort and money into improving the detection, and subsequent reduction, of cardiovascular risk factors in the population. For example, in England, the National Service Framework (NSF) for Coronary Heart Disease (CHD) has established national standards and introduced performance management into the National Health Service. In addition, the new General Medical Services (GMS) contract measures the performance of general practices across a range of different clinical and organisational areas, which includes the detection and management of high blood pressure. Good quality care will be financially rewarded and it is clear that doctors respond well to financial incentives. I expect to see a great improvement in blood pressure control in the UK population, and in the next few years I hope that we will be the best in the world in managing this serious problem.

## What should patients expect from their GP?

All adults should have their blood pressure checked regularly and at the very least once every 5 years. Anyone with raised blood pressure should have it repeatedly measured to check that it actually is raised. If high blood pressure has been diagnosed, then all other risk factors for cardiovascular disease should be identified and managed appropriately. High quality lifestyle advice should be given to assist with any behavioural changes that are deemed necessary. After a joint decision is made between the doctor and patient that drug treatment is the best way forward, the choice of drugs should be tailored according to the patient's needs, and the patient should fully understand the treatment plan. The patient should be entered on a hypertension register and reviewed regularly to check that all is well and that their blood pressure is well controlled.

This is an ideal scenario and will only be achieved if there is a well informed and open relationship between the doctor/nurse and their patient. The patient should be encouraged to adopt a more active role in this process, rather than the passive doctor–patient relationship that previously prevailed in traditional general practice. Given government, professional and public support, I fully expect the reduction in cardiovascular deaths to continue.

*All adults should have their blood pressure checked regularly and at the very least once every 5 years.*

# Glossary

$\alpha_2$-adrenoceptors – Proteins on the surface of cells that mediate the biological effects of adrenaline and/or noradrenaline. Adrenoceptors are divided into $\alpha$ and $\beta$ subtypes, with $\alpha$ receptors further subdivided into $\alpha_1$ and $\alpha_2$ receptors.

**Absorption** – The movement and uptake of a drug into cells or across tissues (such as the skin, intestine and kidney).

**Acromegaly** – A disease in which the head, jaw, hands and feet are abnormally enlarged. The disease is caused by the excessive secretion of growth hormone from the pituitary gland in the brain.

**Acute** – A relatively short course of drug treatment lasting days or weeks rather than months. Can also refer to the duration of a disease or condition.

**Adrenal** – Pertaining to the adrenal glands.

**Adrenal cortex** – The outer section of the adrenal glands, two triangular-shaped glands located above the kidneys. The adrenal cortex secretes the corticosteroid hormones – aldosterone, hydrocortisone and corticosterone – which play an important role in the regulation of fat, protein and carbohydrate metabolism, and inflammatory reactions.

**Adrenal glands** – Two triangular-shaped glands located above the kidneys. The adrenal glands secrete the hormones aldosterone, hydrocortisone and corticosterone (see Adrenal cortex). The adrenal glands also secrete adrenaline and noradrenaline, two chemicals involved in the transmission of nervous impulses in the sympathetic nervous system.

**Adrenaline** – Secreted from the adrenal glands, adrenaline is one of the neurotransmitters of the sympathetic nervous system. Binds to and exerts its actions through adrenoceptors.

**Adverse event** – An unwanted reaction to a medical treatment.

**Aetiology** – The specific causes or origins of a disease, usually a result of both genetic and environmental factors.

**Agonist activity** – Mimicking or promoting the effects of another chemical (e.g. a hormone or neurotransmitter) by stimulating the receptor or target site for that particular chemical.

**Agonistic** – Showing agonist activity.

**Agranulocytosis** – A disorder of the blood characterised by a dramatic reduction in the number of granulocytes (a type of white blood cell). As a result, the patient has little resistance to infection. The disorder is commonly caused by radiation therapy and the use of certain drugs (e.g. sulphonamides). Treatment involves the use of antibiotics and steroids, and blood transfusions to supply white blood cells.

**Alanine aminotransferase** – An enzyme produced in the liver that catalyses the conversion of one amino acid into another. Alanine aminotransferase leaks into the bloodstream when the liver is damaged. Thus, levels of the enzyme in the bloodstream can be used as an indicator of liver damage.

**Albumin** – The major protein found in the blood plasma.

**Albumin excretion rate** – The amount of albumin excreted into the urine over a certain period of time. Provides an indication of the extent of kidney disease, and is usually expressed as micrograms ($\mu$g) per minute or milligrams (mg) per 24 hours.

**Albuminuria** – The presence of albumin in the urine. Usually an indication of kidney disease.

**Aldosterone** – A hormone secreted by the adrenal glands, which plays an important role in the control of blood pressure and the balance of salt within the body. Aldosterone stimulates the kidneys to retain sodium and secrete potassium. The presence of sodium in the blood and body tissues attracts water, thereby increasing the volume of fluid in the blood vessels and increasing blood pressure.

**Aldosterone-mediated sodium** – Sodium that has been retained in the body due to the action of aldosterone on the kidneys.

**Ambulatory** – Able to walk around freely.

**Angina (pectoris)** – Brief, recurring attacks of chest pain caused by an insufficient flow of blood and hence an insufficient supply of oxygen to the heart muscle. Caused by narrowed or blocked coronary arteries (the arteries that supply the heart muscle). Angina may be stable or unstable. The pain associated with stable angina tends to occur following exertion or when the person is under stress and can usually be relieved with rest or medication. The pain of unstable angina is usually more prolonged and severe, and may even occur when the person is resting. A person with unstable angina is at high risk of having a heart attack (myocardial infarction).

**Angioedema** – Large swellings in the skin, larynx (voice box) and other areas of the body that appear suddenly and are caused by allergic reactions to food, drugs, insect bites or stings, infections, animals and pollen. Angioedema may cause sudden difficulty in breathing, speaking and swallowing, and may be life-threatening if the swelling blocks the airways. The swelling may persist for several hours or days if it is not treated.

**Angioplasty** – A non-surgical technique used to unblock clogged coronary arteries (the arteries that supply blood to the heart). A balloon catheter is threaded into the blocked artery and inflated in the area of the blockage to open up the artery and restore blood flow.

**Angiotensin I** – A small, inactive protein formed in blood plasma when renin interacts with angiotensinogen.

**Angiotensin II** – The active form of angiotensin, produced by the action of angiotensin-converting enzyme (ACE) on angiotensin I. Angiotensin II increases blood pressure by controlling the constriction, or narrowing, of blood vessels.

**Angiotensin-converting enzyme (ACE)** – An enzyme that converts angiotensin I to angiotensin II.

**Angiotensin-converting enzyme (ACE) inhibitors** – Drugs that block the action of angiotensin-converting enzyme (ACE). This relaxes the blood vessels and consequently reduces blood pressure. ACE inhibitors are used to treat hypertension and heart failure.

**Angiotensin II receptor antagonist** – An agent that blocks the action of angiotensin II, thereby lowering blood pressure. Also called angiotensin receptor blockers.

**Antagonists** – Substances (e.g. drugs) that block the action of other substances by binding to specific cell receptors without eliciting a biological response (see Reader's Guide).

**Aorta** – The large artery that carries oxygenated blood from the left ventricle of the heart to the other arteries of the body.

**Aortic smooth muscle cell** – One of the many cells that make up the layer of smooth muscle in the walls of the aorta. Smooth muscle cells are long, spindle-shaped cells that are arranged in bundles. Contraction and relaxation of smooth muscle is controlled by the autonomic nervous system.

**Aortic stenosis** – Narrowing or constriction of the aorta, the large artery that carries oxygenated blood from the left side of the heart to the other arteries throughout the body.

**Arterial compliance** – The stiffness or stretchability of an artery in response to the pressure exerted by the blood flowing through it.

**Arteriolar vasoconstriction** – Narrowing (constriction) of the arterioles due to contraction of the smooth muscle in the walls of these vessels.

**Arteriole** – The smallest arteries of the circulatory system. Any artery with a diameter less than 0.5 mm is considered to be an arteriole.

**Artery** – A blood vessel that carries oxygenated blood away from the heart.

**Arthralgia** – Pain in the joints.

**Asymptomatic** – No symptoms.

**Atherosclerosis** – The deposition of fatty substances (mainly cholesterol) in the inner lining of an artery leading to the build-up of a substance known as an atheroma or plaque (also known as atherogenesis).

**Atherosclerotic plaque** – Another name for an atheroma.

**Atrial natriuretic peptide (ANP)** – A protein produced in the walls of the upper chambers of the heart (atria) in response to an increase in atrial muscle tension (as occurs in some types of hypertension and in heart failure), high sodium concentrations in the blood or a high volume of blood. ANP helps to lower blood pressure by decreasing the volume of water in the blood vessels and by widening the blood vessels so that blood can flow more easily.

**Atrioventricular** – Pertaining to a group of cells located between the atria (upper chambers) and ventricles (lower chambers) of the heart. Atrioventricular cells conduct electrical impulses (which control the beating of the heart) from the atria to the ventricles.

**Autonomic nervous system** – The part of the nervous system that controls the automatic and involuntary functions of the body, such as breathing, digestion and the beating of the heart. The autonomic nervous system is divided into the sympathetic and parasympathetic systems.

**β-adrenoceptor** – Proteins on the surface of cells that mediate the biological effects of adrenaline and noradrenaline. β-adrenoceptors are subdivided into $\beta_1$, $\beta_2$ and $\beta_3$ receptors. β-adrenoceptors mediate the relaxation of bronchial and vascular smooth muscle and control heart rate.

**β-blockers** – Drugs that block the β-adrenoceptors in the heart, circulatory system, lungs, pancreas and liver, thereby inhibiting the effects of the neurotransmitters, adrenaline and noradrenaline. This can reduce blood pressure and heart rate, and also stabilises the heart beat. β-blockers are commonly used to treat hypertension, irregular heart beats (cardiac arrhythmias) and angina pectoris.

**β-blocker therapy** – Treatment with β-blockers.

**Baroceptor reflex sensitivity** – Sensitivity of the baroceptor reflex, a system that helps to regulate blood pressure within the body. Baroceptors (or baroreceptors) can detect the pressure of blood flowing through the vessels. If blood pressure falls, the baroceptors send signals to the brain, which, in turn, sends signals to the smooth muscle in the walls of the blood vessels, causing it to contract. The brain also sends signals to the heart muscle, causing it to beat faster and with more force. These changes lead to an overall increase in blood pressure, restoring it to normal values. The converse occurs if blood pressure increases.

**Baseline** – The starting point to which all subsequent measurements are compared. Used as a means of assessing improvement or deterioration during the course of a clinical trial.

**Bile** – A yellow/green fluid produced by the liver. Bile is stored in the gallbladder and released into the small intestine at the time of eating, where it breaks down food, especially fats.

**Biliary** – Pertaining to the bile ducts and gallbladder.

**Biliary obstruction** – An obstruction occurring in the bile ducts or gallbladder. The bile ducts are a system of ducts that carry bile from the liver (where it is produced) to the gallbladder (where it is stored), and from the gallbladder to the small intestine (where it helps to break down fats).

**Biliary route** – Referring to the removal of a compound from the body via the bile ducts and gallbladder, and from there into the small intestine.

**Bilirubin levels** – The concentration of bilirubin in blood. Bilirubin is the yellow pigment found in bile. It is formed by the breakdown of haemoglobin, the pigment found in red blood cells.

**Bioavailability** – The amount of a drug that enters the bloodstream and hence reaches the tissues and organs of the body. Usually expressed as a percentage of the dose given.

**Biochemical disturbance** – The disruption of a chemical reaction or process within the body.

**Blinded endpoint design** – Pertaining to a clinical trial in which the investigator who assesses the endpoints (or outcomes) of the trial is unaware of what treatment each patient has received.

**Blood glucose** – Sugar present in the blood that is used by the body as an energy source.

**Body mass** – The amount of matter in the body, usually expressed in kilograms.

**Brachial-ankle pulse wave velocity (baPWV)** – The speed at which pulse waves travel between two points (the brachial artery in the upper arms and the posterior tibial artery in the ankles) in the body's system of arteries. Pulse waves are produced by inflating and deflating blood pressure cuffs placed around the upper arm and just above the ankle. Pulse wave velocity provides an indication of the extent of atherosclerosis (hardening of the arteries due to the deposition of fatty substances in the artery walls) and the future risk of cardiovascular disease.

**Bradycardia** – An abnormally slow heart rate of less than 60 beats per minute.

**Bradykinin** – A protein produced by blood vessels, the gut wall, damaged tissues and, during an asthma attack, mast cells. Bradykinin is a potent dilator of blood vessels, increases vessel permeability, causes contraction of non-vascular smooth muscle and induces pain.

**Bronchi** – Branched tubes of the respiratory system, located between the trachea (windpipe) and the bronchioles of the lungs.

**Bronchoconstriction** – Reduction of the diameter of the smaller airways in the lungs, which impedes the flow of air through the lungs.

**Bronchospasm** – The sudden narrowing of the airways in response to the rapid contraction of the smooth muscle in the airway walls. This makes it difficult for air to move in and out of the lungs and can lead to breathing difficulties.

**Calcium ions (Ca$^{2+}$)** – Atoms of calcium that carry a double positive electrical charge due to the loss of two negatively charged electrons.

**Calcium-channel blocker** – Drugs that block the calcium channels in cell membranes, thus preventing calcium ions (Ca$^{2+}$) from flowing into cells. Prevents the smooth muscle cells in the walls of blood vessels from contracting, thereby keeping the blood vessels dilated and reducing blood pressure. Calcium-channel blockers are effective in the treatment of hypertension.

**Capillary permeability** – The ability of various substances to pass through the walls of the capillaries, the smallest blood vessels in the body. Oxygen and nutrients pass from the blood in the capillaries into the tissues of the body, while carbon dioxide and other waste products pass from the tissues into the blood.

**Carbonic anhydrase inhibitor** – Drugs (e.g. acetazolamide, dichlorphenamide, methazolamide) that reduce the secretion of H$^+$ ions by the kidney tubules through the inhibition of the carbonic anhydrase enzyme. Not used routinely as diuretics, carbonic anhydrase inhibitors are most frequently used in the treatment of glaucoma.

**Carboxylesterase** – A family of enzymes that promote the breakdown or synthesis of carboxylic ester compounds (organic compounds). Carboxylesterases are involved in the metabolic pathways that lead to the production of energy in the body.

**Cardiac myocytes** – The cells that make up the heart muscle.

**Cardiovascular** – Pertaining to the heart and/or circulatory system.

**Cardiovascular disease (CVD)** – Disease of the heart and/or circulatory system. Stroke, coronary heart disease, atherosclerosis, hypertension, angina pectoris, cardiac arrhythmias and hypercholesterolaemia are all types of cardiovascular disease which represents the leading cause of death in the western world.

**Cardiovascular homeostasis** – The regulation of blood pressure and the general functioning of the heart and circulatory system.

**Carotid artery** – Referring to one of the two carotid arteries, the two main arteries that supply blood to the head.

**Carotid bruits** – The sounds made in the carotid arteries when the blood flow through them is abnormal, due to narrowing or widening of the arteries. These sounds can be heard through a stethoscope.

**Catecholamines** – A group of structurally related compounds occurring naturally in the body that act as hormones and/or neurotransmitters. Examples include dopamine, adrenaline and noradrenaline.

**Chronic** – A prolonged course of drug treatment lasting months rather than weeks. Can also refer to the duration of a disease or condition.

**Circadian** – Occurring approximately every 24 hours.

**Cirrhosis** – A disease in which the liver accumulates scar tissue and fat and, as a consequence, is unable to function properly. Long-term alcohol abuse and infections (e.g. hepatitis) are the most common causes of cirrhosis.

**Co-administration** – The simultaneous administration of more than one type of medication.

**Coarctation of the aorta** – Abnormal narrowing of the aorta in the part of the vessel that supplies blood to the lower part of the body, including the legs. As a result, the heart has to work harder to supply blood to the lower part of the body. This causes hypertension in the upper body but blood pressure in the lower part of the body remains normal or low. Coarctation of the aorta is a congenital condition (i.e. it is present at birth).

**Collagen vascular disease** – A general term for diseases in which the immune system malfunctions and affects the structures in the body containing collagen (a glue-like protein), including tendons, bones and connective tissue. Examples of collagen vascular diseases include rheumatoid arthritis (inflammation of the connective tissue in the joints), systemic lupus erythematosus (inflammation of the skin, joints and many of the body's internal organs) and scleroderma (hardening of the connective tissue in the skin, blood vessels, muscles and internal organs).

**Comorbid** – A co-existing medical condition.

**Congenital hyperplasia** – A condition present at birth that is characterised by insufficient amounts of the enzymes necessary for the synthesis of the hormones cortisol and aldosterone. As a result, the adrenal glands are unable to produce sufficient quantities of these hormones. This leads to an inability to fight off infections, insufficient salt in the body and blood pressure problems. In women, it can cause masculine features and the presence of male genitalia.

**Congestive heart failure** – Failure of the heart to pump an adequate amount of blood around the body. Blood pools in the veins because the heart does not pump efficiently enough to allow it to return, and this results in the accumulation of fluid in the lungs and other body tissues. This, in turn, can lead to breathing difficulties.

**Contra-indication** – Specific circumstances under which a drug should not be prescribed, for example, certain drugs should not be given simultaneously.

**Coronary heart disease (CHD)** – The gradual reduction in the blood supply to the heart muscle caused by narrowing or blocking of the coronary arteries. As a result, the heart is deprived of oxygen and is unable to function properly. In the short-term, this can cause angina pectoris, and in the long-term, it can lead to a heart attack (myocardial infarction).

**Crossover study** – A clinical trial in which every subject receives each treatment being tested, in a random order. In this type of trial, subjects act as their own control.

**Curve of contractile response** – A graphical plot of the dose of a drug that causes muscle contraction, against the extent to which the muscle contracts. This is also known as a dose–response curve.

**Cushing's syndrome** – A hormonal disorder caused by abnormally high levels of corticosteroid hormones in the blood, owing to overactivity of the adrenal glands or pituitary gland, or by the prolonged use of corticosteroid drugs. Patients with Cushing's syndrome have a characteristic round, red face, an obese trunk, a humped upper back, and wasted limbs.

**Diabetic nephropathy** – Damage to the kidneys caused by diabetes. The high blood sugar levels associated with diabetes cause damage to the blood vessels within the kidneys, leading to kidney malfunction. Diabetic nephropathy occurs in the later stages of diabetes, and is characterised by protein leaking from the kidneys into the urine (albuminuria) and high blood pressure. The development of diabetic nephropathy can be delayed by the strict control of blood glucose (sugar) levels.

**Dialysis** – The artificial filtering of blood from patients whose kidneys do not function properly in order to remove waste products from the blood that are normally removed by the kidneys.

**Diastolic blood pressure (DBP)** – The lower number of a blood pressure reading. It represents the force of blood pushing against the walls of the arteries when the heart is at rest between consecutive beats.

**Dissecting aneurysm** – A split in the lining of the wall of an artery (usually the aorta), which then expands. The artery becomes weakened and may rupture.

**Distal convoluted tubule** – A portion of the long, twisted tubules found in the kidneys. The tubules regulate the amount of water and ions in the body by filtering them out from the blood and reabsorbing (taking up) anything that should be kept. The distal convoluted tubule is the portion of tubule between the Loop of Henle and the collecting duct. Its main function is to reabsorb calcium, sodium and bicarbonate ions from the urine, and to secrete potassium and hydrogen ions into the urine.

**Diuresis** – The increased secretion of urine by the kidneys. This occurs after drinking more fluid than the body requires and after taking a diuretic drug. It is also a symptom of diabetes.

**Diuretics** – A group of drugs that remove excess water from the body by increasing the production of urine. Diuretics are used to treat many conditions associated with water retention, including heart failure, certain kidney and liver disorders, high blood pressure, glaucoma and premenstrual syndrome.

**Diurnal variation** – A biological pattern that fluctuates according to the time of day (e.g. cortisol secretion).

**Dose-response curve** – see Curve of contractile response.

**Double-blind** – A clinical trial in which neither the doctor nor the patient are aware of the treatment allocation.

**Double dummy** – The use of two different types of placebo in a clinical trial so that participants do not know which treatment they are receiving. If the mode of administration of the two active treatments is different, participants will be able to deduce which treatment they are receiving.

**Drug interactions** – In which the action of one drug interferes with that of another, with potentially hazardous consequences. Interactions are particularly common when the patient is taking more than one form of medication for the treatment of multiple disease states or conditions.

**Dyslipidaemia** – Abnormal levels of lipids or lipoproteins in the blood.

**Echocardiography** – A diagnostic technique whereby an image of the heart is obtained using ultrasound. High frequency sound waves are fired at the heart, and the echoes reflected back are picked up by a detector and displayed graphically. The resulting 'picture' can be used to detect structural abnormalities of the heart and associated blood vessels.

**Efficacy** – The effectiveness of a drug against the disease or condition it was designed to treat.

**Electrocardiogram (ECG)** – A recording of the electrical activity of the heart. Useful for diagnosing disorders of the heart, many of which cause abnormal electrical patterns.

**Electrolyte** – A substance that dissolves in water to form ions which are able to conduct electricity. Examples of electrolytes are sodium and potassium salts. These dissolve in water to produce sodium and potassium ions, respectively.

**Endocrine** – Pertaining to hormones, chemicals produced by certain organs in the body that have an effect on cells and tissues elsewhere in the body.

**End-organ damage** – Damage to organs in the body as a result of a particular disease. For example, hypertension causes changes to the thickness of the wall of the left ventricle of the heart and the wall of the carotid artery, the deposition of atherosclerotic plaques (fatty deposits) in the carotid artery wall and changes in renal function.

**Endothelial cells** – Multifunctional cells that line blood vessels. Endothelial cells act as a barrier between the blood and other body tissues, attract white blood cells to the site of an infection, regulate blood flow and blood clotting, and control the contraction and relaxation of veins. The endothelial cells are collectively called the endothelium of a blood vessel.

**Endothelin** – A substance produced by the cells lining the blood vessels (endothelial cells) that causes contraction of the vascular smooth muscle and hence narrowing of the blood vessels. This, in turn, leads to a rise in blood pressure and may contribute to hypertension and heart failure. Endothelin also stimulates the production of aldosterone and atrial natriuretic peptide (ANP), and reduces blood filtration in the kidneys.

**Endothelium-derived relaxing factor (EDRF)** – A substance produced by the cells lining blood vessels (endothelial cells) that causes relaxation of the vascular smooth muscle and hence widening of the blood vessels. This, in turn, leads to a fall in blood pressure. Synonymous with nitric oxide (NO).

**Endpoint** – A recognised stage in the disease process, used to compare the outcome in the different treatment arms of clinical trials. Endpoints can mark improvement or deterioration of the patient and signify the end of the trial.

**End-stage** – Complete or near failure of an organ or the late, fully developed phase of a disease.

**Enzymatic** – Pertaining to the involvement of enzymes.

**Enzymatic processes** – Biochemical reactions in the body that are regulated by enzymes.

**Enzyme** – A protein produced by cells in the body that catalyses (increases the rate of) a specific biochemical reaction and is itself not destroyed in the process.

**Epidemiology** – The incidence or distribution of a disease within a population.

**Exacerbation** – A period during which the symptoms of a disease recur or become worse. The term exacerbation is commonly used to describe an asthma attack.

**Excretion** – The elimination of a drug or substance from the body as a waste product, for example, in the urine or faeces.

**Exudate** – Fluid that seeps from blood vessels into tissue or onto the surface of tissue during the inflammatory response.

**Factorial-design study** – A clinical or experimental study in which at least two variables or factors are investigated at two or more different levels. This design allows any interaction between factors to be examined.

**First-dose hypotension** – Abnormally low blood pressure that may occur immediately after taking the first dose of a blood pressure-lowering drug. This is a common side-effect of angiotensin converting enzyme (ACE) inhibitors, which are used to treat high blood pressure. Patients particularly at risk of developing first-dose hypotension are those taking diuretics, those who are fluid-depleted and the elderly.

**Fluid volume status** – The amount of fluid in the body.

**Fundal haemorrhages** – Bleeding in the main cavity of the eye due to the rupture of a blood vessel. Such haemorrhages are often a sign of raised pressure in the blood vessels supplying the subarachnoid space (the fluid-filled space surrounding the brain).

**Genetic predisposition** – An individuals' susceptibility to developing a disease or condition as a result of their genetic make-up.

**Glomerular** – Pertaining to the glomeruli (singular, glomerulus) – the filtering units of the kidneys. Substances to be cleared from the blood pass from the glomeruli into the kidney tubules, where urine is formed.

**Gouty arthritis** – Arthritis caused by gout. Gout is a metabolic disorder characterised by excessive uric acid in the blood. This leads to the formation of uric acid crystals in the joints, and ultimately, joint inflammation and pain. Gouty arthritis usually affects a single joint, commonly in the big toe or foot.

**Haemodialysis** – The artificial filtering of blood outside the body using a dialysis machine in order to remove waste products from the blood. Dialysis is commonly performed in patients whose kidneys are not functioning properly.

**Haemostatic-fibrinolytic balance** – The normal balance between haemostatis, the arrest of bleeding, and fibrinolysis, the removal of the blood clot that caused the bleeding to stop.

**Hepatic** – Pertaining to the liver.

**Hepatic cytochrome** – A group of enzymes in the liver that act as electron carriers and play an important role in many biochemical reactions that occur in the body, such as the production of energy.

**Hepato-** – Pertaining to the liver.

**Heterocyclic** – Ring compounds having atoms other than carbon in their nuclei.

**Heterogeneity** – Diversity; variety.

**High density lipoprotein cholesterol (HDL-C)** – Cholesterol that is carried in the blood by high density lipoprotein (HDL). Around 20–30% of blood cholesterol is carried in this way. HDL-C is known as 'good' cholesterol because high levels appear to protect against heart disease.

**Histamine** – An inflammatory substance that is released from mast cells during an allergic reaction. Histamine is one of the substances responsible for the swelling and redness associated with inflammation. Other effects include narrowing of the airways, itching and the stimulation of acid production in the stomach. The effects of histamine can be counteracted with antihistamine drugs (e.g. cetirizine, desloratadine and loratadine).

**Hydrochlorothiazide add-on therapy** – The addition of hydrochlorothiazide to a treatment regimen for hypertension. Hydrochlorothiazide is a diuretic drug, which means that it removes excess water from the body by increasing the production of urine. It enhances the effectiveness of many of the drugs used to treat hypertension, and is therefore often used in combination with these drugs.

**Hyperparathyroidism** – Overactivity of the parathyroid glands – pea-sized glands located in the thyroid gland in the neck. This leads to the overproduction of parathyroid hormone (which controls the level of calcium in the body), and hence high blood calcium levels (hypercalcaemia). Hyperparathyroidism is most commonly caused by a benign (non-cancerous) tumour in the parathyroid glands.

**Hypertensive retinopathy** – Damage to the retina of the eye as a result of high blood pressure.

**Hypertriglyceridaemia** – Excessively high levels of triglycerides in the blood. The condition may be inherited (familial hypertriglyceridaemia) or it may occur as a result of another condition, such as diabetes or kidney failure.

**Hyperuricaemia** – Abnormally high levels of uric acid in the blood. Hyperuricaemia may cause gout (joint inflammation and pain) due to the deposition of uric acid crystals in the joints and may also lead to the development of kidney stones (hardened crystal deposits in the kidneys).

**Hypokalaemia** – Abnormally low levels of potassium in the blood. Hypokalaemia can cause muscle weakness and abnormal heart rhythms.

**Hypotension** – Abnormally low blood pressure.

**Idiopathic** – A disease or condition of unknown cause.

**Imidazole group** – Three carbon atoms, four hydrogen atoms and two nitrogen atoms. Imidazole compounds inhibit the production of histamine in the body (the chemical released from cells during an allergic reaction).

**Imidazole moiety** – See Imidazole group.

**Inotropic** – Having an effect on the strength of muscular contraction. Positive inotropic agents increase the strength of muscular contraction, whilst negative inotropic agents weaken the strength of muscular contraction. The term is often used to describe the effect of drugs on heart muscle contractility.

**Intima-media** – The wall of an artery. The thickness of the intima-media of the carotid arteries (the arteries that supply blood to the head) is related to a person's risk of developing cardiovascular disease, the thicker the intima-media the greater the risk of disease. Carotid intima-media thickness can be readily measured using ultrasound, and is often used as an indicator of cardiovascular risk.

**Intraglomerular pressure** – The blood pressure in the glomeruli, the filtering units of the kidneys.

**Intrinsic sympathomimetic activity** – Produces effects similar to those of the sympathetic nervous system. These include an increased heart rate, dilation of the airways and the constriction of blood vessels.

**In vivo** – Used with reference to experiments performed within the living cell or organism.

**In vitro** – 'In glass'. Used with reference to experiments performed outside the living system in a laboratory setting.

**Ion channel** – A protein or protein complex in a cell membrane that conducts ions (electrically charged atoms) into or out of cells (e.g. potassium [$K^+$], sodium [$Na^+$] and calcium [$Ca^{2+}$] channels).

**Ischaemia** – Reduced blood supply.

**Ischaemic attack** – A reduction in the blood supply to an organ or tissue, such that insufficient oxygen reaches the organ or tissue. An ischaemic attack in the brain, also known as a stroke, causes symptoms such as disturbed vision, slurred speech and paralysis.

**Isolated systolic hypertension** – A condition in which systolic blood pressure is abnormally high but diastolic blood pressure is normal. If left untreated, isolated systolic hypertension can lead to stroke, myocardial infarction, congestive heart failure, kidney damage and blindness.

**Kaplan–Meier curves** – Graphs constructed using patient survival data gathered from clinical trials. Takes into account the fact that patients participating in a trial are usually followed for different periods of time and provides a measure of the probability that a patient will survive for a specified time interval.

**Kininase II** – See angiotensin converting enzyme (ACE).

**Kinins** – A group of proteins found in blood (e.g. bradykinin) that play a role in inflammation, smooth muscle contraction, the regulation of blood pressure, blood clotting and the perception of pain.

**Left-ventricular ejection fraction (LVEF)** – The volume of blood ejected from the left ventricle of the heart when it contracts expressed as a percentage of the total amount of blood in the ventricle at each heartbeat. LVEF can be measured using echocardiography and provides an indication of how well the heart is functioning.

**Left ventricular hypertrophy (LVH)** – Enlargement of the left ventricle of the heart, the most common cause of which is high blood pressure.

**Left ventricular mass (LVM)** – The amount of muscle in the left ventricle of the heart. It can be measured using echocardiography and is usually quantified as grams per square metre of body surface area ($g/m^2$). Left ventricular mass is commonly increased in patients with left ventricular hypertrophy and can be a sign of heart disease.

**Left ventricular stroke volume** – The volume of blood ejected from the left ventricle of the heart when it contracts. It can be measured using echocardiography and provides an indication of how well the heart is functioning.

**Lipid solubility** – The extent to which a substance dissolves in lipids (fats).

**Lipophilic** – Having a tendency to dissolve in fat. The term literally means 'fat-loving'. Examples of lipophilic molecules include oils and fats.

**Lipophilic benzimidazole group** – A 'fat-loving' molecular group consisting of seven carbon atoms, six hydrogen atoms and two nitrogen atoms that are arranged in two rings.

**Lipophilicity** – The extent to which a molecule or part of a molecule is lipophilic or 'fat-loving'.

**Loop diuretics** – Drugs (e.g. furosemide, bumetanide) that act on the loop of Henle in the kidneys to inhibit the reabsorption of sodium and chloride ions from the urine. Most frequently used in the treatment of pulmonary oedema due to left ventricular failure and in patients with chronic heart failure.

**Loop of Henle** – A hairpin-like bend in the long, convoluted tubules of the kidneys, that takes up (reabsorbs) water and sodium, chloride and potassium ions from the urine that flows through the tubule.

**Low density lipoprotein cholesterol (LDL-cholesterol)** – Cholesterol that is carried in the blood by the lipid–protein complex, low density lipoprotein (LDL). LDL-C is known as 'bad' cholesterol because high levels increase the risk of heart disease.

**L-type calcium channels** – One of six types of voltage-gated calcium channels (T, L, N, P, Q and R). These are proteins or protein complexes in cell membranes that conduct calcium ions into or out of cells and opens or closes in response to a change in the voltage across the cell membrane (the difference between the electrical charge inside the cell and that on the outside of the cell). L-type channels are found in all excitable cells, including those in blood vessels and the heart muscle. Many of the drugs used to treat hypertension (e.g. verapamil, nifedipine, felodipine, isradipine and diltiazem) interact with L-type calcium channels.

**Lumen diameter** – The diameter of a hollow organ (e.g. blood vessel) or tube (e.g. hollow needle or catheter).

**Markov model** – A statistical model that is commonly used to analyse systems that may exist in different states. The model measures the probability of the system being in a given state at a given time point, the amount of time the system spends in a given state and the expected number of transitions between different states.

**Mechanism of action** – The manner in which a drug exerts its therapeutic effects.

**Meta-analysis** – A set of statistical procedures designed to amalgamate the results from a number of different clinical studies. Meta-analyses provide a more accurate representation of a particular clinical situation than is provided by individual clinical studies.

**Metabolism** – The process by which a drug is broken down within the body.

**Metabolites** – The products of metabolism.

**Microalbuminuria** – The excretion of albumin (a protein) in the urine at a relatively low rate (30–300 mg in 24 hours).

**Microscopy** – The use of a microscope to view small objects. A microscope produces a magnified image of objects, enabling the visualisation of features that cannot be seen with the naked eye.

**Monotherapy** – Treatment with a single drug.

**Morbidity** – A diseased condition or state or the incidence of a disease within a population.

**Mortality** – The death rate of a population. The ratio of the total number of deaths to the total population.

**Multicentre** – A clinical trial conducted across a number of treatment centres, either abroad or in the same country.

**Multifactorial** – A disease or state arising from more than one causative element.

**Muscarinic** – Pertaining to the neurotransmitter acetylcholine. Describes a substance that produces or mediates the effects of acetylcholine.

**Muscarinic receptor** – A receptor that responds to acetylcholine and related compounds, including the mushroom poison, muscarine. Located on smooth muscle, cardiac muscle, some nerve cells in the central nervous system (CNS) and glands.

**Myocardial contractility** – The ability of heart muscle to undergo contraction.

**Myocardial infarction (MI)** – Commonly known as a heart attack, MI is defined as permanent damage to an area of heart muscle caused by a lack of blood supply and hence an inadequate supply of oxygen. The most common cause is a blood clot that blocks the coronary arteries. The characteristic symptom of an MI is a crushing pain in the chest that radiates into the shoulders or arms. One out of every five deaths is due to a heart attack.

**Nanomolar affinity** – Being active at very low (nanomolar) concentrations. A nanomole is one billionth of a mole, and a mole is the weight of one molecule of a substance expressed in grams. The term may be used to describe the ability of a drug to bind to its biological target (e.g. receptor or enzyme).

**Nasopharyngitis** – Inflammation of the nasopharynx, the passage connecting the nasal cavity to the top of the throat.

**Negatively chronotropic** – Having the effect of slowing the rate of the heartbeat.

**Negatively inotropic** – Having the effect of weakening the strength of muscular contraction. The term is often used to describe the effect of drugs on heart muscle contractility.

**Nephropathy** – Diseased or damaged kidneys.

**Nephrosclerosis** – The formation of scar tissue in the kidneys, leading to hardening of the kidneys and ultimately kidney failure. The condition is usually associated with hypertension.

**Neurohormone** – A hormone involved in the functioning of the nervous system.

**Neurotransmitter** – A chemical that transmits nervous impulses from one nerve cell to another, or from nerve cells to muscles.

**Nifedipine** – A drug that blocks calcium channels in cell membranes, thereby preventing the contraction of the smooth muscle in the walls of blood vessels. Calcium-channel blockers help to keep blood vessels dilated and ultimately lower blood pressure. Nifedipine is used to treat angina pectoris, hypertension and other disorders of the circulatory system. Possible side-effects include fluid accumulation in the tissues (oedema), flushing, headache and dizziness.

**Nodal conduction** – The transmission of electrical impulses that control the beating of the heart via the atrioventricular or sinoatrial nodes.

**Non-ACE pathways** – Biochemical reactions that are not dependent on angiotensin-converting enzyme (ACE).

**Non-biphenyl** – Not resembling a biphenyl, a toxic chemical consisting of carbon and hydrogen atoms that is used as a solvent in the production of many drugs.

**Non-planar, acetylated amino acid** – An amino acid that has had an acetyl group ($COCH_3$) added to its structure and displays a bent or kinked orientation.

**Non-tetrazole** – Not resembling a tetrazole, a chemical consisting of one carbon atom, two hydrogen atoms and four nitrogen atoms arranged in a ring structure.

**Noradrenaline** – A monoamine neurotransmitter. It is also a hormone produced by the adrenal glands that stimulates the sympathetic nervous system. This results in an increased heart rate, the release of energy from fat and the release of glucose from the liver.

**Noradrenaline release** – The release of noradrenaline from nerve endings or the adrenal glands.

**Normoalbuminuria** – Normal amounts of the protein, albumin, in the urine. That is, less than 20 mg/L of urine. Higher levels than this indicate the possibility of kidney disease.

**Normotensive** – Normal blood pressure.

**Open-label** – A clinical trial in which all participants (i.e. the doctor and the patient) are aware of the treatment allocation.

**Ouabain** – A drug used to improve the performance of the heart by increasing the force of contraction of the heart muscle. It works by preventing calcium ions from leaving the muscle cells, thus improving muscular contraction.

***p*-value** – In statistical analysis, a measure of the probability that a given result occurred by chance. If the *p*-value is less than or equal to 0.05 then the result is usually considered to be statistically significant, and not due to chance.

**Pancreatitis** – Inflammation of the pancreas. Acute pancreatitis may be caused by infections (e.g. mumps), gallstones, alcohol abuse, the use of certain drugs (e.g. steroids), duodenal ulcers and pregnancy. Symptoms include severe abdominal pain, nausea, vomiting and loss of appetite. Chronic pancreatitis is caused by repeated attacks of acute pancreatitis, as a result of alcoholism or diseases of the biliary tract. Symptoms include persistent abdominal pain, severe nausea, chronic diarrhoea and diabetes. Treatment involves the use of pain relief, intravenous fluids, replacement pancreatic enzymes and insulin if necessary.

**Pathophysiology** – The functional changes that accompany a particular syndrome or disease.

**Papilloedema** – Swelling of the optic disc in the eye. The optic disc is the circular area where the optic nerve connects to the retina. Papilloedema usually occurs as a result of raised pressure inside the skull.

**Parenchymal disease** – Disease of the parenchymal tissue of an organ; the functioning or essential tissue as opposed to the supporting or structural tissue.

**Pathogenesis** – The processes involved in the development of a particular disease.

**Peptide vasodilator** – A small protein that widens (dilates) blood vessels by relaxing the smooth muscle in the blood vessel walls.

**Peripheral arteriolar resistance** – The cumulative resistance of the arterioles (the smallest arteries in the body) in the periphery of the body (e.g. the arms and legs). Resistance refers to the force in the arterioles opposing the flow of blood, which is essentially the stiffness of the arteriole walls.

**Peripheral oedema** – The abnormal accumulation of fluid in the peripheral (away from the central core of the body) tissues or cavities of the body, such as the legs.

**Peripheral vasculature** – Blood vessels in the periphery (away from the central core) of the body, such as those in the arms and legs.

**Phaeochromocytoma** – A tumour of the adrenal glands, leading to the oversecretion of adrenaline and noradrenaline, which in turn, causes hypertension. Symptoms can include headaches, palpitations, flushing, nausea and vomiting.

**Pharmacodynamics** – The physiological and biological effects of a drug, including its mechanism of action – the process by which it exerts its therapeutic effects.

**Pharmacokinetics** – The activity of the drug within the body over a period of time.

**Pharmacology** – The branch of science that deals with the origin, nature, chemistry, effects and uses of drugs.

**Pharyngitis** – Inflammation of the pharynx (throat), the main symptom of which is a sore throat. Most often caused by a viral infection, pharyngitis may also be caused by a bacterial infection.

**Phaechromocytoma** – A tumour of the adrenal glands, leading to the oversecretion of adrenaline and noradrenaline, which in turn, causes hypertension. Symptoms can include headaches, palpitations, flushing, nausea and vomiting.

**Placebo** – An inert substance with no specific pharmacological activity.

**Placebo-controlled** – A clinical trial in which a proportion of patients are given placebo in place of the active drug.

**Plasma protein binding** – The binding of substances that circulate in the blood (e.g. a drug or hormone) to proteins present in the fluid component of blood (plasma), such as albumin.

**Plasma renin activity** – The amount of renin in the fluid portion of the blood. Plasma renin activity is measured to screen for high blood pressure as a result of malfunctioning kidneys and to test for excess secretion of aldosterone (a hormone produced by the adrenal glands that increases blood pressure).

**Pooled analysis** – The amalgamation and processing of data derived from multiple clinical trials.

**Portal vein preparations** – Strips of portal vein (the main vein that drains blood from the digestive system and carries it to the liver) derived from animals. These strips can be used experimentally to evaluate the effects of different substances on venous tissue, particularly the smooth muscle.

*Post hoc* **analysis** – Analysis of the data from a completed clinical study to see if any results were obtained that were not specified at the start of the study (i.e. coincidental results).

**Postsynaptic** – Occurring after a synapse; the junction of two nerve cells.

**Postsynaptic AT$_1$ receptor** – Angiotensin II type 1 receptors located on the postsynaptic membrane of nerve cells.

**Potassium-sparing** – Having the effect of limiting the amount of potassium lost from the body. Potassium-sparing diuretics (e.g. amoloride, triamterene, spironolactone) inhibit the secretion of potassium ions by the distal convoluted tubules in the kidneys, thus reducing the amount of potassium lost in the urine. They have a mild diuretic effect, and are useful in patients in whom low potassium levels could be dangerous (e.g. those with cirrhosis of the liver).

**Presynaptic** – Occurring before a synapse; the junction between two nerve cells.

**Presynaptic AT$_1$ receptor** – Angiotensin II type 1 receptors located on the presynaptic membrane of nerve cells.

**Primary hyperaldosteronism** – A metabolic disorder resulting from overproduction of the aldosterone hormone by the adrenal glands. Ultimately leads to the retention of too much sodium in the body, which, in turn, causes an increase in blood pressure. Symptoms include tiredness, muscle weakness and impaired kidney function.

**Prodrug** – An inactive form of a drug that has to be activated within the body through a metabolic process before it can exert its biological effect.

**Prostaglandins** – Naturally occurring chemicals in the body that act as hormones. Prostaglandins are found in many different tissues and have a wide range of effects in the body, including causing pain and inflammation in damaged tissues and the development of fever.

**Proteinuria** – The excretion of protein in the urine.

**Proteinuric renal disease** – Kidney disease characterised by the excretion of protein in the urine.

**Proteolytic action** – Describing the cleavage, or break down, of proteins by protease enzymes.

**Protocol drugs** – Those drugs being tested in a clinical trial under controlled conditions.

**Pulmonary** – Pertaining to the lungs.

**Pulmonary artery** – Carries deoxygenated blood from the right ventricle of the heart to the lungs, where it is oxygenated.

**Pulmonary oedema** – The abnormal accumulation of fluid in the tissues and air spaces of the lungs. This leads to difficulty in breathing and is potentially fatal if left untreated.

**Radiograph** – An X-ray. Shows the image of a bodily structure on photographic film. The image is produced by exposing the body to X-rays. Any X-rays that are not absorbed by the body are detected by the photographic film.

**Radiolabelled plasma** – Blood plasma that has been tagged with a radioactive substance. Commonly used to visualise biological processes *in vivo*.

**Raynaud's syndrome** – A painful condition in which the small arteries in the fingers and toes go into spasm when exposed to cold temperatures or following emotional upset. The fingers and toes become pale, cold and numb due to the loss of their blood supply. In extreme cases, the person may develop gangrene that is severe enough to warrant amputation.

**Receptor selectivity** – The specificity of a drug or other substance for a particular receptor. For example, dopamine and dopamine-like drugs show a high selectivity for dopamine receptors.

**Rebound hypertension** – The return of blood pressure to dangerously high levels after missing doses of, or abruptly stopping treatment with, a drug used to treat high blood pressure.

**Renal** – Pertaining to the kidneys.

**Renal failure** – Failure of the kidneys to function properly.

**Renal haemodynamics** – The movement of blood through the kidneys.

**Renin** – An enzyme produced by the kidneys that helps to control the body's sodium–potassium balance, fluid volume and blood pressure. Catalyses the formation of angiotensin I.

**Renin–angiotensin cascade** – A series of reactions in the body that restores blood pressure to normal. A decrease in blood pressure stimulates the kidneys to produce the enzyme renin. This converts the inactive protein angiotensinogen into another inactive protein, angiotensin I, which is rapidly converted into the vasodilatory protein, angiotensin II, by angiotensin-converting enzyme (ACE). Drugs that affect any part of the renin–angiotensin system can be used to treat high blood pressure (e.g. ACE inhibitors).

**Renin–angiotensin system** – See Renin–angiotensin cascade.

**Renin-producing tumour** – An abnormal mass of tissue that secretes the renin enzyme. This ultimately causes hypertension through the stimulation of the renin–angiotensin cascade.

**Renovascular disease** – Disease affecting the blood vessels that supply the kidneys.

**Rhinitis** – Inflammation of the mucous membrane lining the nose. Symptoms include sneezing, a runny, itchy nose and nasal congestion (blocked nose). Rhinitis is commonly caused by an allergy to an airborne substance, such as pollen or dust. Hay fever is rhinitis caused by an allergy to grass pollen.

**Safety and tolerability** – The side-effects associated with a particular drug and the likelihood that patients will tolerate a drug treatment regimen.

**Seated trough blood pressure** – The lowest blood pressure reading acquired when the patient is seated.

**Serum** – The clear, straw-coloured, fluid component of blood, after the clotting agents (e.g. fibrinogen and prothrombin) have been removed.

**Serum creatinine** – The amount of creatinine in the fluid portion of blood.

**Serum lipid profile** – The proportion of various lipids (fats) in the fluid portion of blood. Measurement of the serum lipid profile provides an indication of how susceptible a person is to heart disease.

**Serum potassium** – The amount of potassium in the fluid portion of blood. Serum potassium levels can be used to screen patients for irregular heart rhythms (arrhythmias), neuromuscular disorders and kidney disease.

**Serum total cholesterol** – The total amount of cholesterol in the fluid portion of blood. Provides an indication of how susceptible a person is to heart disease.

**Serum uric acid** – The amount of uric acid present in the fluid portion of blood. Serum uric acid levels are measured to screen for gout (painful, inflamed joints due to the accumulation of uric acid crystals).

**Single-blind** – A clinical trial in which only the patient is unaware of the treatment allocation.

**Sinoatrial** – Pertaining to a group of cells located in the wall of the right atrium (upper chamber) of the heart. Sinoatrial cells generate the electrical impulses that control the beating of the heart.

**Sinusitis** – Inflammation of the membrane lining the facial sinuses (hollow cavities behind the forehead and cheekbones) due to a bacterial or viral infection, or an allergic reaction. Symptoms include pain in the face, headache, a blocked or runny nose, sensitive teeth and swelling around the eyes. The condition may be treated with decongestants (drugs that reduce nasal congestion) and, in the case of a bacterial infection, antibiotics.

**Smooth muscle** – The muscle found in the walls of internal organs, such as the bladder, blood vessels and the digestive tract. It consists of thin layers of muscle cells and is not under conscious control (the person is not aware that the muscle is contracting or relaxing).

**Socioeconomic impact** – Social and economic factors that characterise the influence of a disease. Incorporates the financial cost incurred by the healthcare provider, patient and/or their employer.

**Sodium–potassium exchange** – The simultaneous pumping of sodium ions out of a cell and potassium ions into a cell via an enzyme located in the cell membrane of virtually every cell in the body. The technical name for this enzyme is sodium–potassium ATPase, but it is commonly known as the sodium–potassium pump or the sodium–potassium exchanger. The process helps to maintain an electrical charge across the cell membrane and to regulate the amount of fluid in a cell.

**Statin** – A drug that lowers blood cholesterol levels by inhibiting the enzyme HMG-CoA reductase, which plays a crucial role in the synthesis of cholesterol in the liver. Examples include atorvastatin, pravastatin, rosuvastatin and simvastatin.

**Statistical significance** – A measure of the probability that a given result derived from a clinical trial – be it an improvement or a decline in the health of the patient – is due to a specific effect of drug treatment, rather than a chance occurrence.

**Suboptimal** – Below optimum.

**Substance P** – A neuropeptide that functions as a neurotransmitter. Substance P is involved in the transmission of pain and is important in many inflammatory diseases (e.g. arthritis, asthma, hay fever, inflammatory bowel disease and migraine).

**Substrate** – A substance that is involved in a biochemical reaction and upon which an enzyme acts.

**Surrogate markers** – Laboratory or physical parameters that are used as a substitute for a direct biological measurement, such as how a patient feels, or how effective a particular treatment is.

**Sympathetic nervous system** – The part of the autonomic nervous system that controls the automatic functions of the body, such as breathing, digestion and the beating of the heart. Most sympathetic nerve cells (but not all) use noradrenaline as a neurotransmitter.

**Sympathetic neurotransmission** – The transmission of nervous impulses within the sympathetic nervous system.

**Systemic vascular tone** – The extent of muscle contraction in the walls of the peripheral blood vessels (excluding those supplying the lungs). Essentially, the resistance of the walls of the peripheral blood vessels to blood flow.

**Systolic blood pressure (SBP)** – The higher number of a blood pressure reading. It represents the force of blood pushing against the walls of the arteries when the heart contracts.

**Tachykinin** – A family of structurally similar, biologically active peptides (small proteins) that play diverse roles in the central nervous system, and the cardiovascular, genitourinary, respiratory and gastrointestinal systems. Examples of tachykinins include neurokinins A and B, and substance P.

**Target-organ damage** – Damage to organs in the body as a result of a particular disease. For example, hypertension can cause damage to the brain (stroke and dementia), heart (angina and myocardial infarction), blood vessels (atherosclerosis) and kidneys.

**Terminal half-life (t$_{1/2}$)** – The time required for half the original amount of a drug to be eliminated from the body by natural processes (see Reader's Guide).

**Thiazide** – A type of diuretic (e.g. hydrochlorothiazide, bendrofluazide). Thiazide diuretics act on the distal convoluted tubules in the kidneys to inhibit the uptake of sodium ions and water, which ultimately leads to a moderate increase in urine production.

**Thyroid disease** – Disease of the thyroid gland. Any disease affecting the thyroid gland has the potential to upset the body's metabolic state.

**Thyroid gland** – An endocrine (hormone-producing) gland situated at the front of the neck just below the larynx (voice box). Produces the hormones thyroxine (T4) and tri-iodothyronine (T3) which play an important role in regulating metabolism.

**Titrated** – Having undergone titration. Dose titration describes the determination of the lowest dose of a particular drug that will give the desired effect.

**Tracheobronchitis** – Inflammation of the trachea (the windpipe) and bronchi (the largest air passages in the lungs) due to infection.

**Transient ischaemic attack (TIA)** – A temporary reduction in blood supply to the brain, causing symptoms that last for less than 24 hours, and which may include visual disturbances, slurred speech and paralysis. A TIA is usually a sign of diseased blood vessels.

**Triglyceride** – The chemical form in which most fats exist in the body and in food. A triglyceride consists of one molecule of glycerol and three fatty acids.

**Trough** – The lowest value of a given parameter.

**Type 2 diabetes mellitus** – A disease in which the body is unable to regulate the amount of glucose in the blood because it no longer responds to insulin or the amount of insulin produced is too low. As a result, blood glucose levels become abnormally high. Type 2 diabetes usually develops later in life, and is also known as late-onset diabetes or non-insulin dependent diabetes mellitus (NIDDM). In most cases, insulin injections are unnecessary and the disease can be controlled simply by appropriate diet, weight loss and oral medication.

**Type I diabetic nephropathy** – Damage to the kidneys caused by type 1 diabetes. In this type of diabetes, the body does not produce sufficient insulin to control blood glucose (sugar) levels.

**Type II diabetic nephropathy** – Damage to the kidneys caused by type 2 diabetes. In this type of diabetes, the body produces insulin but is unable to respond to it (insulin resistance).

**Uric acid** – A substance found in blood and urine that is a waste product of protein breakdown. High blood levels of uric acid may lead to deposits of uric acid in the joints, a painful condition called gout.

**Uric acid excretion** – The removal of uric acid from the body via the kidneys and urine.

**Urine albumin excretion rate (UAER)** – The rate at which protein albumin is excreted from the kidneys into the urine. Expressed as the amount of albumin in the urine per time unit of urine collection, usually milligrams (mg) per 24 hours or micrograms (μg) per minute. The UAER provides an indication of the extent of renal disease and also acts as a marker of cardiovascular disease. For a person with a well functioning kidney, the UAER is less than 20 μg per minute.

**Vascular** – Pertaining to the blood vessels.

**Vascular smooth muscle cell** – One smooth muscle cell out of the many that make up the layer of smooth muscle in the walls of blood vessels. Smooth muscle cells are long, spindle-shaped cells that are arranged in bundles. Contraction and relaxation of smooth muscle is controlled by the autonomic nervous system.

**Vasoactive pathway** – A series of biochemical reactions that affects the calibre (lumen diameter) of blood vessels.

**Vasoactive prostaglandins** – Prostaglandins that affect the calibre (or lumen diameter) of blood vessels. Prostaglandins are naturally occurring chemicals in the body that act in the same way as hormones. They are found in many different tissues and have a wide range of effects in the body, including causing pain, fever and inflammation in damaged tissue and protecting the lining of the stomach against acid attack.

**Vasoconstricting** – Causing narrowing (constriction) of the blood vessels due to contraction of the smooth muscle in the blood vessel walls.

**Vasodilation** – Widening (dilation) of the blood vessels due to relaxation of the smooth muscle in the blood vessel walls.

**Wash-out** – A period of time during a clinical trial when the participants do not receive any treatment so that the variables being evaluated (e.g. blood pressure) can return to their normal values.

# Useful contacts

The organisations listed below represent an accurate cross-section of what we believe to be reliable and up-to-date sources of information on hypertension, its prevention and its management.

## • British Hypertension Society

Blood Pressure Unit
Department of Physiological Medicine
St George's Hospital Medical School
Cranmer Terrace
London
SW17 0RE
Email: *bhsis@sghms.ac.uk*
Tel: 020 8725 3412
Website: *http://www.hyp.ac.uk/bhs/*
**Registered charity**

## • High Blood Pressure Foundation

Department of Medical Sciences
Western General Hospital
Edinburgh
EH4 2XU
Email: *hbpf@hbpf.org.uk*
Tel: 0131 332 9211
Website: *http://www.hbpf.org.uk*
**Registered charity**

## • Blood Pressure Association

60 Cranmer Terrace
London
SW17 0QS
Tel: 020 8772 4994.
Website: *http://www.bpassoc.org.uk/*
**Registered charity**

## • Best Treatments UK

Website: *http://www.besttreatments.co.uk/btuk/home.html*
**Produced by the British Medical Association**
**NHS Direct**
Website: *http://www.nhsdirect.nhs.uk/*

## • The British Heart Foundation

14 Fitzhardinge Street
London
W1H 6DH
Heart Information Line: 08450 70 80 70
Tel: 020 7935 0185
Website: *http://www.bhf.org.uk/*
**Registered charity**

## • National Heart Forum

Tavistock House South
Tavistock Square
London
WC1H 9LG
Email: *webenquiry@heartforum.org.uk*
Tel: 020 7383 7638
Website: *http://www.heartforum.org.uk*
**Registered charity**

## • The Stroke Association

240 City Road
London
EC1V 2PR
Email: *info@stroke.org.uk*
National Stroke Helpline: 0845 30 33 100
Tel: 020 7566 0300
Website: *http://www.stroke.org.uk/*
**Registered charity**

# Index

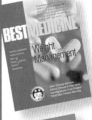
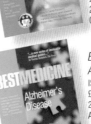
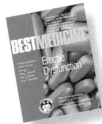
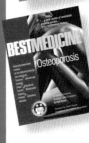
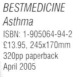
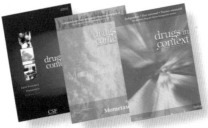